What Your Patients Need to Know About Psychiatric Medications

Second Edition

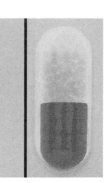

What Your Patients Need to Know About Psychiatric Medications

Second Edition

Robert H. Chew, Pharm.D.

Robert E. Hales, M.D., M.B.A.

Stuart C. Yudofsky, M.D.

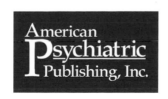

Washington, DC
London, England

Copyright © 2009 American Psychiatric Publishing, Inc.
ALL RIGHTS RESERVED

Manufactured in the United States of America on acid-free paper
13   12   11   10   09   5   4   3   2   1
Second Edition

Typeset in Adobe's Janson Text and AG Book Rounded

American Psychiatric Publishing, Inc.
1000 Wilson Boulevard
Arlington, VA 22209-3901
www.appi.org

Library of Congress Cataloging-in-Publication Data
Chew, Robert H., 1949–
    What your patients need to know about psychiatric medications / by Robert H. Chew, Robert E. Hales, Stuart C. Yudofsky. — 2nd ed.
        p. ; cm.
    Robert E. Hales' name appears first on the earlier ed.
    Includes bibliographical references and index.
    ISBN 978-1-58562-356-3 (alk. paper)
    1. Psychotropic drugs—Popular works. I. Hales, Robert E. II. Yudofsky, Stuart C. III. Title.
[DNLM: 1. Psychotropic Drugs. 2. Patient Education as Topic. QV 77.2 C529w 2009]
    RM315.H328 2009
    615′.788—dc22

                                                                                                    2008048565

British Library Cataloguing in Publication Data
A CIP record is available from the British Library.

Contents

Introduction

Not infrequently, one of our patients will tell us the following during a follow-up office visit:

> "At my last appointment, you spent a long time discussing my new medication with me. Even though you asked me several times if I had any questions about my new drug, none occurred to me at the time. However, I had many more questions about the medication once I got home than I had in your office."

We have pondered this paradox over the years and have concluded that there are several key reasons that patients often require much more information about their psychiatric medications than they take away from their prescribing physicians—even under ideal circumstances. We believe that the following are some of the reasons for this important discrepancy:

1. **Anxiety.** Despite most physicians' efforts to be supportive, empathic, communicative, and where appropriate, reassuring, many patients remain highly anxious in their doctors' offices. Specialists in internal medicine have documented that the blood pressure of many patients becomes elevated because they feel stressed by being in the medical environment—a phenomenon called "the white coat effect." The anxiety of many patients upon being told that they require a psychiatric medication can interfere with their ability to concentrate and absorb the information being imparted their physicians. During their appointments, they may feel so nervous that they "draw blanks" when their doctors ask if they have any questions about their medications. It is only later—on the drive home or after the prescription has been filled—that many important questions and concerns occur to them.

2. **Psychiatric disorders may impair attention and concentration.** The acute symptoms associated with many—if not most—psychiatric disorders impair patients' ability to absorb and process information. For example, patients with obsessive-compulsive disorder might be preoccupied by intrusive and distracting concerns or worries during the entirety of their office visits. Similarly, people with psychotic disorders might be focusing on fearful delusions or auditory hallucinations at the exact moment that their psychiatrists are explaining how to take their medications. Prototypically, major depression affects the brains of many people with this condition, and they are unable to pay attention or concentrate at their usual levels. The minds of people with mania often are racing to such a degree that they are unable to slow down sufficiently to listen to the advice and instruction of their physicians. The net result is that people with these and many other psychiatric conditions often are not in the states of mind to attend to or process their doctors' information about their medications.

3. **Learning differences.** As educators, we understand that people acquire and retain new information (i.e., "learn") in different ways. Certain individuals are "auditory learners," and these individuals often do quite well during office visits in retaining important data about their medications imparted by their psychiatrists. Other patients, however, find having more visual stimuli and written information is helpful for them to learn optimally, and these patients will benefit from well-organized and succinct information about their medications.

4. **Stigma.** The stigmatization of people with mental illnesses—and of those of us in the caring professions who are devoted to helping them—has important ramifications for the transmission of information about psychiatric disorders. Many people with psychiatric illnesses are reluctant to accept that they have these conditions. For these individuals, the idea that they must take a psychiatric medication is a tangible "admission" that they have a mental illness. When told by their physician that they must take a psychiatric medication, their resistance and denial may be so strong that they do not pay close attention to the specifics of the doctor's explanations and recommendations.

5. **Skepticism.** Even when patients acknowledge that they do, in fact, have a mental illness, they might not believe that "something they swallow" can elevate their mood, help them think more rationally, or make them feel more like themselves. The specific symptoms of many mental illnesses may also reinforce the patients' disbelief in the benefit of psychiatric medications. For example, people with major depression often feel hopeless and are especially pessimistic that anything can change their sad feelings and self-deprecating beliefs. Individuals with paranoid disorders are often distrustful of those, such as physicians, who they believe might want to influence or control them with drugs. Often, people with mania enjoy their grandiose ideas and inflated mood and therefore, do not want medications to "bring them down." The net result is that they do not accept what their physicians tell them about psychiatric medications and may even believe that such drugs will bring them great harm.

6. **Time.** Physicians are usually very busy, and there is often limited time available (or reimbursed) to review the *full* range of information related to the new medication being prescribed. In addition, responding to patients' concerns about the efficacy and side effects of prescribed medications can take a great deal of professional time. Primary care physicians, in particular, commonly prescribe psychiatric medications but often have only brief periods of time to spend with each patient. Patients sense this time pressure and may feel uncomfortable asking their physicians for clarification or additional information about their medications. We have had patients tell us that they feel "stupid" because they do not understand certain scientific information conveyed to them about their psychiatric medications. Others have said that they do not want to "bother" us with their "dumb questions." Thus patients are bereft of information that may have made them feel more confident about the safety and benefits of their medications, and they may even be confused about our prescribing information.

7. **Complexities of the human brain and psychiatric medications.** The human brain is our most complex organ, and arguably, its most important functions involve regulation of mood, thinking, perceptions, impulses, and behavior. The mechanisms of action, benefits, and side effects of psychiatric medications—as they alter the brain to treat psychiatric disorders—are also difficult to describe and understand. Our patients acquire new information in many disparate ways. Some patients learn best through dialogue with physicians, whereas others are "visual learners" and may prefer to read about and think through new ideas in the quiet of their own homes.

Understanding these varying needs and differences among our patients, the authors undertook to write the first edition of *What Your Patients Need to Know About Psychiatric Medications*. Drs. Hales and Yudofsky have active clinical practices, and we have provided for most of our patients supplemental information from the book about the medications that we prescribe. Our patients have been uniform in their feedback to us that the information in these forms has been most helpful to them, and we believe that their compliance with medications has also improved significantly. Additionally, the information that we imparted to our patients from the first edition of *What Your Patients Need to Know About Psychiatric Medications* has improved our communication with our patients. For example, they are much more proactive in informing us about medication side effects. For these reasons, because so many new psychiatric medications have become available since we published the first edition of the book, and because new data have emerged about the safety, side effects, and effectiveness of psychiatric medications over this time, we have decided that it would be worthwhile to update the information in a second edition of the text.

What Your Patients Need to Know About Psychiatric Medications has been written by two psychiatrists and a pharmacist with many decades of experience as clinicians, educators, and authors. Based on this experience, we have endeavored to write a book that addresses the barriers to optimal psychopharmacological treatment as enumerated above. We have attempted to complement the work of the treating physician by writing a book that provides patients with relevant, easy-to-use, and easy-to-understand information about psychiatric medications. The book has been conceptualized and organized to answer the most common questions that patients have about their psychiatric medications—including how to take their medications and the benefits and side effects of those medications. Emphasis is placed on the clarity, accuracy, and accessibility of information offered. We have prioritized information that is evidence-based and that enhances the safe and effective use of psychiatric medications. We believe that the more informed our patients are about their psychiatric disorders and their medication-based treatments, the greater the degree of their compliance, safety, and treatment response. We hope that we have written a book that physicians will "prescribe" to their patients receiving psychiatric medications. We also hope that *What Your Patients Need to Know About Psychiatric Medications* will enhance patients' understanding of why they need to take medication and will increase their motivation to comply with their physicians' treatment recommendations. We believe that the book will also help improve patient–physician communication regarding psychiatric medications.

Instructions on How to Use This Book

This book provides essential information about all the major classes of psychiatric medications as well as more detailed information about specific medications. When prescribing a medication for one of your patients, you may wish to photocopy or download from the CD-ROM both general information about the class of medication and more detailed information about the specific agent. For instance, if you are prescribing Zoloft, a general discussion of selective serotonin reuptake inhibitors is found on pages 73–76 and specific information on Zoloft is found on pages 103–106.

Each medication is presented in a standard format. The various sections and a brief discussion of each are as follows:

Brand Name: The trade name the manufacturer has given the medication for marketing to the consumer

Generic Name: The chemical or pharmaceutical name of the medication

Available Strengths: The dosages and available formulations

Available in Generic: Whether the medication is available in a generic form

Drug Class: The classification of the medication (e.g., tricyclic antidepressant), applicable to a group of medications similar in chemical formulation, mode of action, or general uses

General Information: An overview of the medication, including how it works, why it was developed, and its general advantages and disadvantages

Dosing Information: Concise information about how the medication is prescribed, including dosage forms and strengths, when it should be taken, and how doses should be increased

Common Side Effects: The most common side effects noted during clinical trials and in clinical practice (Because additional side effects may occur, patients should be instructed to report these to their physicians.)

Adverse Reactions and Precautions: Cautionary advice concerning the medication itself and other medications to be avoided

Use in Pregnancy and Breastfeeding: Whether the medication should be taken by women who are or may become pregnant and women who are breastfeeding, as well as the U.S. Food and Drug Administration's (FDA) categorization of the drug (A, B, C, D, or X)

Psychotropic medications are almost never systematically studied in pregnant women; potential effects on humans are usually drawn from research conducted in mice or other animals. Category A means that controlled studies show no risk to humans. Most psychotropic medications have been classified by the FDA as Category B, meaning no evidence of risk in humans has been found but that adequate human studies have not been performed, or as Category C, meaning that risk to humans cannot be ruled out. Category D drugs have proven risk to humans, but the risk of potential harm to the fetus may be outweighed by the potential benefit to the mother. Category X medications should not be used during pregnancy because of positive evidence of fetal abnormalities.

Possible Drug Interactions: Other medications that may be of concern or that should be avoided altogether when taking the medication in question

Overdose: General information concerning the signs and symptoms of overdose and what to do if someone takes too much of the prescribed medication

Special Considerations: Special considerations to be aware of with the medication in question, including concise review of the medication discussed and a summary of its unique advantages and disadvantages; *warnings*; and general advice concerning what to do if a dose is missed, whether the tablet or capsule may be cut or crushed, whether the medication should be taken with food, and how to store the medications

Notes: Space provided for the patient to write down 1) side effects that the patient may have experienced so he or she can discuss them with the physician at the next visit and 2) questions the patient or a family member may have about the medication, such as dosing, side effects, or potential drug interactions with existing medications

Web Sites

There are several helpful Web sites for physicians and patients. The following may be especially helpful:

Internet Mental Health (www.mentalhealth.com): An excellent forum for diagnosis and treatment of mental disorders

Drug Information Online (www.drugs.com): Prescription drug information (also in Spanish) for consumers and professionals

U.S. Library of Medicine and National Institutes of Health (www.nlm.nih.gov/medlineplus): Health information for consumers

Recommended Reading

Listed below are several books with more detailed information about the medications contained in this book.

1. Dulcan MK: *Helping Parents, Youth, and Teachers Understand Medications for Behavioral and Emotional Problems: A Resource Book of Medication Information Handouts*, 3rd Edition. Washington, DC, American Psychiatric Publishing, 2007
2. Findling RL (ed): *Clinical Manual of Child and Adolescent Psychopharmacology*. Washington, DC, American Psychiatric Publishing, 2008
3. Hales RE, Shahrokh NC, Schatzberg AF, Nemeroff CB: *Study Guide to Psychopharmacology: A Companion to The American Psychiatric Publishing Textbook of Psychopharmacology, Fourth Edition*. Washington, DC, American Psychiatric Publishing, 2009
4. Jacobson SA, Pies RW, Katz IR: *Clinical Manual of Geriatric Psychopharmacology*. Washington, DC, American Psychiatric Publishing, 2007
5. Kranzler HR, Ciraulo DA (eds): *Clinical Manual of Addiction Psychopharmacology*. Washington, DC, American Psychiatric Publishing, 2005
6. Marangell LB, Martinez JM, Silver JM, Yudofsky SC: *Concise Guide to Psychopharmacology*, 2nd Edition. Washington, DC, American Psychiatric Publishing, 2006
7. Pies RW: *Handbook of Essential Psychopharmacology*, 2nd Edition. Washington, DC, American Psychiatric Publishing, 2005
8. Schatzberg AF, Cole JO, DeBattista C: *Manual of Clinical Psychopharmacology*, 6th Edition. Washington, DC, American Psychiatric Publishing, 2007
9. Schatzberg AF, Nemeroff CB: *The American Psychiatric Publishing Textbook of Psychopharmacology*, 4th Edition. Washington, DC, American Psychiatric Publishing, 2009
10. Wynn GH, Oesterheld JR, Cozza KL, Armstrong SC: *Clinical Manual of Drug Interaction Principles for Medical Practice*. Washington, DC, American Psychiatric Publishing, 2008

Medications in Pregnancy

Historical Perspective

At one time, it was widely held by most physicians that the uterus afforded a protective environment for the fetus, and the placenta served as a protective shield from the external environment. This belief was questioned in 1941 by Dr. N.M. Gregg, an Australian physician, who observed a high incidence of birth defects in women who contracted German measles (rubella) during the first 3 months (first trimester) of pregnancy. The susceptibility of the developing fetus to medications became tragically evident when women who took **thalidomide** in the first trimester of pregnancy gave birth to infants with limb defects. Thalidomide, a sedative, was marketed in Europe and Canada in the 1950s and prescribed to pregnant women to treat morning sickness. Fortunately, it was not introduced in the United States because the U.S. Food and Drug Administration (FDA) was not convinced of its safety. It was later found that thalidomide caused infants to be born with missing limbs or short, flipper-like limbs, and the drug was subsequently banned worldwide. The FDA's cautious approach probably prevented thousands of similar birth defects in this country.

Overview

Many medications and chemicals can cross the placenta and, depending on their properties, can attain varying levels in the embryo and fetus. If the fetus is exposed to certain medications and chemicals, or a virus such as rubella, these agents can cause abnormal cell formation and growth. Something that causes cellular damage or abnormal cell formation in the fetus is **teratogenic,** and the term *teratogenesis* refers to the production of congenital malformations, such as cleft lip and abnormal limbs, from in utero exposure to a **teratogen.**

In the absence of clinical studies of drugs in pregnant women, much of our information about the risks of medications in pregnancy comes from animal testing, empirical evaluation, and collection of data from reported cases. Although animal studies are useful and provide some insight into the potential adverse effects in humans, they by no means guarantee that a drug found to be safe in animals is also safe for humans.

Since 1975, the FDA has required pharmaceutical companies to include in their labeling a section on the drug's ability to cause birth defects and other effects on reproduction and pregnancy. Moreover, all medications must be classified under one of the five categories that the FDA assigned as risk factors for drugs in pregnancy (see table on p. xiv).

Psychotropic Medications in Pregnancy

All psychotropic medications cross the placenta in varying degrees. If administered during pregnancy, particularly during the first trimester, there is risk of teratogenesis with certain medications. Lithium has been associated with cardiac defects, and Depakote (divalproex sodium), used in the treatment of bipolar disorder, has

Risk categories for medications used in pregnancy

Category	Description
A	Controlled studies show no risk to humans.
B	Animal studies have revealed no evidence of harm to the fetus; however, there are no adequate and well-controlled studies in pregnant women.
C	Animal studies have shown an adverse effect, but there are no adequate and well-controlled studies in pregnant women. Therefore, the risk to humans cannot be ruled out.
D	Studies or observations have demonstrated positive evidence of risk to the fetus. The benefits of therapy may outweigh the potential risks.
X	Studies or observations have demonstrated positive evidence of fetal abnormalities, and the use is contraindicated in women who are or may become pregnant.

a 1%–2% risk of spina bifida (incomplete formation of the spinal cord); these medications are assigned to the high-risk Category D. The benzodiazepines used for treating sleep disorders, including Halcion (triazolam), Dalmane (flurazepam), Restoril (temazepam), and ProSom (estazolam), are in Category X and contraindicated in pregnancy. Most psychotropic medications, however, are assigned to Category C and have not been observed to cause birth defects, but risks in humans have not been ruled out.

Psychotropic medications can also affect labor and delivery. The adverse side effects of these medications may complicate pregnancy or affect the infant. For example, infants born to mothers taking benzodiazepines (e.g., Valium) may undergo withdrawal symptoms shortly after birth. These newborns are often observed to be flaccid and slow to respond after delivery.

Medications should be avoided, if possible, during pregnancy. However, when medications are discontinued, symptoms frequently recur, worsening preexisting psychiatric conditions. The physician and patient often face the dilemma of restarting the medication or seeking a safer, but perhaps less effective, alternative treatment during pregnancy. Not treating the mental condition during pregnancy also has significant risks for the mother and the unborn infant.

Treatment Considerations

The decision to administer medication during pregnancy must be based on informed consent from the patient. The physician should inform the woman of the potential risks of the medication and offer safer alternative treatment options, which may not include medications. Ultimately, the benefits of therapy must outweigh any potential risks.

Patients should be referred to the pregnancy section of the handout for the medication they are taking. In addition, patients can learn more about medications in pregnancy and breastfeeding at the following Web sites:

Perinatology.com (www.perinatology.com/exposures/druglist.htm)
American Council for Drug Education (www.acde.org/parent/Pregnant.htm)
Organization of Teratology Information Specialists (www.otispregnancy.org)

About the CD-ROM

The forms and protocols are included on the enclosed CD-ROM in Adobe's Portable Document Format (PDF). The PDF files are essentially pictures of the book pages, and they will allow you to view and print the forms exactly as they appear in the book. You need Adobe's Acrobat Reader 6.0.1 or higher to view and print the PDF files; if Acrobat or Adobe Reader is not already installed on your computer, the CD-ROM will prompt you to install this free program. (Adobe Reader 9 is included on the CD-ROM.) Please note that you can only view and print the PDF files with the Acrobat Reader; you cannot modify them.

Minimum System Requirements

Windows

- Intel® Pentium® III or equivalent processor
- Microsoft® Windows 2000 with Service Pack 4, Windows Server 2003, Windows XP Professional or Home Edition, or Windows XP Tablet PC Edition with Service Pack 2 or 3, Windows Vista with or without Service Pack 1
- 128MB of RAM
- 170MB of available hard-disk space
- Microsoft Internet Explorer 5 or higher
- Safari 2.0.2 or higher

Macintosh

- PowerPC® G3 processor
- Mac OS X v10.4.11–10.5.5
- 128MB of RAM
- 170MB of available hard-disk space
- Safari 2.0.2 or higher

Customer Support

Customer support is available:

9:00 A.M. to 5:30 P.M. (EST) Monday through Friday

Contact:
Telephone: (800) 368-5777
E-mail: appi@psych.org

Acknowledgments

The authors would like to thank John McDuffie, Editorial Director at American Psychiatric Publishing, Inc., for his strong support of this project, and Bob Pursell and his exceptional marketing team for developing an excellent marketing plan. In addition, Greg Kuny, Managing Editor of the Books Department, completed the detailed editorial review of the manuscript in his usual meticulous fashion. Tammy Cordova, Graphic Design Manager, designed the cover, incorporating artwork by Peter Shahrokh, and Judy Castagna managed the manufacturing of the book and accompanying CD-ROM.

Antianxiety Medications

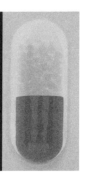

Benzodiazepines

Ativan (lorazepam)
Librium (chlordiazepoxide)
Klonopin (clonazepam)
Serax (oxazepam)
Tranxene (clorazepate)
Valium (diazepam)
Xanax (alprazolam)

Nonbenzodiazepines

BuSpar (buspirone)

Antianxiety medications, also commonly called minor *tranquilizers*, are used for treating anxiety disorders, which present in different forms. An individual has a specific **phobia** when the anxiety involves undue fears of certain objects or situations and a social disorder when the fear is related to social situations or interactions. **Panic attacks** are episodic and sudden, and the individual is overcome with unexplainable terror reactions, triggering rapid heart rate and breathing, sweating, and an intense state of fear and anxiety. In **generalized anxiety disorder** (GAD), the patient experiences chronic anxiety that causes distress and impairment and is often accompanied with depression. Individuals with **posttraumatic stress disorder** (PTSD) have experienced traumatic and life-threatening events that they relive in recurring dreams and flashbacks. Often the patient is seized with terror, anxiety, and guilt. People who experience reoccurring and new disturbing thoughts and who act out repetitive and compulsive behaviors to relieve these distressing thoughts have **obsessive-compulsive disorder** (OCD).

Before the introduction of benzodiazepines, the **barbiturates** were widely used for treating anxiety and sleep disorders. Phenobarbital and other similar long-acting barbiturates were commonly used to treat anxiety and to assist in bedtime sleep. With the introduction of Valium (diazepam) and Librium (chlordiazepoxide) in the 1960s, the benzodiazepines replaced the barbiturates for the treatment of anxiety and sleep disorders because they are safer than the barbiturates. However, benzodiazepines are associated with abuse, dependence, and withdrawal symptoms and thus are regulated under state and federal laws as controlled substances.

BuSpar (buspirone), a nonbenzodiazepine, is another agent used for treatment of anxiety. Unlike the benzodiazepines, buspirone is not associated with dependence and withdrawal symptoms and is not regulated as a controlled substance.

Antidepressants also are effective for treating various anxiety disorders, such as panic disorder, GAD, PTSD, and OCD.

Benzodiazepines

Valium and Librium are the most familiar benzodiazepines of the antianxiety medications. Other benzodiazepines, such as Dalmane (flurazepam) and Halcion (triazolam), are marketed primarily for treating insomnia. The distinction of a benzodiazepine for use as an **anxiolytic** (i.e., a medication that relieves anxiety) or **hypnotic** (i.e., a medication that induces sleep) is somewhat arbitrary because any benzodiazepine can be used to treat anxiety or insomnia, depending on the dose. Benzodiazepines prescribed primarily for sleep are discussed in separate handouts in the section on **sedative-hypnotics** (see "Medications for Treatment of Insomnia").

The benzodiazepines' effectiveness for treating anxiety may be attributed to their pharmacological action in the brain at specific receptor sites. *Receptors* are specific sites on the nerve cell membrane that receive signals from a neurochemical called the **neurotransmitter.** Once a neurotransmitter locks in on the receptor, the neurochemical signal is changed to an electrical or another chemical signal and travels down the neuron. The receptor sites in which benzodiazepines elicit their action are found in various regions of the brain, and the specific receptors are known as γ**-aminobutyric acid** (GABA) receptors. The coupled reaction of benzodiazepines to GABA receptors is inhibitory in that region of the brain. Benzodiazepines' action on GABA receptors appears to produce their anxiolytic, sedative, and anticonvulsant actions. Valium, for example, is an effective anxiolytic, hypnotic (e.g., anesthesia), and antiseizure medication.

Nonbenzodiazepine Agent: BuSpar (Buspirone)

BuSpar (buspirone) is the only nonbenzodiazepine antianxiety medication available in the United States. It is believed that BuSpar exerts its anxiolytic action through its effects on a specific serotonin receptor, much as with **selective serotonin reuptake inhibitor** (SSRI) antidepressants. It may have some effect on GABA receptors, but unlike the benzodiazepines, BuSpar does not have antiseizure activity. BuSpar's advantage is that it does not produce dependence and withdrawal symptoms with chronic use, as occurs with benzodiazepines.

Antidepressants

SSRIs, as well as some other antidepressants such as Effexor (venlafaxine), are effective for treating anxiety disorders. For example, in addition to carrying an indication for depression, Paxil (paroxetine) has U.S. Food and Drug Administration indications for the treatment of GAD, social anxiety disorder, OCD, panic disorder, and PTSD. Effexor XR is approved for treating GAD, social anxiety disorder, and panic disorder. Zoloft (sertraline), an SSRI, is indicated for treating panic disorder, OCD, and PTSD. Anafranil (clomipramine), a tricyclic antidepressant, is highly effective for treating OCD, whereas other tricyclics and SSRIs are effective in treating panic attacks.

For more information on the use of antidepressants, refer to the individual handouts on antidepressants.

From Chew RH, Hales RE, Yudofsky SC: *What Your Patients Need to Know About Psychiatric Medications*, Second Edition. Washington, DC, American Psychiatric Publishing, 2009

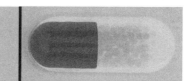

Ativan (lorazepam)

Generic name: Lorazepam
Available strengths: 0.5 mg, 1 mg, 2 mg tablets;
   2 mg/mL oral solution; 2 mg/mL, 4 mg/mL injection
Available in generic: Yes
Drug class: Benzodiazepine/anxiolytic; sedative-hypnotic

General Information

Ativan (lorazepam) is a benzodiazepine indicated for management of anxiety disorders or short-term relief of symptoms of anxiety. The use of a medication for its approved indications is called its *labeled use*. In clinical practice, however, physicians often prescribe medications for *unlabeled* ("off-label") uses when published clinical studies, case reports, or their own clinical experiences support the efficacy and safety of those treatments. Physicians may use Ativan outside its approved indications to treat social phobia, posttraumatic stress disorder, agitation in acute mania and psychosis, acute alcohol withdrawal, and other conditions. Like other benzodiazepines, Ativan is associated with dependence and abuse and is therefore regulated as a controlled substance by state and federal laws.

Ativan's effectiveness for treating anxiety may be explained by its pharmacological action in the brain at specific receptor sites. *Receptors* are specific sites on the nerve cell membrane that receive a signal from a neurochemical called the **neurotransmitter.** Once a neurotransmitter locks in on the receptor, the neurochemical signal is changed to an electrical or another chemical signal and travels down the neuron. The receptor sites in which benzodiazepines elicit their action are found in various regions of the brain, and the specific receptors are also known as **benzodiazepine receptors.** The coupled reaction of benzodiazepines to the receptors facilitates the inhibitory action of the neurotransmitter γ-**aminobutyric acid** (GABA) in that region of the brain. Benzodiazepines' action on GABA receptors appears to produce their anxiolytic, sedative, and anticonvulsant actions. Ativan, for example, is an effective anxiolytic, hypnotic, and antiseizure medication.

Dosing Information

The usual starting dosage of Ativan is 0.5 mg three times a day, with an increase to a therapeutic dosage of 4–6 mg/day administered in divided doses. Depending on the severity of symptoms, the dosage may be increased to a maximum of 8 mg/day.

Common Side Effects

The most common side effects reported with Ativan are sedation and drowsiness, especially shortly after initiating therapy. Other frequent symptoms are impaired concentration and memory, feeling of dissociation ("spacey"), and impaired coordination.

Adverse Reactions and Precautions

Ativan affects alertness and coordination, and patients should exercise caution when driving or performing other tasks requiring alertness while taking this medication. Seniors may be more adversely affected, because it may affect their coordination and reflexes and lead to falls and injury. Taking Ativan with other central nervous system (CNS) depressants such as alcohol, narcotics, and barbiturates may compound these CNS effects.

Prolonged use of benzodiazepines can lead to dependence. When the medication is abruptly withdrawn, symptoms of withdrawal may occur. Withdrawal symptoms include headache, vomiting, impaired concentration, confusion, tremor, muscle cramps, and seizures.

Benzodiazepines are centrally acting depressants, and they can depress respiration. This is particularly problematic for patients with chronic obstructive pulmonary disease and emphysema. Patients with sleep apnea—a sleep disorder in which respiration is interrupted by long pauses during the sleep cycle—should not take Ativan or other benzodiazepines. The respiratory depressant effect of benzodiazepines may further suppress the respiratory drive in these patients and put them at risk for respiratory depression and death.

Benzodiazepines may induce **paradoxical reactions** in susceptible individuals. Instead of the expected depressant effects, the medication produces excitement, aggression, anger, uninhibited behavior, and rage in susceptible individuals. These reactions are more likely to occur in seniors, people with brain damage, and individuals with personality and impulse-control disorders.

Use in Pregnancy and Breastfeeding: Pregnancy Category D

Benzodiazepines and their metabolites are known to cross the placenta and accumulate in the fetal circulation. They are associated with a risk of congenital malformations when used during pregnancy, causing cleft lip and heart deformities in the fetus. Benzodiazepines should be avoided during pregnancy, particularly in the first trimester. The use of benzodiazepines during pregnancy should be considered only when the need for the medication outweighs its risk and alternative therapies have failed.

Nursing mothers should not take Ativan, because it will pass into breast milk and be ingested by the baby. If stopping the drug is not an alternative, breastfeeding should not be started or should be discontinued.

Possible Drug Interactions

The drug interactions reported with Ativan are summarized in the table on the next page.

Patients taking Ativan should not consume alcohol because the combination may increase sedation and drowsiness.

CNS depressants (e.g., alcohol, narcotics, barbiturates, hypnotics) and antihistamines	Combination of Ativan and another CNS depressant may impair coordination and breathing and increase sedation.
Oral contraceptives	Clearance rate of Ativan may be increased when it is taken concurrently with oral contraceptives, which may decrease the effectiveness of Ativan.
Lanoxin (digoxin)	Ativan may increase the blood levels of Lanoxin, and toxicity may occur. Patients taking Ativan and Lanoxin should have their Lanoxin levels monitored closely.

Overdose

Overdoses from oral ingestion of benzodiazepines alone are generally not fatal. Most fatalities reported with benzodiazepines involve multiple medication ingestion, particularly the combination of a benzodiazepine with other CNS depressants, such as alcohol, narcotics, and barbiturates.

Mild symptoms of benzodiazepine overdose include drowsiness, confusion, somnolence, tiredness, impaired coordination, clumsiness in walking (ataxia), and slow reflexes. Benzodiazepine overdose, when these agents are taken alone, is rarely fatal. When multiple medications are implicated in benzodiazepine overdose, severe symptoms include difficulty breathing, slowed heart rate, low blood pressure, loss of coordination, and loss of consciousness leading to coma and, potentially, death.

Any suspected overdose should be treated as an emergency. The person should be taken to the emergency room for observation and treatment. The prescription bottle of medication (and any other medication suspected in the overdose) should be brought as well, because the information on the prescription label can be helpful to the treating physician in determining the number of pills ingested.

Special Considerations

- Ativan should be discontinued gradually by tapering the dose. Stopping the medication abruptly, especially after taking it regularly for long periods, may trigger withdrawal symptoms, including irritability, agitation, tension, and insomnia.
- If you miss a dose, take it as soon as possible. If it is close to the next scheduled dose, skip the missed dose and continue on your regular dosing schedule. Do not take double doses.
- Ativan may be taken with or without food.
- Ativan may cause sedation and drowsiness, especially during initiation of therapy, and impair your alertness. Use caution when driving or performing tasks that require alertness. Avoid alcohol when taking Ativan, because alcohol may intensify these effects.
- Store the medication in its originally labeled, light-resistant container, away from heat and moisture. Heat and moisture may precipitate breakdown of your medication, and the medication may lose its therapeutic effects.
- Keep your medication out of reach of children.

If you have any questions about your medication, consult your physician or pharmacist.

Notes

_____

_____

_____

_____

_____

_____

_____

_____

_____

_____

From Chew RH, Hales RE, Yudofsky SC: *What Your Patients Need to Know About Psychiatric Medications*, Second Edition. Washington, DC, American Psychiatric Publishing, 2009

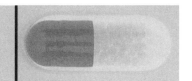

Librium (chlordiazepoxide)

Generic name: Chlordiazepoxide
Available strengths: 5 mg, 10 mg, 25 mg capsules;
    100 mg/2 mL injection
Available in generic: Yes
Drug class: Benzodiazepine/anxiolytic; sedative-hypnotic

General Information

Librium (chlordiazepoxide) is a benzodiazepine indicated for management of anxiety disorders or short-term relief of symptoms of anxiety and acute alcohol withdrawal. The use of a medication for its approved indications is called its *labeled use*. In clinical practice, however, physicians often prescribe medications for *unlabeled* ("off-label") uses when published clinical studies, case reports, or their own clinical experiences support the efficacy and safety of those treatments. Physicians may use Librium outside its approved indications to treat social phobia, posttraumatic stress disorder, insomnia, premenstrual syndrome, and other conditions. As with other benzodiazepines, Librium is associated with dependence and abuse and is therefore regulated as a controlled substance by state and federal laws.

Librium's effectiveness for treating anxiety may be explained by its pharmacological action in the brain at specific receptor sites. *Receptors* are specific sites on the nerve cell membrane that receive a signal from a neurochemical called the **neurotransmitter.** Once a neurotransmitter locks in on the receptor, the neurochemical signal is changed to an electrical or another chemical signal and travels down the neuron. The receptor sites in which benzodiazepines elicit their action are found in various regions of the brain, and the specific receptors are also known as **benzodiazepine receptors.** The coupled reaction of benzodiazepines to the receptors facilitates the inhibitory action of the neurotransmitter γ-**aminobutyric acid** (GABA) in that region of the brain. Benzodiazepines' action on GABA receptors appears to produce their anxiolytic, sedative, and anticonvulsant actions. Librium, for example, is an effective anxiolytic and hypnotic medication.

Dosing Information

For mild to moderate anxiety, smaller dosages of 5–10 mg three or four times a day are effective. For severe symptoms and for treatment of alcohol withdrawal, larger dosages of Librium are required. For severe anxiety, the usual starting dosage is 25 mg two or three times a day, with increases in dosage as needed to control symptoms. However, the maximum dosage of Librium should not exceed 300 mg/day.

7

Common Side Effects

The most common side effects reported with Librium are sedation and drowsiness, especially shortly after initiating therapy. Other frequent symptoms are impaired concentration and memory, feeling of dissociation ("spacey"), and impaired coordination.

Adverse Reactions and Precautions

Librium affects alertness and coordination, and patients should exercise caution when driving or performing other tasks requiring alertness while taking this medication. Seniors may be more adversely affected, because it may affect their coordination and reflexes and lead to falls and injury. Taking Librium with other central nervous system (CNS) depressants such as alcohol, narcotics, and barbiturates may compound these CNS effects.

Prolonged use of benzodiazepines can lead to dependence. When the medication is abruptly withdrawn, symptoms of withdrawal may occur. Withdrawal symptoms include headache, vomiting, impaired concentration, confusion, tremor, muscle cramps, and seizures. Because Librium has a long duration of action, withdrawal symptoms are generally milder than with shorter-acting benzodiazepines such as Xanax (alprazolam).

Benzodiazepines are centrally acting depressants, and they can depress respiration. This is particularly problematic for patients with chronic obstructive pulmonary disease and emphysema. Patients with sleep apnea—a sleep disorder in which respiration is interrupted by long pauses during the sleep cycle—should not take Librium or other benzodiazepines. The respiratory depressant effect of benzodiazepines may further suppress the respiratory drive of these patients and put them at risk for respiratory depression and death.

Benzodiazepines may induce **paradoxical reactions** in susceptible individuals. Instead of the expected depressant effects, the medication produces excitement, aggression, anger, uninhibited behavior, and rage in susceptible individuals. These reactions are more likely to occur in seniors, people with brain damage, and individuals with personality and impulse-control disorders.

Use in Pregnancy and Breastfeeding: Pregnancy Category D

Benzodiazepines and their metabolites are known to cross the placenta and accumulate in the fetal circulation. They are associated with risk of congenital malformations when used during pregnancy, causing cleft lip and heart deformities in the fetus. Benzodiazepines should be avoided during pregnancy, particularly in the first trimester. The use of benzodiazepines during pregnancy should be considered only when the need for the medication outweighs its risk and alternative therapies have failed.

Nursing mothers should not take Librium, because it will pass into breast milk and be ingested by the baby. If stopping the drug is not an alternative, breastfeeding should not be started or should be discontinued.

Possible Drug Interactions

A number of significant drug interactions have been reported with Librium; these are summarized in the table on the next page.

Patients taking Librium should not consume alcohol because the combination may increase sedation and drowsiness.

CNS depressants (e.g., alcohol, narcotics, barbiturates, hypnotics) and antihistamines	Combination of Librium and another CNS depressant may impair coordination and breathing and increase sedation.
Tagamet (cimetidine), oral contraceptives, Prozac (fluoxetine), Nizoral (ketoconazole), Inderal (propranolol), Depakote (divalproex sodium), Darvon (propoxyphene), Antabuse (disulfiram)	These medications may inhibit the metabolism of Librium, thus increasing the level and pharmacological effects of Librium and producing excessive sedation and other adverse CNS effects.
Lanoxin (digoxin)	Librium may increase the blood levels of Lanoxin, and toxicity may occur. Patients taking Librium and Lanoxin should have their Lanoxin levels monitored closely.

Overdose

Overdoses from oral ingestion of benzodiazepines alone are generally not fatal. Most fatalities reported with benzodiazepines involve multiple medication ingestion, particularly the combination of a benzodiazepine with other CNS depressants, such as alcohol, narcotics, and barbiturates.

Mild symptoms of benzodiazepine overdose include drowsiness, confusion, somnolence, tiredness, impaired coordination, clumsiness in walking (ataxia), and slow reflexes. Benzodiazepine overdose, when these agents are taken alone, is rarely fatal. When multiple medications are implicated in benzodiazepine overdose, severe symptoms include difficulty breathing, slowed heart rate, low blood pressure, loss of coordination, and loss of consciousness leading to coma and, potentially, death.

Any suspected overdose should be treated as an emergency. The person should be taken to the emergency room for observation and treatment. The prescription bottle of medication (and any other medication suspected in the overdose) should be brought as well, because the information on the prescription label can be helpful to the treating physician in determining the number of pills ingested.

Special Considerations

- Librium should be discontinued gradually by tapering the dose. Stopping the medication abruptly, especially after taking it regularly for long periods, may trigger withdrawal symptoms, including irritability, agitation, tension, and insomnia.
- If you miss a dose, take it as soon as possible. If it is close to the next scheduled dose, skip the missed dose and continue on your regular dosing schedule. Do not take double doses.
- Librium may be taken with or without food.
- Librium may cause sedation and drowsiness, especially during initiation of therapy, and impair your alertness. Use caution when driving or performing tasks that require alertness. Avoid alcohol when taking Librium, because alcohol may intensify these effects.
- Store the medication in its originally labeled, light-resistant container, away from heat and moisture. Heat and moisture may precipitate breakdown of your medication, and the medication may lose its therapeutic effects.
- Keep your medication out of reach of children.

If you have any questions about your medication, consult your physician or pharmacist.

Notes

_____

_____

_____

_____

_____

_____

_____

_____

_____

_____

_____

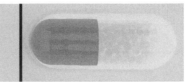

Klonopin (clonazepam)

Generic name: Clonazepam
Available strengths: 0.5 mg, 1 mg, 2 mg tablets;
   0.125 mg, 0.25 mg, 0.5 mg, 1 mg, 2 mg rapid-dissolving tablets
Available in generic: Yes
Drug class: Benzodiazepine/anxiolytic; sedative-hypnotic

General Information

Klonopin (clonazepam) is a benzodiazepine indicated for management of seizure disorders and panic disorder. The use of a medication for its approved indications is called its *labeled use*. In clinical practice, however, physicians often prescribe medications for *unlabeled* ("off-label") uses when published clinical studies, case reports, or their own clinical experiences support the efficacy and safety of those treatments. Physicians may use Klonopin outside its approved indications to treat social anxiety disorder, posttraumatic stress disorder, agitation in acute psychosis and mania, and premenstrual syndrome. As with other benzodiazepines, Klonopin is associated with dependence and abuse and is therefore regulated as a controlled substance by state and federal laws.

Klonopin's effectiveness for treating anxiety may be explained by its pharmacological action in the brain at specific receptor sites. *Receptors* are specific sites on the nerve cell membrane that receive a signal from a neurochemical called the **neurotransmitter.** Once a neurotransmitter locks in on the receptor, the neurochemical signal is changed to an electrical or another chemical signal and travels down the neuron. The receptor sites in which benzodiazepines elicit their action are found in various regions of the brain, and the specific receptors are also known as **benzodiazepine receptors.** The coupled reaction of benzodiazepines to the receptors facilitates the inhibitory action of the neurotransmitter γ-**aminobutyric acid** (GABA) in that region of the brain. Benzodiazepines' action on GABA receptors appears to produce their anxiolytic, sedative, and anticonvulsant actions. Klonopin, for example, is an effective anxiolytic, hypnotic, and antiseizure medication.

Dosing Information

The usual starting dosage of Klonopin is 0.5 mg two to three times a day, with increases to a therapeutic dosage of 1–4 mg/day administered in divided doses. Depending on the severity of symptoms, the dosage may be increased to a maximum of 6–8 mg/day.

Common Side Effects

The most common side effects reported with Klonopin are sedation and drowsiness, especially shortly after initiating therapy. Other frequent symptoms are impaired concentration and memory, feeling of dissociation ("spacey"), and impaired coordination.

Adverse Reactions and Precautions

Klonopin affects alertness and coordination, and patients should exercise caution when driving or performing other tasks requiring alertness while taking this medication. Seniors may be more adversely affected, because it may affect their coordination and reflexes and lead to falls and injury. Taking Klonopin with other central nervous system (CNS) depressants such as alcohol, narcotics, and barbiturates may compound these CNS effects.

Prolonged use of benzodiazepines can lead to dependence. When the medication is abruptly withdrawn, symptoms of withdrawal may occur. Withdrawal symptoms include headache, vomiting, impaired concentration, confusion, tremor, muscle cramps, and seizures. However, because Klonopin has a longer duration of action than some other benzodiazepines, such as Xanax (alprazolam), it rarely induces withdrawal reactions.

Benzodiazepines are centrally acting depressants, and they can depress respiration. This is particularly problematic for patients with chronic obstructive pulmonary disease and emphysema. Patients with sleep apnea—a sleep disorder in which respiration is interrupted by long pauses during the sleep cycle—should not take Klonopin or other benzodiazepines. The respiratory depressant effect of benzodiazepines may further suppress the respiratory drive in these patients and put them at risk for respiratory depression and death.

Benzodiazepines may induce **paradoxical reactions** in susceptible individuals. Instead of the expected depressant effects, the medication produces excitement, aggression, anger, uninhibited behavior, and rage in susceptible individuals. These reactions are more likely to occur in seniors, people with brain damage, and individuals with personality and impulse-control disorders.

Use in Pregnancy and Breastfeeding: Pregnancy Category D

Benzodiazepines and their metabolites are known to cross the placenta and accumulate in the fetal circulation. They are associated with risk of congenital malformations when used during pregnancy, causing cleft lip and heart deformities in the fetus. Benzodiazepines should be avoided during pregnancy, particularly in the first trimester. The use of benzodiazepines during pregnancy should be considered only when the need for the medication outweighs its risk and alternative therapies have failed.

Nursing mothers should not take Klonopin, because it will pass into breast milk and be ingested by the baby. If stopping the drug is not an alternative, breastfeeding should not be started or should be discontinued.

Possible Drug Interactions

The drug interactions reported with Klonopin are summarized in the table on the next page.

Patients taking Klonopin should not consume alcohol because the combination may increase sedation and drowsiness.

CNS depressants (e.g., alcohol, narcotics, barbiturates, hypnotics) and antihistamines	Combination of Klonopin and another CNS depressant may impair coordination and breathing and increase sedation.
Serzone (nefazodone), erythromycin, Nizoral (ketoconazole), Sporanox (itraconazole), Cipro (ciprofloxacin)	When any of these medications are taken concurrently with Klonopin, they may inhibit the metabolism of Klonopin and increase its blood levels and side effects (especially sedation and drowsiness).

Overdose

Overdoses from oral ingestion of benzodiazepines alone are generally not fatal. Most fatalities reported with benzodiazepines involve multiple medication ingestion, particularly the combination of a benzodiazepine with other CNS depressants, such as alcohol, narcotics, and barbiturates.

Mild symptoms of benzodiazepine overdose include drowsiness, confusion, somnolence, tiredness, impaired coordination, clumsiness in walking (ataxia), and slow reflexes. Benzodiazepine overdose, when these agents are taken alone, is rarely fatal. When multiple medications are implicated in benzodiazepine overdose, severe symptoms include difficulty breathing, slowed heart rate, low blood pressure, loss of coordination, and loss of consciousness leading to coma and, potentially, death.

Any suspected overdose should be treated as an emergency. The person should be taken to the emergency room for observation and treatment. The prescription bottle of medication (and any other medication suspected in the overdose) should be brought as well, because the information on the prescription label can be helpful to the treating physician in determining the number of pills ingested.

Special Considerations

- Klonopin should be discontinued gradually by tapering the dose. Stopping the medication abruptly, especially after taking it regularly for long periods, may trigger withdrawal symptoms, including irritability, agitation, tension, and insomnia.
- If you miss a dose, take it as soon as possible. If it is close to the next scheduled dose, skip the missed dose and continue on your regular dosing schedule. Do not take double doses.
- Klonopin may be taken with or without food.
- Klonopin may cause sedation and drowsiness, especially during initiation of therapy, and impair your alertness. Use caution when driving or performing tasks that require alertness. Avoid alcohol when taking Klonopin, because alcohol may intensify these effects.
- Store the medication in its originally labeled, light-resistant container, away from heat and moisture. Heat and moisture may precipitate breakdown of your medication, and the medication may lose its therapeutic effects.
- Keep your medication out of reach of children.

If you have any questions about your medication, consult your physician or pharmacist.

Notes

_____

_____

_____

_____

_____

_____

_____

_____

_____

_____

_____

_____

_____

_____

_____

From Chew RH, Hales RE, Yudofsky SC: _What Your Patients Need to Know About Psychiatric Medications_, Second Edition. Washington, DC, American Psychiatric Publishing, 2009

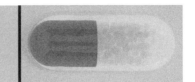

Serax (oxazepam)

Generic name: Oxazepam
Available strengths: 10 mg, 15 mg, 30 mg capsules
Available in generic: Yes
Drug class: Benzodiazepine/anxiolytic; sedative-hypnotic

General Information

Serax (oxazepam) is a benzodiazepine indicated for management of anxiety disorders or short-term relief of symptoms of anxiety and acute alcohol withdrawal. The use of a medication for its approved indications is called its *labeled use*. In clinical practice, however, physicians often prescribe medications for *unlabeled* ("off-label") uses when published clinical studies, case reports, or their own clinical experiences support the efficacy and safety of those treatments. Physicians may use Serax outside its approved indications to treat social phobia, posttraumatic stress disorder, insomnia, premenstrual syndrome, and other conditions. As with other benzodiazepines, Serax is associated with dependence and abuse and is therefore regulated as a controlled substance by state and federal laws.

Serax's effectiveness for treating anxiety may be explained by its pharmacological action in the brain at specific receptor sites. *Receptors* are specific sites on the nerve cell membrane that receive a signal from a neurochemical called the **neurotransmitter.** Once a neurotransmitter locks in on the receptor, the neurochemical signal is changed to an electrical or another chemical signal and travels down the neuron. The receptor sites in which benzodiazepines elicit their action are found in various regions of the brain, and the specific receptors are also known as **benzodiazepine receptors.** The coupled reaction of benzodiazepines to the receptors facilitates the inhibitory action of the neurotransmitter γ-**aminobutyric acid** (GABA) in that region of the brain. Benzodiazepines' action on GABA receptors appears to produce their anxiolytic, sedative, and anticonvulsant actions. Serax is an effective anxiolytic and hypnotic medication.

Dosing Information

For mild to moderate anxiety, the usual starting dosage of Serax is 10–15 mg three to four times a day. For severe anxiety and in management of acute alcohol withdrawal, the usual dosage is 15–30 mg given three to four times daily. Seniors may need smaller dosages, and Serax should be started at 10 mg three times daily, with gradual increases in dosage as necessary.

Common Side Effects

The most common side effects reported with Serax are sedation and drowsiness, especially shortly after initiating therapy. Other frequent symptoms are impaired concentration and memory, feeling of dissociation ("spacey"), and impaired coordination.

Adverse Reactions and Precautions

Serax affects alertness and coordination, and patients should exercise caution when driving or performing other tasks requiring alertness while taking this medication. Seniors may be more adversely affected, because it may affect their coordination and reflexes and lead to falls and injury. Taking Serax with other central nervous system (CNS) depressants such as alcohol, narcotics, and barbiturates may compound these CNS effects.

Prolonged use of benzodiazepines can lead to dependence. When the medication is abruptly withdrawn, symptoms of withdrawal may occur. Withdrawal symptoms include headache, vomiting, impaired concentration, confusion, tremor, muscle cramps, and seizures.

Benzodiazepines are centrally acting depressants, and they can depress respiration. This is particularly problematic for patients with chronic obstructive pulmonary disease and emphysema. Patients with sleep apnea—a sleep disorder in which respiration is interrupted by long pauses during the sleep cycle—should not take Serax or other benzodiazepines. The respiratory depressant effect of benzodiazepines may further suppress the respiratory drive in these patients and put them at risk for respiratory depression and death.

Benzodiazepines may induce **paradoxical reactions** in susceptible individuals. Instead of the expected depressant effects, the medication produces excitement, aggression, anger, uninhibited behavior, and rage in susceptible individuals. These reactions are more likely to occur in seniors, people with brain damage, and individuals with personality and impulse-control disorders.

Use in Pregnancy and Breastfeeding: Pregnancy Category D

Benzodiazepines and their metabolites are known to cross the placenta and accumulate in the fetal circulation. They are associated with risk of congenital malformations when used during pregnancy, causing cleft lip and heart deformities in the fetus. Benzodiazepines should be avoided during pregnancy, particularly in the first trimester. The use of benzodiazepines during pregnancy should be considered only when the need for the medication outweighs its risk and alternative therapies have failed.

Nursing mothers should not take Serax because it will pass into breast milk and be ingested by the baby. If stopping the drug is not an alternative, breastfeeding should not be started or should be discontinued.

Possible Drug Interactions

The drug interactions reported with Serax are summarized in the table on the next page.

Patients taking Serax should not consume alcohol because the combination may increase sedation and drowsiness.

CNS depressants (e.g., alcohol, narcotics, barbiturates, hypnotics) and antihistamines	Combination of Serax and another CNS depressant may impair coordination and breathing and increase sedation.
Oral contraceptives	The clearance rate of Serax may be increased when it is taken concurrently with oral contraceptives, which may decrease the effectiveness of Serax.
Lanoxin (digoxin)	Serax may increase the blood levels of Lanoxin, and toxicity may occur. Patients taking Serax and Lanoxin should have their Lanoxin levels monitored closely.
Theophylline (e.g., Theo-Dur)	Theophylline-containing medications may diminish the therapeutic effect of Serax.

Overdose

Overdoses from oral ingestion of benzodiazepines alone are generally not fatal. Most fatalities reported with benzodiazepines involve multiple medication ingestion, particularly the combination of a benzodiazepine with other CNS depressants, such as alcohol, narcotics, and barbiturates.

Mild symptoms of benzodiazepine overdose include drowsiness, confusion, somnolence, tiredness, impaired coordination, clumsiness in walking (ataxia), and slow reflexes. Benzodiazepine overdose, when these agents are taken alone, is rarely fatal. When multiple medications are implicated in benzodiazepine overdose, severe symptoms include difficulty breathing, slowed heart rate, low blood pressure, loss of coordination, and loss of consciousness leading to coma and, potentially, death.

Any suspected overdose should be treated as an emergency. The person should be taken to the emergency room for observation and treatment. The prescription bottle of medication (and any other medication suspected in the overdose) should be brought as well, because the information on the prescription label can be helpful to the treating physician in determining the number of pills ingested.

Special Considerations

- Serax should be discontinued gradually by tapering the dose. Stopping the medication abruptly, especially after taking it regularly for long periods, may trigger withdrawal symptoms, including irritability, agitation, tension, and insomnia.
- If you miss a dose, take it as soon as possible. But if it is close to the next scheduled dose, skip the missed dose and continue on your regular dosing schedule. Do not take double doses.
- Serax may be taken with or without food.
- Serax may cause sedation and drowsiness, especially during initiation of therapy, and impair your alertness. Use caution when driving or performing tasks that require alertness. Avoid alcohol when taking Serax, because alcohol may intensify these effects.
- Store the medication in its originally labeled, light-resistant container, away from heat and moisture. Heat and moisture may precipitate breakdown of your medication, and the medication may lose its therapeutic effects.
- Keep your medication out of reach of children.

If you have any questions about your medication, consult your physician or pharmacist.

Notes

_____

_____

_____

_____

_____

_____

_____

_____

_____

_____

_____

_____

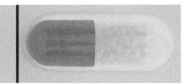

Tranxene (clorazepate)

Generic name: Clorazepate
Available strengths: 3.75 mg, 7.5 mg, 15 mg capsules or tablets;
    11.25 mg (Tranxene-SD Half Strength), 22.5 mg (Tranxene-SD)
Available in generic: Yes, except Tranxene-SD
Drug class: Benzodiazepine/anxiolytic; sedative-hypnotic

General Information

Tranxene (clorazepate) is a benzodiazepine indicated for treatment of anxiety disorders or short-term relief of symptoms of anxiety, alcohol withdrawal, and seizure disorders. The use of a medication for its approved indications is called its *labeled use*. In clinical practice, however, physicians often prescribe medications for *unlabeled* ("off-label") uses when published clinical studies, case reports, or their own clinical experiences support the efficacy and safety of those treatments. Physicians may use Tranxene outside its approved indications to treat social phobia, posttraumatic stress disorder, insomnia, and premenstrual syndrome. As with other benzodiazepines, Tranxene is associated with dependence and abuse and is therefore regulated as a controlled substance by state and federal laws.

Tranxene's effectiveness for treating anxiety may be explained by its pharmacological action in the brain at specific receptor sites. *Receptors* are specific sites on the nerve cell membrane that receive a signal from a neurochemical called the **neurotransmitter.** Once a neurotransmitter locks in on the receptor, the neurochemical signal is changed to an electrical or another chemical signal and travels down the neuron. The receptor sites in which benzodiazepines elicit their action are found in various regions of the brain, and the specific receptors are also known as **benzodiazepine receptors.** The coupled reaction of benzodiazepines to the receptors facilitates the inhibitory action of the neurotransmitter γ-**aminobutyric acid** (GABA) in that region of the brain. Benzodiazepines' action on GABA receptors appears to produce their anxiolytic, sedative, and anticonvulsant actions. Tranxene is an effective anxiolytic and hypnotic medication.

Dosing Information

For treatment of anxiety, the usual starting dosage of Tranxene is 3.75 mg three times a day (11.25 mg/day), which can be administered in a single dose once a day with Tranxene-SD Half Strength in the 11.25 mg tablet. The dosage may be increased to 7.5 mg two or three times a day (15–22.5 mg/day). Patients whose symptoms are stabilized with 7.5 mg three times a day may have their medication switched to Tranxene-SD 22.5 mg tablet administered once a day. The therapeutic dosage for treating anxiety is generally in the range of 15–60 mg/day administered in divided doses. For severe anxiety and in management of acute alcohol withdrawal, the usual dosage is 15–30 mg given three to four times daily.

Common Side Effects

The most common side effects reported with Tranxene are sedation and drowsiness, especially shortly after initiating therapy. Other frequent symptoms are impaired concentration and memory, feeling of dissociation ("spacey"), and impaired coordination.

Adverse Reactions and Precautions

Tranxene affects alertness and coordination, and patients should exercise caution when driving or performing other tasks requiring alertness while taking this medication. Seniors may be more adversely affected, because it may affect their coordination and reflexes and lead to falls and injury. Taking Tranxene with other central nervous system (CNS) depressants such as alcohol, narcotics, and barbiturates may compound these CNS effects.

Prolonged use of benzodiazepines can lead to dependence. When the medication is abruptly withdrawn, symptoms of withdrawal may occur. Withdrawal symptoms include headache, vomiting, impaired concentration, confusion, tremor, muscle cramps, and seizures.

Benzodiazepines are centrally acting depressants, and they can depress respiration. This is particularly problematic for patients with chronic obstructive pulmonary disease and emphysema. Patients with sleep apnea—a sleep disorder in which respiration is interrupted by long pauses during the sleep cycle—should not take Tranxene or other benzodiazepines. The respiratory depressant effect of benzodiazepines may further suppress the respiratory drive in these patients and put them at risk for respiratory depression and death.

Benzodiazepines may induce **paradoxical reactions** in susceptible individuals. Instead of the expected depressant effects, the medication may produce excitement, aggression, anger, uninhibited behavior, and rage in susceptible individuals. These reactions are more likely to occur in seniors, people with brain damage, and individuals with personality and impulse-control disorders.

Use in Pregnancy and Breastfeeding: Pregnancy Category D

Benzodiazepines and their metabolites are known to cross the placenta and accumulate in the fetal circulation. They are associated with risk of congenital malformations when used during pregnancy, causing cleft lip and heart deformities in the fetus. Benzodiazepines should be avoided during pregnancy, particularly in the first trimester. The use of benzodiazepines during pregnancy should be considered only when the need for the medication outweighs its risk and alternative therapies have failed.

Nursing mothers should not take Tranxene, because it will pass into breast milk and be ingested by the baby. If stopping the drug is not an alternative, breastfeeding should not be started or should be discontinued.

Possible Drug Interactions

The significant drug interactions reported with Tranxene are summarized in the table on the next page.

Patients taking Tranxene should not consume alcohol because the combination may increase sedation and drowsiness.

CNS depressants (e.g., alcohol, narcotics, barbiturates, hypnotics) and antihistamines	Combination of Tranxene and another CNS depressant may impair coordination and breathing and increase sedation.
Tagamet (cimetidine), Serzone (nefazodone), erythromycin, Biaxin (clarithromycin), TAO (troleandomycin), Antabuse (disulfiram), Prozac (fluoxetine), Luvox (fluvoxamine), isoniazid (e.g., INH), Diflucan (fluconazole), Nizoral (ketoconazole), Sporanox (itraconazole), Cipro (ciprofloxacin), protease inhibitors (e.g., Crixivan, Norvir, Fortovase), grapefruit juice	When any of these medications, or grapefruit juice, are taken concurrently with Tranxene, they may inhibit the metabolism of Tranxene and increase its levels. This may enhance the adverse effects (e.g., sedation, drowsiness, respiratory depression) of the benzodiazepine. If the medication is administered concurrently with Tranxene, a dosage reduction for Tranxene may be necessary.
Oral contraceptives	The metabolism of Tranxene may be increased when taken concurrently with oral contraceptives, which may decrease the effectiveness of Tranxene.
Lanoxin (digoxin)	Tranxene may increase the blood levels of Lanoxin, and toxicity may occur. Patients taking Tranxene and Lanoxin should have their Lanoxin levels monitored closely.
Theophylline (e.g., Theo-Dur)	Theophylline-containing medications may diminish the therapeutic effect of Tranxene.

Overdose

Overdoses from oral ingestion of benzodiazepines alone are generally not fatal. Most fatalities reported with benzodiazepines involve multiple medication ingestion, particularly the combination of a benzodiazepine with other CNS depressants, such as alcohol, narcotics, and barbiturates.

Mild symptoms of benzodiazepine overdose include drowsiness, confusion, somnolence, tiredness, impaired coordination, clumsiness in walking (ataxia), and slow reflexes. Benzodiazepine overdose, when these agents are taken alone, is rarely fatal. When multiple medications are implicated in benzodiazepine overdose, severe symptoms include difficulty breathing, slowed heart rate, low blood pressure, loss of coordination, and loss of consciousness leading to coma and, potentially, death.

Any suspected overdose should be treated as an emergency. The person should be taken to the emergency room for observation and treatment. The prescription bottle of medication (and any other medication suspected in the overdose) should be brought as well, because the information on the prescription label can be helpful to the treating physician in determining the number of pills ingested.

Special Considerations

- Tranxene should be discontinued gradually by tapering the dose. Stopping the medication abruptly, especially after taking it regularly for long periods, may trigger withdrawal symptoms, including irritability, agitation, tension, and insomnia.
- If you miss a dose, take it as soon as possible. But if it is close to the next scheduled dose, skip the missed dose and continue on your regular dosing schedule. Do not take double doses.
- Tranxene may be taken with or without food.

21

- Tranxene may cause sedation and drowsiness, especially during initiation of therapy, and impair your alertness. Use caution when driving or performing tasks that require alertness. Avoid alcohol when taking Tranxene, because alcohol may intensify these effects.
- Store the medication in its originally labeled, light-resistant container, away from heat and moisture. Heat and moisture may precipitate breakdown of your medication, and the medication may lose its therapeutic effects.
- Keep your medication out of reach of children.

If you have any questions about your medication, consult your physician or pharmacist.

Notes

_____

_____

_____

_____

_____

_____

_____

_____

_____

From Chew RH, Hales RE, Yudofsky SC: *What Your Patients Need to Know About Psychiatric Medications*, Second Edition. Washington, DC, American Psychiatric Publishing, 2009

Valium (diazepam)

Generic name: Diazepam
Available strengths: 2 mg, 5 mg, 10 mg tablets;
   5 mg/5 mL oral solution; 2 mg/1 mL injection
Available in generic: Yes
Drug class: Benzodiazepine/anxiolytic; sedative-hypnotic

General Information

Valium (diazepam) is a benzodiazepine indicated for treatment of anxiety disorders or short-term relief of symptoms of anxiety, seizure disorder, and skeletal muscle spasms as a muscle relaxant. The use of a medication for its approved indications is called its *labeled use.* In clinical practice, however, physicians often prescribe medications for *unlabeled* ("off-label") uses when published clinical studies, case reports, or their own clinical experiences support the efficacy and safety of those treatments. Physicians may use Valium outside its approved indications to treat social phobia, posttraumatic stress disorder, panic attacks, insomnia, premenstrual syndrome, and other conditions. As with other benzodiazepines, Valium is associated with dependence and abuse and is therefore regulated as a controlled substance by state and federal laws.

Valium's effectiveness for treating anxiety may be explained by its pharmacological action in the brain at specific receptor sites. *Receptors* are specific sites on the nerve cell membrane that receive the signal from a neurochemical called the **neurotransmitter.** Once a neurotransmitter locks in on the receptor, the neurochemical signal is changed to an electrical or another chemical signal and travels down the neuron. The receptor sites in which benzodiazepines elicit their action are found in various regions of the brain, and the specific receptors are also known as **benzodiazepine receptors.** The coupled reaction of benzodiazepines to the receptors facilitates the inhibitory action of the neurotransmitter γ-**aminobutyric acid** (GABA) in that region of the brain. Benzodiazepines' action on GABA receptors appears to produce their anxiolytic, sedative, and anticonvulsant actions. Valium, for example, is an effective anxiolytic, hypnotic (e.g., used in anesthesia), and antiseizure medication.

Dosing Information

The usual starting dosage of Valium is 2–5 mg two or three times a day. Depending on the severity of symptoms, the dosage may range from 4 mg/day to 40 mg/day, administered in divided doses. Diazepam breaks down to an active metabolite in the body. In seniors who have decreased metabolism, diazepam and its metabolite may be eliminated more slowly and thus can accumulate. The initial dosage for elderly persons should be small, and the dosage should be increased gradually to prevent any untoward reactions.

Common Side Effects

The most common side effects reported with Valium are sedation and drowsiness, especially shortly after initiating therapy. Other frequent symptoms are impaired concentration and memory, feeling of dissociation ("spacey"), and impaired coordination.

Adverse Reactions and Precautions

Valium affects alertness and coordination, and patients should exercise caution when driving or performing other tasks requiring alertness while taking this medication. Seniors may be more adversely affected, because it may affect their coordination and reflexes and lead to falls and injury. Taking Valium with other central nervous system (CNS) depressants such as alcohol, narcotics, and barbiturates may compound these CNS effects.

Prolonged use of benzodiazepines can lead to dependence. When the medication is abruptly withdrawn, symptoms of withdrawal may occur. Withdrawal symptoms include headache, vomiting, impaired concentration, confusion, tremor, muscle cramps, and seizures. Because Valium has a longer duration of action, withdrawal symptoms are generally milder than with shorter-acting benzodiazepines such as Xanax (alprazolam).

Benzodiazepines are centrally acting depressants, and they can depress respiration. This is particularly problematic for patients with chronic obstructive pulmonary disease and emphysema. Patients with sleep apnea—a sleep disorder in which respiration is interrupted by long pauses during the sleep cycle—should not take Valium or other benzodiazepines. The respiratory depressant effect of benzodiazepines may further suppress the respiratory drive in these patients and put them at risk for respiratory depression and death.

Benzodiazepines may induce **paradoxical reactions** in susceptible individuals. Instead of the expected depressant effects, the medication produces excitement, aggression, anger, uninhibited behavior, and rage in susceptible individuals. These reactions are more likely to occur in seniors, people with brain damage, and individuals with personality and impulse-control disorders.

Use in Pregnancy and Breastfeeding: Pregnancy Category D

Benzodiazepines and their metabolites are known to cross the placenta and accumulate in the fetal circulation. They are associated with risk of congenital malformations when used during pregnancy, causing cleft lip and heart deformities in the fetus. Benzodiazepines should be avoided during pregnancy, particularly in the first trimester. The use of benzodiazepines during pregnancy should be considered only when the need for the medication outweighs its risk and alternative therapies have failed.

Nursing mothers should not take Valium, because it will pass into breast milk and be ingested by the baby. If stopping the drug is not an alternative, breastfeeding should not be started or should be discontinued.

Possible Drug Interactions

A number of significant drug interactions have been reported with Valium; these are summarized in the table on the next page.

Patients taking Valium should not consume alcohol because the combination may increase sedation and drowsiness.

CNS depressants (e.g., alcohol, narcotics, barbiturates, hypnotics) and antihistamines	Combination of Valium and another CNS depressant may impair coordination and breathing and increase sedation.
Tagamet (cimetidine), oral contraceptives, Prozac (fluoxetine), Nizoral (ketoconazole), Inderal (propranolol), Depakote (divalproex sodium), Darvon (propoxyphene), Antabuse (disulfiram)	Any of these medications may increase the pharmacological effects of Valium and produce excessive sedation and other adverse CNS effects. These medications are known to inhibit the metabolism of Valium, thus increasing the medication level.
Lanoxin (digoxin)	Valium may increase the blood levels of Lanoxin, and toxicity may occur. Patients taking Valium and Lanoxin should have their Lanoxin levels monitored closely.
Antacids (e.g., Maalox)	The combination of antacids and Valium may decrease the therapeutic effect of Valium.

Overdose

Overdoses from oral ingestion of benzodiazepines alone are generally not fatal. Most fatalities reported with benzodiazepines involve multiple medication ingestion, particularly the combination of a benzodiazepine with other CNS depressants, such as alcohol, narcotics, and barbiturates.

Mild symptoms of benzodiazepine overdose include drowsiness, confusion, somnolence, tiredness, impaired coordination, clumsiness in walking (ataxia), and slow reflexes. Benzodiazepine overdose, when these agents are taken alone, is rarely fatal. When multiple medications are implicated in benzodiazepine overdose, severe symptoms include difficulty breathing, slowed heart rate, low blood pressure, loss of coordination, and loss of consciousness leading to coma and, potentially, death.

Any suspected overdose should be treated as an emergency. The person should be taken to the emergency room for observation and treatment. The prescription bottle of medication (and any other medication suspected in the overdose) should be brought as well, because the information on the prescription label can be helpful to the treating physician in determining the number of pills ingested.

Special Considerations

- Valium should be discontinued gradually by tapering the dose. Stopping the medication abruptly, especially after taking it regularly for long periods, may trigger withdrawal symptoms, including irritability, agitation, tension, and insomnia.
- If you miss a dose, take it as soon as possible. But if it is close to the next scheduled dose, skip the missed dose and continue on your regular dosing schedule. Do not take double doses.
- Valium may be taken with or without food.
- Valium should not be taken with antacids, which may delay or alter the absorption of Valium. Separate the dosing of Valium from the antacid by 2–3 hours.
- Valium may cause sedation and drowsiness, especially during initiation of therapy, and impair your alertness. Use caution when driving or performing tasks that require alertness. Avoid alcohol when taking Valium, because alcohol may intensify these effects.

- Store the medication in its originally labeled, light-resistant container, away from heat and moisture. Heat and moisture may precipitate breakdown of your medication, and the medication may lose its therapeutic effects.
- Keep your medication out of reach of children.

If you have any questions about your medication, consult your physician or pharmacist.

Notes

From Chew RH, Hales RE, Yudofsky SC: *What Your Patients Need to Know About Psychiatric Medications,* Second Edition. Washington, DC, American Psychiatric Publishing, 2009

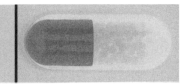

Xanax (alprazolam)

Generic name: Alprazolam
Available strengths: 0.25 mg, 0.5 mg, 1 mg, 2 mg tablets;
    0.5 mg, 1 mg, 2 mg, 3 mg extended-release tablets (Xanax XR);
    0.25 mg, 0.5 mg, 1 mg, 2 mg rapidly disintegrating tablets
    1 mg/mL oral solution
Available in generic: Yes, except Xanax XR
Drug class: Benzodiazepine/anxiolytic; sedative-hypnotic

General Information

Xanax (alprazolam) is a benzodiazepine indicated for management of anxiety disorders or short-term relief of symptoms of anxiety and for the treatment of panic attacks. The use of a medication for its approved indications is called its *labeled use*. In clinical practice, however, physicians often prescribe medications for *unlabeled* ("off-label") uses when published clinical studies, case reports, or their own clinical experiences support the efficacy and safety of those treatments. Physicians may use Xanax outside its approved indications to treat social phobia, depression, and premenstrual syndrome. As with other benzodiazepines, Xanax is associated with dependence and abuse and is therefore regulated as a controlled substance by state and federal laws.

Xanax's effectiveness for treating anxiety may be explained by its pharmacological action in the brain at specific receptor sites. *Receptors* are specific sites on the nerve cell membrane that receive a signal from a neurochemical called the **neurotransmitter.** Once a neurotransmitter locks in on the receptor, the neurochemical signal is changed to an electrical or another chemical signal and travels down the neuron. The receptor sites in which benzodiazepines elicit their action are found in various regions of the brain, and the specific receptors are also known as **benzodiazepine receptors.** The coupled reaction of benzodiazepines to the receptors facilitates the inhibitory action of the neurotransmitter γ-**aminobutyric acid** (GABA) in that region of the brain. Benzodiazepines' action on GABA receptors appears to produce their anxiolytic, sedative, and anticonvulsant actions. Xanax is an effective anxiolytic and hypnotic medication.

Dosing Information

The usual starting dosage of Xanax in treating anxiety disorders is 0.25–0.5 mg three times a day. The dosage may be gradually increased to a therapeutic range of 1–4 mg/day. The maximum dosage should not exceed 4 mg/day.

For treatment of panic disorder, higher dosages may be required. The initial dosage is 0.5 mg three times a day, with increases at intervals of 3–4 days in increments of no more than 1 mg/day. The average dosage for treating panic disorder is approximately 6 mg/day, but some patients may require dosages of up to 8 mg/day to achieve a successful response. Xanax is also available in extended-release tablets that may be taken once a day.

Common Side Effects

The most common side effects reported with Xanax are sedation and drowsiness, especially shortly after initiation of therapy. Other frequent symptoms are impaired concentration and memory, feeling of dissociation ("spacey"), and impaired coordination.

Adverse Reactions and Precautions

Xanax affects alertness and coordination, and patients should exercise caution when driving or performing other tasks requiring alertness while taking this medication. Seniors may be more adversely affected, because it may affect their coordination and reflexes and lead to falls and injury. Taking Xanax with other central nervous system (CNS) depressants such as alcohol, narcotics, and barbiturates may compound these CNS effects.

Prolonged use of benzodiazepines can lead to dependence, particularly with Xanax, which is associated with abuse. When the medication is abruptly withdrawn, symptoms of withdrawal may occur. Withdrawal symptoms include headache, vomiting, impaired concentration, confusion, tremor, muscle cramps, and seizures. In patients who have received Xanax for more than several months or at high dosages (e.g., 4 mg/day or greater), abrupt discontinuation of the medication should be avoided because they may be susceptible to withdrawal symptoms. Xanax has also been associated with seizures after abrupt withdrawal. The risk of seizures appears to be greatest 24–72 hours after discontinuation. Gradual tapering of the daily dosage reduces the risk of withdrawal symptoms and seizures. One recommended tapering schedule is to decrease Xanax by no more than 0.5 mg every 3 days. If withdrawal symptoms emerge, the patient should be placed back on the previous dosage. Some patients may require a much slower dosage reduction over several months or longer.

Benzodiazepines are centrally acting depressants, and they can depress respiration. This is particularly problematic for patients with chronic obstructive pulmonary disease and emphysema. Patients with sleep apnea—a sleep disorder in which respiration is interrupted by long pauses during the sleep cycle—should not take Xanax or other benzodiazepines. The respiratory depressant effect of benzodiazepines may further suppress the respiratory drive in these patients and put them at risk for respiratory depression and death.

Benzodiazepines may induce **paradoxical reactions** in susceptible individuals. Instead of the expected depressant effects, the medication produces excitement, aggression, anger, uninhibited behavior, and rage in susceptible individuals. These reactions are more likely to occur in seniors, people with brain damage, and individuals with personality and impulse-control disorders.

Use in Pregnancy and Breastfeeding: Pregnancy Category D

Benzodiazepines and their metabolites are known to cross the placenta and accumulate in the fetal circulation. They have been associated with increased risk of congenital malformations when used during pregnancy, causing cleft lip and heart deformities in the fetus. Benzodiazepines should be avoided during pregnancy, particularly in the first trimester. The use of benzodiazepines during pregnancy should be considered only when the need for the medication outweighs its risk and alternative therapies have failed.

Nursing mothers should not take Xanax, because it will pass into breast milk and be ingested by the baby. If stopping the drug is not an alternative, breastfeeding should not be started or should be discontinued.

Possible Drug Interactions

A number of drug interactions have been reported with Xanax; these are summarized in the table below.

CNS depressants (e.g., alcohol, narcotics, barbiturates, hypnotics), antihistamines, kava (herbal supplement)	Combination of Xanax and another CNS depressant or an antihistamine may impair coordination and breathing and increase sedation.
Tagamet (cimetidine), Serzone (nefazodone), erythromycin, Biaxin (clarithromycin), TAO (troleandomycin), oral contraceptives, Antabuse (disulfiram), Prozac (fluoxetine), Luvox (fluvoxamine), isoniazid (e.g., INH), Diflucan (fluconazole), Nizoral (ketoconazole), Sporanox (itraconazole), Cipro (ciprofloxacin), protease inhibitors (e.g., Crixivan, Norvir, Fortovase), grapefruit juice	When any of these medications, or grapefruit juice, are taken concurrently with Xanax, they may inhibit the metabolism of Xanax and increase its levels. This may enhance the adverse effects (e.g., sedation, drowsiness, respiratory depression) of the benzodiazepine. If the medication is administered concurrently with Xanax, a dosage reduction for Xanax may be necessary.
Antacids (e.g., Maalox), Tegretol (carbamazepine), theophylline (e.g., Theo-Dur), St. John's wort	The combination of any of these medications may decrease the therapeutic effect of Xanax.

Patients taking Xanax should not consume alcohol because the combination may increase sedation and drowsiness.

Overdose

Overdoses from oral ingestion of benzodiazepines alone are generally not fatal. Most fatalities reported with benzodiazepines involve multiple medication ingestion, particularly the combination of a benzodiazepine with other CNS depressants, such as alcohol, narcotics, and barbiturates.

Mild symptoms of benzodiazepine overdose include drowsiness, confusion, somnolence, tiredness, impaired coordination, clumsiness in walking (ataxia), and slow reflexes. Benzodiazepine overdose, when these agents are taken alone, is rarely fatal. When multiple medications are implicated in benzodiazepine overdose, severe symptoms include difficulty breathing, slowed heart rate, low blood pressure, loss of coordination, and loss of consciousness leading to coma and, potentially, death.

Any suspected overdose should be treated as an emergency. The person should be taken to the emergency room for observation and treatment. The prescription bottle of medication (and any other medication suspected in the overdose) should be brought as well, because the information on the prescription label can be helpful to the treating physician in determining the number of pills ingested.

Special Considerations

- Xanax should be discontinued gradually by tapering the dose. Stopping the medication abruptly, especially after taking it regularly for long periods, may trigger withdrawal symptoms, including irritability, agitation, tension, and insomnia.

- If you miss a dose, take it as soon as possible. But if it is close to the next scheduled dose, skip the missed dose and continue on your regular dosing schedule. Do not take double doses.
- Xanax may be taken with or without food.
- Xanax should not be taken with antacids, which may delay or alter the absorption of Xanax. Separate the dosing of Xanax from the antacid by 2–3 hours.
- Do not drink grapefruit juice while taking Xanax because it may decrease the metabolism and enhance the adverse effects of the medication.
- Xanax may cause sedation and drowsiness, especially during initiation of therapy, and impair your alertness. Use caution when driving or performing tasks that require alertness. Avoid alcohol when taking Xanax, because alcohol may intensify these effects.
- Store the medication in its originally labeled, light-resistant container, away from heat and moisture. Heat and moisture may precipitate breakdown of your medication, and the medication may lose its therapeutic effects.
- Keep your medication out of reach of children.

If you have any questions about your medication, consult your physician or pharmacist.

Notes

_____

_____

_____

_____

_____

_____

_____

From Chew RH, Hales RE, Yudofsky SC: *What Your Patients Need to Know About Psychiatric Medications*, Second Edition. Washington, DC, American Psychiatric Publishing, 2009

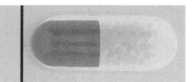

BuSpar (buspirone)

Generic name: Buspirone
Available strengths: 5 mg, 7.5 mg, 15 mg, 30 mg tablets
Available in generic: Yes
Drug class: Nonbenzodiazepine/antianxiety agent

General Information

BuSpar (buspirone) is an antianxiety medication indicated for management of selected anxiety disorders or for short-term relief of anxiety symptoms. It is not chemically related to the benzodiazepines (e.g., Valium) or barbiturates. In addition, unlike those medications, BuSpar neither produces prominent sedation nor significantly interferes with memory or cognition. The major advantage of BuSpar is its low abuse potential. It is not regulated as a controlled medication like the benzodiazepines and barbiturates. It does not appear to induce dependence, making it the better choice for individuals with a history of alcoholism and substance abuse. Moreover, unlike benzodiazepines, BuSpar does not require gradual tapering before discontinuation and may be abruptly stopped without withdrawal symptoms.

BuSpar's effectiveness for treating anxiety may be explained by its pharmacological action in the brain at specific receptor sites. *Receptors* are specific sites on the nerve cell membrane that receive a signal from a neurochemical called the **neurotransmitter.** Once a neurotransmitter locks in on the receptor, the neurochemical signal is changed to an electrical or another chemical signal and travels down the neuron. BuSpar's ability to relieve anxiety may be due to its action on serotonin receptors, by altering serotonin-receptor sensitivity at a specific serotonin receptor subtype ($5\text{-}HT_{1A}$). In contrast to benzodiazepines, which affect other types of receptors (in particular, γ-**aminobutyric acid** [GABA]), BuSpar does not have anticonvulsant or muscle relaxant effects.

Dosing Information

The usual starting dosage of BuSpar is 5 mg two or three times a day (10–15 mg/day), with increases of 5 mg/day at intervals of 2–3 days to an optimal therapeutic dosage of 20–30 mg/day in divided doses. The maximum dosage should not exceed 60 mg/day.

Common Side Effects

The common side effects associated with BuSpar are headaches, dizziness, and drowsiness. These side effects occur frequently shortly after initiating therapy but usually subside in about 1 week of therapy. Unlike benzodiazepines, BuSpar is less sedating and does not appear to impair cognition and coordination. However, some individuals who may be particularly sensitive to the central nervous system (CNS) effects of the medication or who metabolize it slowly may experience nervousness and excitement. Overall, BuSpar has very few troublesome side effects and is generally well tolerated.

Adverse Reactions and Precautions

Individuals, particularly seniors, should be aware of how BuSpar affects their alertness and coordination and observe caution while driving or performing other tasks requiring alertness. Some individuals may be especially sensitive to the CNS adverse effects (e.g., dizziness) of the medication.

Prolonged use of BuSpar is not known to lead to dependence. The medication may be abruptly withdrawn without inducing withdrawal symptoms. For most people, BuSpar does not appear to have any significant interaction with alcohol and does not intensify alcohol's sedative effects. Unlike benzodiazepines, which are centrally acting depressants and can depress respiration, BuSpar does not have this effect and will not affect respiration. It is safe for patients with chronic obstructive pulmonary disease and emphysema, as well as for patients with sleep apnea—a sleep disorder in which respiration is interrupted by long pauses during the sleep cycle.

BuSpar should not be taken with a type of antidepressant called **monoamine oxidase inhibitors** (MAOIs). The combination can precipitate a dangerous elevation of blood pressure.

Use in Pregnancy and Breastfeeding: Pregnancy Category B

The use of BuSpar during pregnancy has not been clinically studied, and our understanding of its risks is limited. BuSpar should be avoided during pregnancy, especially in the first trimester. The use of BuSpar during pregnancy should be considered only when the need for the medication outweighs its risk and alternative therapies have failed.

Nursing mothers should not take BuSpar, because it will pass into breast milk and be ingested by the baby. If stopping the drug is not an alternative, breastfeeding should not be started or should be discontinued.

Possible Drug Interactions

There are few significant drug interactions reported with BuSpar; those reported are summarized in the table on the next page.

Overdose

No deaths have been reported from overdoses with BuSpar alone. Nausea, vomiting, drowsiness, and stomach upset were reported by patients who took more than five times the maximum dosage of BuSpar. However, the combination of BuSpar with other CNS depressants in overdose may result in more severe symptoms.

erythromycin, Biaxin (clarithromycin), TAO (troleandomycin)	The combination of BuSpar and these antibiotics may inhibit the metabolism of BuSpar and lead to adverse side effects.
Nizoral (ketoconazole), Sporanox (itraconazole)	The combination of BuSpar and these antifungal agents may inhibit the metabolism of BuSpar and increase the likelihood of adverse side effects.
Serzone (nefazodone)	Serzone may markedly increase the blood levels of BuSpar and increase the likelihood of adverse side effects.
MAOIs (e.g., Marplan, Parnate, and Nardil)	MAOIs should not be combined with BuSpar. There have been reports of elevated blood pressure when BuSpar was added to medication regimens including an MAOI.

Any suspected overdose should be treated as an emergency. The person should be taken to the emergency room for observation and treatment. The prescription bottle of medication (and any other medication suspected in the overdose) should be brought as well, because the information on the prescription label can be helpful to the treating physician in determining the number of pills ingested.

Special Considerations

- If you miss a dose, take it as soon as possible. But if it is close to the next scheduled dose, skip the missed dose and continue on your regular dosing schedule. Do not take double doses.
- BuSpar may be taken with or without food.
- BuSpar may cause sedation and drowsiness, especially during initiation of therapy, and impair your alertness. Use caution when driving or performing tasks that require alertness. Avoid alcohol when taking BuSpar, because alcohol may intensify these effects.
- Store the medication in its originally labeled, light-resistant container, away from heat and moisture. Heat and moisture may precipitate breakdown of your medication, and the medication may lose its therapeutic effects.
- Keep your medication out of reach of children.

If you have any questions about your medication, consult your physician or pharmacist.

Notes

_____

_____

_____

_____

_____

_____

_____

_____

_____

_____

_____

From Chew RH, Hales RE, Yudofsky SC: *What Your Patients Need to Know About Psychiatric Medications*, Second Edition. Washington, DC, American Psychiatric Publishing, 2009

Medications for Treatment of Insomnia

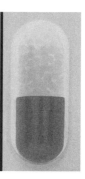

Benzodiazepines

Dalmane (flurazepam)
Halcion (triazolam)
ProSom (estazolam)
Restoril (temazepam)

Nonbenzodiazepines

Ambien (zolpidem)
Lunesta (eszopiclone)
Rozerem (ramelteon)
Sonata (zaleplon)
Trazodone (Desyrel)

Medications for treating **insomnia** are known as **sedative-hypnotics,** or simply **hypnotics.** With insomnia, the person may have difficulty falling asleep or staying asleep or may not feel rested after sleeping. Frequently, insomnia is caused by worry, tension, and stress of daily life. Sleep difficulties may occur with physical pain, discomfort, or illness. Certain medications and substances, including alcohol, stimulants, caffeine, selective serotonin reuptake inhibitor (SSRI) antidepressants, and illicit drugs can cause insomnia or upset sleep rhythm and disturb the quality of sleep. Some individuals may have a primary sleep disorder that causes sleep disruption, resulting in excessive sleepiness during the day and wakefulness at night. **Sleep apnea,** for example, is a breathing-related sleep disorder in which the sleeping patient stops breathing during the respiratory cycle and then suddenly snorts and gasps for air the next moment. This stop/start breathing rhythm prevents the person from getting a restful sleep. Insomnia may also be a symptom of an underlying mental disorder. Insomnia is a common symptom of depression, anxiety disorders, schizophrenia, and bipolar disorder. Depressed individuals, for example, have characteristic changes in their sleep pattern, and they may have marked difficulty falling asleep, sleep too much, sleep fitfully after falling asleep, or experience early-morning awakening.

Commonly, individuals treat their insomnia early on with nonprescription, over-the-counter sleep aids and then see their physician when their insomnia becomes unmanageable. Antihistamines are the primary hypnotic ingredients in over-the-counter sleep aids, such as Sominex (diphenhydramine) and Unisom (doxylamine), and many of these products come in combination with a mild analgesic, acetaminophen, to reduce minor aches and pains.

When individuals seek medical help for their insomnia, the physician evaluates the cause of their troublesome insomnia to determine whether it is related to an underlying mental disorder or physical condition. It is not simply a matter of prescribing a sleep medication for the patient but rather diagnosing and treating the underlying problem causing the insomnia.

The sedative-hypnotic medications frequently prescribed by physicians can be broadly divided into two categories: the **benzodiazepines** and the **nonbenzodiazepines.** The benzodiazepines denote a chemical class of medications with similar chemical structure and pharmacological action. The nonbenzodiazepine hypnotics include medications other than the benzodiazepines used for sleep. Physicians frequently prescribe medications not officially approved for hypnotic use and exploit a medication's sedating effects when it has been shown to be safe in treating insomnia. The antidepressant trazodone, for example, is widely used in low doses to induce sleep, especially when sleep difficulty is caused by SSRIs. Antihistamines, including Benadryl (diphenhydramine) and Atarax or Vistaril (hydroxyzine), are also commonly used as sedative-hypnotics.

At one time, barbiturates were widely used for sleep. However, barbiturates have a number of serious problems. Barbiturates can be lethal in overdose or when mixed with other depressants, such as alcohol. With chronic use of barbiturates, patients may develop tolerance to the barbiturate, requiring higher and higher doses to achieve sleep, which may lead to dependence. With the introduction of safer benzodiazepines and other hypnotics, physicians today rarely prescribe barbiturates for sleep. Moreover, other older sedative-hypnotics, such as chloral hydrate (Noctec) and glutethimide (Doriden), have fallen by the wayside as safer hypnotics have been introduced.

Benzodiazepines

The distinction of a benzodiazepine for use as an **anxiolytic** (i.e., a medication that relieves anxiety) or **hypnotic** (i.e., a medication that induces sleep) is somewhat arbitrary because any benzodiazepine can be used to treat anxiety or sleep problems, depending on the dosage. Valium (diazepam), for example, is well known for its use in treating anxiety but can also be used to treat insomnia. Benzodiazepines prescribed primarily for anxiety are discussed in separate handouts under "Antianxiety Medications."

Nonbenzodiazepine Hypnotics

In the group of nonbenzodiazepine hypnotics, Ambien (zolpidem), Lunesta (eszopiclone), Rozerem (ramelteon), and Sonata (zaleplon) have official approval from the U.S. Food and Drug Administration for treatment of insomnia. Except for Lunesta, which can be effective for up to 6 months, the other hypnotics are indicated for short-term use, generally not recommended for more than 2–3 weeks.

Antidepressants

Antidepressants with sedating effects are frequently prescribed at bedtime to induce sleep. Besides trazodone, which was discussed earlier, tricyclic antidepressants (TCAs) such as amitriptyline and Sinequan (doxepin) are often prescribed to help overcome insomnia, especially when the underlying cause is depression. Remeron (mirtazapine) is sedating at low dosages and can also be used for insomnia.

Antipsychotics

When treating patients with schizophrenia or bipolar disorder whose insomnia is due to agitation, the administration of a sedating antipsychotic at bedtime, in conjunction with routine psychotropic medications, may provide the dual benefits of antipsychotic and hypnotic effects to manage the patient's mental disorder. Chlorpromazine is widely used for its sedative effects at bedtime to induce sleep in agitated patients. Seroquel (quetiapine) at low doses is effective for treating insomnia in patients with schizophrenia.

For more information on a specific medication used to treat insomnia, refer to the handout on that medication.

From Chew RH, Hales RE, Yudofsky SC: *What Your Patients Need to Know About Psychiatric Medications*, Second Edition. Washington, DC, American Psychiatric Publishing, 2009

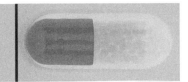

Dalmane (flurazepam)

Generic name: Flurazepam
Available strengths: 15 mg, 30 mg capsules
Available in generic: Yes
Drug class: Benzodiazepine/sedative-hypnotic

General Information

Dalmane (flurazepam) is a benzodiazepine sedative-hypnotic medication approved for the short-term treatment of insomnia. Similar to other benzodiazepines, Dalmane has anxiolytic effects (i.e., relieves anxiety), but it is seldom prescribed for this use. Because it has a long duration of action, the medication builds up in the body with continuous use. This may lead to daytime sedation, drowsiness, and memory disturbance. Generally, Dalmane should not be used for longer than 1 week. However, longer use occasionally may be necessary for some patients; in such cases, careful monitoring is needed to prevent physical or psychological dependence. As with other benzodiazepines, Dalmane is associated with dependence and abuse and is therefore regulated as a controlled substance by federal and state laws.

Dosing Information

The usual dose of Dalmane is 15 mg at bedtime. The dose may be increased to 30 mg if needed but should not exceed this amount. Seniors should not take more than 15 mg/day, because they may be more susceptible to the side effects of the medication.

Common Side Effects

The most common side effects reported with Dalmane are daytime drowsiness and sedation, especially shortly after initiating therapy. Other frequent complaints are impaired concentration and memory, feeling of dissociation ("spacey"), and impaired coordination.

Adverse Reactions and Precautions

Dalmane may affect alertness and coordination the next day after taking a single bedtime dose. Patients should exercise caution when driving or performing other tasks requiring alertness while taking this medication. Seniors may be more adversely affected, because it may affect their coordination and reflexes and lead to falls and injury. Taking Dalmane with other central nervous system (CNS) depressants such as alcohol, narcotics, and barbiturates may compound these CNS effects.

Prolonged use of benzodiazepines can lead to dependence. When the medication is abruptly withdrawn, symptoms of withdrawal may occur. Withdrawal symptoms include headache, vomiting, impaired concentration, confusion, tremor, muscle cramps, and seizures.

Benzodiazepines are centrally acting depressants, and they can depress respiration. This can affect patients with chronic obstructive pulmonary disease and emphysema by decreasing their "respiratory drive" or their ability to breathe. Patients with sleep apnea—a sleep disorder in which respiration is interrupted by long pauses during the sleep cycle—should not take Dalmane or other benzodiazepines. The respiratory depressant effect of benzodiazepines may further suppress the respiratory drive in these patients and put them at risk for respiratory depression.

Benzodiazepines may induce **paradoxical reactions** in susceptible individuals. Instead of the expected depressant effects, the medication produces excitement, aggression, anger, uninhibited behavior, and rage in susceptible individuals. These reactions are more likely to occur in seniors, people with brain damage, and individuals with personality and impulse-control disorders.

Use in Pregnancy and Breastfeeding: Pregnancy Category X

Benzodiazepines and their metabolites are known to cross the placenta and accumulate in the fetal circulation. They are associated with increased risk of congenital malformations when used during pregnancy, causing cleft lip and heart deformities in the fetus. Benzodiazepines should be avoided during pregnancy, particularly in the first trimester. The use of benzodiazepines during pregnancy should be considered only when the need for the medication outweighs its risk and alternative therapies have failed.

Nursing mothers should not take Dalmane, because it will pass into breast milk and be ingested by the baby. If stopping the drug is not an alternative, breastfeeding should not be started or should be discontinued.

Possible Drug Interactions

The potential drug interactions with Dalmane are summarized in the table below.

CNS depressants (e.g., alcohol, narcotics, barbiturates, hypnotics) and antihistamines	Combination of Dalmane and another CNS depressant may impair coordination and breathing, increase sedation, and produce other CNS depressant effects.
Tagamet (cimetidine), Serzone (nefazodone), oral contraceptives, Antabuse (disulfiram), Prozac (fluoxetine), Luvox (fluvoxamine), isoniazid (e.g., INH), Diflucan (fluconazole), Nizoral (ketoconazole), Sporanox (itraconazole), protease inhibitors (e.g., Crixivan, Norvir, Fortovase)	When any of these medications are taken concurrently with Dalmane, they may inhibit its metabolism and increase its blood levels. This may increase the likelihood of adverse side effects from Dalmane (e.g., sedation, drowsiness).

Patients taking Dalmane should not consume alcohol because the combination may increase sedation and drowsiness.

Overdose

Overdoses from oral ingestion of benzodiazepines alone are generally not fatal. Most fatalities reported with benzodiazepines involve multiple medication ingestion, particularly the combination of a benzodiazepine with other CNS depressants, such as alcohol, narcotics, and barbiturates.

Mild symptoms of benzodiazepine overdose include drowsiness, confusion, somnolence, tiredness, impaired coordination, clumsiness in walking (ataxia), and slow reflexes. Benzodiazepine overdose, when these agents are taken alone, is rarely fatal. When multiple medications are implicated in benzodiazepine overdose, severe symptoms include difficulty breathing, slowed heart rate, low blood pressure, loss of coordination, and loss of consciousness leading to coma and, potentially, death.

Any suspected overdose should be treated as an emergency. The person should be taken to the emergency room for observation and treatment. The prescription bottle of medication (and any other medication suspected in the overdose) should be brought as well, because the information on the prescription label can be helpful to the treating physician in determining the number of pills ingested.

Special Considerations

- Dalmane should only be taken when needed for sleep. Do not take more than the prescribed dose.
- Dalmane may cause sedation and drowsiness, especially during initiation of therapy, and impair your alertness. Use caution when driving or performing tasks that require alertness. Avoid alcohol when taking Dalmane, because alcohol may intensify these effects.
- Store the medication in its originally labeled, light-resistant container, away from heat and moisture. Heat and moisture may precipitate breakdown of your medication, and the medication may lose its therapeutic effects.
- Keep your medication out of reach of children.
- Dalmane should be discontinued gradually by tapering the dose. Stopping the medication abruptly, especially after taking it regularly for long periods, may trigger withdrawal symptoms, including irritability, agitation, tension, and insomnia.

If you have any questions about your medication, consult your physician or pharmacist.

Notes

_____

_____

_____

_____

_____

_____

_____

_____

_____

_____

_____

_____

From Chew RH, Hales RE, Yudofsky SC: *What Your Patients Need to Know About Psychiatric Medications*, Second Edition. Washington, DC, American Psychiatric Publishing, 2009

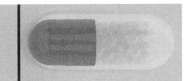

Halcion (triazolam)

Generic name: Triazolam
Available strengths: 0.125 mg, 0.25 mg tablets
Available in generic: Yes
Drug class: Benzodiazepine/sedative-hypnotic

General Information

Halcion (triazolam) is a benzodiazepine sedative-hypnotic medication approved for short-term treatment of insomnia. Similar to other benzodiazepines, Halcion has anxiolytic effects (i.e., relieves anxiety), but it is seldom prescribed for this use. It has a short duration of action (i.e., half-life around 3 hours) and no active metabolite. Consequently, Halcion is unlikely to produce daytime sedation and drowsiness. For this reason Halcion has been widely prescribed for international travelers requiring a sleep aid as they cross different time zones. Generally, Halcion should be used for brief treatment of insomnia for not longer than 1 week. However, longer use occasionally may be necessary for some patients; in such cases, careful monitoring is needed to prevent physical or psychological dependence. As with other benzodiazepines, Halcion is associated with dependence and abuse and is therefore regulated as a controlled substance by federal and state laws.

Dosing Information

The starting dose of Halcion should be the lowest possible, which is usually 0.125 mg at bedtime. The dose may be increased to the next higher strength of 0.25 mg if needed, but it should not exceed this amount. When Halcion was first introduced, it was widely prescribed in a dose of 0.5 mg. At this and higher doses, Halcion was associated with bizarre behavior, violence, and amnesia. Since then, the 0.5 mg formulation has been taken off the market, and physicians have become more cautious, prescribing Halcion at lower doses.

Common Side Effects

The most common side effects reported with Halcion are memory disturbance, drowsiness, and sedation. Because of its short half-life, Halcion is less likely to produce daytime sedation than longer acting agents, such as Dalmane (flurazepam). At higher doses, Halcion has a profound effect on memory and behavior (see "Adverse Reactions and Precautions"). Other frequent complaints are impaired concentration and memory, feeling of dissociation ("spacey"), and impaired coordination.

Adverse Reactions and Precautions

Halcion may affect alertness and coordination the next day after taking a single bedtime dose. Patients should exercise caution when driving or performing other tasks requiring alertness while taking this medication. Seniors may be more adversely affected, because it may affect their coordination and reflexes and lead to falls and injury. Taking Halcion with other central nervous system (CNS) depressants such as alcohol, narcotics, and barbiturates may compound these CNS effects.

Short-term amnesia of varying severity has been reported with Halcion. Those experiencing this effect have no memory of events after taking the hypnotic medication. This occurrence was reported widely with travelers who took the 0.5 mg tablets of Halcion, but it has also been reported with the 0.125 mg and 0.25 mg dosages. A few reports have also been made of individuals taking Halcion committing violent or bizarre acts. Afterward, the individuals had no recollection of their actions.

Prolonged use of Halcion can lead to dependence. When the medication is abruptly withdrawn, symptoms of withdrawal may occur. Withdrawal symptoms include headache, vomiting, impaired concentration, confusion, tremor, muscle cramps, and seizures.

Halcion, as well as other benzodiazepines, are centrally acting depressants, and they can depress respiration. This can affect patients with chronic obstructive pulmonary disease and emphysema by decreasing their "respiratory drive" or their ability to breathe. Patients with sleep apnea—a sleep disorder in which respiration is interrupted by long pauses during the sleep cycle—should not take Halcion or other benzodiazepines. The respiratory depressant effect of benzodiazepines may further suppress the respiratory drive in these patients and put them at risk for respiratory depression.

Benzodiazepines may induce **paradoxical reactions** in susceptible individuals. Instead of the expected depressant effects, the medication produces excitement, aggression, anger, uninhibited behavior, and rage in susceptible individuals. These reactions are more likely to occur in seniors, people with brain damage, and individuals with personality and impulse-control disorders.

Possible Drug Interactions

The potential drug interactions with Halcion are summarized in the table below.

CNS depressants (e.g., alcohol, narcotics, barbiturates, hypnotics) and antihistamines	The combination of Halcion and another CNS depressant may impair coordination and breathing, increase sedation, and produce other CNS depressant effects.
Tagamet (cimetidine); Serzone (nefazodone); oral contraceptives; Antabuse (disulfiram); isoniazid (e.g., INH); Prozac (fluoxetine), Luvox (fluvoxamine), and other selective serotonin uptake inhibitor antidepressants; Diflucan (fluconazole), Nizoral (ketoconazole), and Sporanox (itraconazole); protease inhibitors (e.g., Crixivan, Norvir, Fortovase); grapefruit juice	When any of these medications, or grapefruit juice, are taken concurrently with Halcion, they may inhibit its metabolism and increase its blood levels. This may increase the likelihood of adverse side effects from Halcion (e.g., sedation, drowsiness, amnesia). The dosage of Halcion may need to be reduced when any other of these medications are present in the regimen.

Patients taking Halcion should not consume alcohol because the combination may increase sedation and drowsiness.

Use in Pregnancy and Breastfeeding: Pregnancy Category X

Halcion, as well as other benzodiazepines and their metabolites, is known to cross the placenta and accumulate in the fetal circulation. Reproduction studies in animals demonstrated that Halcion was absorbed into fetal circulation and increased the occurrence of abnormalities. Halcion should not be used during pregnancy.

Nursing mothers should not take Halcion, because it will pass into breast milk and be ingested by the baby. If stopping the drug is not an alternative, breastfeeding should not be started or should be discontinued.

Overdose

Overdoses from oral ingestion of benzodiazepines alone are generally not fatal. Most fatalities reported with benzodiazepines involve multiple medication ingestion, particularly the combination of a benzodiazepine with CNS depressants, including alcohol, narcotics, and barbiturates.

Mild symptoms of benzodiazepine overdose include drowsiness, confusion, somnolence, tiredness, impaired coordination, clumsiness in walking (ataxia), and slow reflexes. Benzodiazepine overdose, when these agents are taken alone, is rarely fatal. When multiple medications are implicated in benzodiazepine overdose, severe symptoms include difficulty breathing, slowed heart rate, low blood pressure, loss of coordination, and loss of consciousness leading to coma and, potentially, death.

Any suspected overdose should be treated as an emergency. The person should be taken to the emergency room for observation and treatment. The prescription bottle of medication (and any other medication suspected in the overdose) should be brought as well, because the information on the prescription label can be helpful to the treating physician in determining the number of pills ingested.

Special Considerations

- Halcion should only be taken when needed for sleep. Do not take more than the prescribed dose.
- Halcion may cause sedation and drowsiness, especially during initiation of therapy, and impair your alertness. Use caution when driving or performing tasks that require alertness. Avoid alcohol when taking Halcion, because alcohol may intensify these effects.
- Store the medication in its originally labeled, light-resistant container, away from heat and moisture. Heat and moisture may precipitate breakdown of your medication, and the medication may lose its therapeutic effects.
- Keep your medication out of reach of children.
- Halcion should be discontinued gradually by tapering the dose. Stopping the medication abruptly, especially after taking it regularly for long periods, may trigger withdrawal symptoms, including irritability, agitation, tension, and insomnia.

If you have any questions about your medication, consult your physician or pharmacist.

Notes

_____

_____

_____

_____

_____

_____

_____

_____

_____

_____

_____

_____

From Chew RH, Hales RE, Yudofsky SC: _What Your Patients Need to Know About Psychiatric Medications_, Second Edition. Washington, DC, American Psychiatric Publishing, 2009

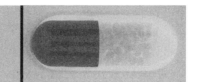

ProSom (estazolam)

Generic name: Estazolam
Available strengths: 1 mg, 2 mg tablets
Available in generic: Yes
Drug class: Benzodiazepine/sedative-hypnotic

General Information

ProSom (estazolam) is a benzodiazepine sedative-hypnotic medication approved for short-term treatment of insomnia. Similar to other benzodiazepines, ProSom has anxiolytic effects (i.e., relieves anxiety), but it is seldom prescribed for this use. It has an intermediate duration of action (i.e., half-life around 16 hours) and no active metabolite. For some patients, a single bedtime dose may lead to daytime sedation and drowsiness. Generally, ProSom should not be used for longer than 1 week. However, longer use occasionally may be necessary for some patients; in such cases, careful monitoring is needed to prevent physical or psychological dependence. As with other benzodiazepines, ProSom is associated with dependence and abuse and is therefore regulated as a controlled substance by federal and state laws.

Dosing Information

The usual dose of ProSom is 1 mg at bedtime. The dose may be increased to 2 mg if needed but should not exceed 2 mg. Seniors may require a lower dose of 1 mg. ProSom should be taken about 1 hour before bedtime to allow for the absorption of the medication.

Common Side Effects

The most common side effects reported with ProSom are daytime drowsiness and sedation, especially shortly after initiating therapy. Other frequent complaints are impaired concentration and memory, feeling of dissociation ("spacey"), and impaired coordination.

Adverse Reactions and Precautions

ProSom may affect alertness and coordination the next day after taking a single bedtime dose. Patients should exercise caution when driving or performing other tasks requiring alertness while taking this medication. Seniors may be more adversely affected, because it may affect their coordination and reflexes and lead to falls and injury. Taking ProSom with other central nervous system (CNS) depressants such as alcohol, narcotics, and barbiturates may compound these CNS effects.

Prolonged use of benzodiazepines can lead to dependence. When the medication is abruptly withdrawn, symptoms of withdrawal may occur. Withdrawal symptoms include headache, vomiting, impaired concentration, confusion, tremor, muscle cramps, and seizures.

Benzodiazepines are centrally acting depressants, and they can depress respiration. This can affect patients with chronic obstructive pulmonary disease and emphysema by decreasing their "respiratory drive" or their ability to breathe. Patients with sleep apnea—a sleep disorder in which respiration is interrupted by long pauses during the sleep cycle—should not take ProSom or other benzodiazepines. The respiratory depressant effect of benzodiazepines may further suppress the respiratory drive in these patients and put them at risk for respiratory depression.

Benzodiazepines may induce **paradoxical reactions** in susceptible individuals. Instead of the expected depressant effects, the medication produces excitement, aggression, anger, uninhibited behavior, and rage in susceptible individuals. These reactions are more likely to occur in seniors, people with brain damage, and individuals with personality and impulse-control disorders.

Use in Pregnancy and Breastfeeding: Pregnancy Category X

Benzodiazepines and their metabolites are known to cross the placenta and accumulate in the fetal circulation. Reproduction studies in animals demonstrated that ProSom was absorbed into fetal circulation and increased the occurrence of abnormalities. ProSom should not be used during pregnancy.

Nursing mothers should not take ProSom, because it will pass into breast milk and be ingested by the baby. If stopping the drug is not an alternative, breastfeeding should not be started or should be discontinued.

Possible Drug Interactions

The potential drug interactions with ProSom are summarized in the table below.

CNS depressants (e.g., alcohol, narcotics, barbiturates, hypnotics) and antihistamines	The combination of ProSom and another CNS depressant may impair coordination and breathing, increase sedation, and produce other CNS depressant effects.
Tagamet (cimetidine), Serzone (nefazodone), Prozac (fluoxetine), Luvox (fluvoxamine), isoniazid (e.g., INH), Diflucan (fluconazole), Nizoral (ketoconazole), Sporanox (itraconazole), protease inhibitors (e.g., Crixivan, Norvir, Fortovase)	When any of these medications are taken concurrently with ProSom, they may inhibit its metabolism and increase its blood levels. This may increase the likelihood of adverse side effects from ProSom (e.g., sedation, drowsiness).

Patients taking ProSom should not consume alcohol because the combination may increase sedation and drowsiness.

Overdose

Overdoses from oral ingestion of benzodiazepines alone are generally not fatal. Most fatalities reported with benzodiazepines involve multiple medication ingestion, particularly the combination of a benzodiazepine with CNS depressants, including alcohol, narcotics, and barbiturates.

Mild symptoms of benzodiazepine overdose include drowsiness, confusion, somnolence, tiredness, impaired coordination, clumsiness in walking (ataxia), and slow reflexes. Benzodiazepine overdose, when these agents are taken alone, is rarely fatal. When multiple medications are implicated in benzodiazepine overdose, severe symptoms include difficulty breathing, slowed heart rate, low blood pressure, loss of coordination, and loss of consciousness leading to coma and, potentially, death.

Any suspected overdose should be treated as an emergency. The person should be taken to the emergency room for observation and treatment. The prescription bottle of medication (and any other medication suspected in the overdose) should be brought as well, because the information on the prescription label can be helpful to the treating physician in determining the number of pills ingested.

Special Considerations

- ProSom should be discontinued gradually by tapering the dose. Stopping the medication abruptly, especially after taking it regularly for long periods, may trigger withdrawal symptoms, including irritability, agitation, tension, and insomnia.
- ProSom should only be taken when needed for sleep. Do not take more than the prescribed dose.
- ProSom may cause daytime sedation and drowsiness, especially during initiation of therapy, and impair your alertness. Use caution when driving or performing tasks that require alertness. Avoid alcohol when taking ProSom, because alcohol may intensify these effects.
- Store the medication in its originally labeled, light-resistant container, away from heat and moisture. Heat and moisture may precipitate breakdown of your medication, and the medication may lose its therapeutic effects.
- Keep your medication out of reach of children.

If you have any questions about your medication, consult your physician or pharmacist.

Notes

_____

_____

_____

_____

_____

_____

_____

_____

_____

_____

_____

_____

From Chew RH, Hales RE, Yudofsky SC: *What Your Patients Need to Know About Psychiatric Medications*, Second Edition. Washington, DC, American Psychiatric Publishing, 2009

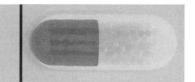

Restoril (temazepam)

Generic name: Temazepam
Available strengths: 7.5 mg, 15 mg, 22.5 mg, 30 mg capsules
Available in generic: Yes
Drug class: Benzodiazepine/sedative-hypnotic

General Information

Restoril (temazepam) is a benzodiazepine sedative-hypnotic medication approved for short-term treatment of insomnia. Similar to other benzodiazepines, Restoril has anxiolytic effects (i.e., relieves anxiety), but it is seldom prescribed for this use. It has an intermediate duration of action (i.e., half-life around 8–12 hours) and no active metabolite. Patients with early morning awakening may find Restoril beneficial because of its intermediate duration of action with little or no daytime drowsiness or grogginess. Generally, Restoril should not be used for longer than 1 week. However, longer use occasionally may be necessary for some patients; in such cases, careful monitoring is needed to prevent physical or psychological dependence. As with other benzodiazepines, Restoril is associated with dependence and abuse and is therefore regulated as a controlled substance by federal and state laws.

Dosing Information

The usual dose of Restoril is 15 mg at bedtime. The dose may be increased to 30 mg if needed but should not exceed this amount. Seniors may require a lower dose of 7.5–15 mg at bedtime. Restoril should be taken about 1 hour before bedtime to allow for the absorption of the medication.

Common Side Effects

The most common side effects reported with Restoril are daytime drowsiness and sedation, especially shortly after initiating therapy. Other frequent complaints are impaired concentration and memory, feeling of dissociation ("spacey"), and impaired coordination.

Adverse Reactions and Precautions

Restoril may affect alertness and coordination the next day after taking a single bedtime dose. Patients should exercise caution when driving or performing other tasks requiring alertness while taking this medication. Seniors may be more adversely affected, because it may affect their coordination and reflexes and lead to falls and injury. Taking Restoril with other central nervous system (CNS) depressants such as alcohol, narcotics, and barbiturates may compound these CNS effects.

Prolonged use of benzodiazepines can lead to dependence. When the medication is abruptly withdrawn, symptoms of withdrawal may occur. Withdrawal symptoms include headache, vomiting, impaired concentration, confusion, tremor, muscle cramps, and seizures.

Benzodiazepines are centrally acting depressants, and they can depress respiration. This can affect patients with chronic obstructive pulmonary disease and emphysema by decreasing their "respiratory drive" or their ability to breathe. Patients with sleep apnea—a sleep disorder in which respiration is interrupted by long pauses during the sleep cycle—should not take Restoril or other benzodiazepines. The respiratory depressant effect of benzodiazepines may further suppress the respiratory drive in these patients and put them at risk for respiratory depression.

Benzodiazepines may induce **paradoxical reactions** in susceptible individuals. Instead of the expected depressant effects, the medication produces excitement, aggression, anger, uninhibited behavior, and rage in susceptible individuals. These reactions are more likely to occur in seniors, people with brain damage, and individuals with personality and impulse-control disorders.

Use in Pregnancy and Breastfeeding: Pregnancy Category X

Benzodiazepines and their metabolites are known to cross the placenta and accumulate in the fetal circulation. Reproduction studies in animals demonstrated that Restoril was absorbed into fetal circulation and increased the occurrence of abnormalities. Restoril should not be used during pregnancy.

Nursing mothers should not take Restoril, because it will pass into breast milk and be ingested by the baby. If stopping the drug is not an alternative, breastfeeding should not be started or should be discontinued.

Possible Drug Interactions

The potential drug interactions with Restoril are summarized in the table below.

CNS depressants (e.g., alcohol, narcotics, barbiturates, hypnotics) and antihistamines	The combination of Restoril and another CNS depressant may impair coordination and breathing, increase sedation, and produce other CNS depressant effects.
Tagamet (cimetidine), Serzone (nefazodone), oral contraceptives, Antabuse (disulfiram), Prozac (fluoxetine), Luvox (fluvoxamine), isoniazid (e.g., INH), Diflucan (fluconazole), Nizoral (ketoconazole), Sporanox (itraconazole), protease inhibitors (e.g., Crixivan, Norvir, Fortovase)	When any of these medications are taken concurrently with Restoril, they may inhibit its metabolism and increase its blood levels. This may increase the likelihood of adverse side effects from Restoril (e.g., sedation, drowsiness).

Patients taking Restoril should not consume alcohol because the combination may increase sedation and drowsiness.

Overdose

Overdoses from oral ingestion of benzodiazepines alone are generally not fatal. Most fatalities reported with benzodiazepines involve multiple medication ingestion, particularly the combination of a benzodiazepine with CNS depressants, including alcohol, narcotics, and barbiturates.

Mild symptoms of benzodiazepine overdose include drowsiness, confusion, somnolence, tiredness, impaired coordination, clumsiness in walking (ataxia), and slow reflexes. Benzodiazepine overdose, when these agents are taken alone, is rarely fatal. When multiple medications are implicated in benzodiazepine overdose, severe symptoms include difficulty breathing, slowed heart rate, low blood pressure, loss of coordination, and loss of consciousness leading to coma and, potentially, death.

Any suspected overdose should be treated as an emergency. The person should be taken to the emergency room for observation and treatment. The prescription bottle of medication (and any other medication suspected in the overdose) should be brought as well, because the information on the prescription label can be helpful to the treating physician in determining the number of pills ingested.

Special Considerations

- Restoril should be discontinued gradually by tapering the dose. Stopping the medication abruptly, especially after taking it regularly for long periods, may trigger withdrawal symptoms, including irritability, agitation, tension, and insomnia.
- Restoril should only be taken when needed for sleep. Do not take more than the prescribed dose.
- Restoril may cause daytime sedation and drowsiness, especially during initiation of therapy, and impair your alertness. Use caution when driving or performing tasks that require alertness. Avoid alcohol when taking Restoril. The combination may increase sedation and drowsiness.
- Store the medication in its originally labeled, light-resistant container, away from heat and moisture. Heat and moisture may precipitate breakdown of your medication, and the medication may lose its therapeutic effects.
- Keep your medication out of reach of children.

If you have any questions about your medication, consult your physician or pharmacist.

Notes

_____

_____

_____

_____

_____

_____

_____

_____

_____

_____

_____

From Chew RH, Hales RE, Yudofsky SC: *What Your Patients Need to Know About Psychiatric Medications*, Second Edition. Washington, DC, American Psychiatric Publishing, 2009

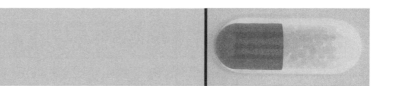

Ambien (zolpidem)

Generic name: Zolpidem
Available strengths: 5 mg, 10 mg tablets;
    6.25 mg, 12.5 mg extended-release tablets (Ambien CR);
    5 mg, 10 mg rapidly disintegrating tablets
Available in generic: Yes, except Ambien CR and
    rapidly disintegrating tablets
Drug class: Nonbenzodiazepine/sedative-hypnotic

General Information

Ambien (zolpidem), a sedative-hypnotic medication, is unrelated to the benzodiazepines or barbiturates and was approved for short-term treatment of insomnia. In contrast to the benzodiazepines, Ambien does not appear to have antianxiety or muscle relaxant effects. Ambien has a short duration of action and no active metabolite and does not appear to cause daytime sedation or drowsiness. For this reason Ambien has been favored by international travelers requiring a sleep aid as they cross different time zones. Generally, Ambien should be used for brief treatment of insomnia for no longer than 1 week. However, longer use occasionally may be necessary for some patients; in such cases, careful monitoring is needed to prevent physical or psychological dependence. Like the benzodiazepines, Ambien may be associated with dependence and abuse and is therefore regulated as a controlled substance by federal and state laws.

Dosing Information

The usual dose of Ambien is 10 mg at bedtime. Patients should not exceed this amount. Seniors may require only 5 mg at bedtime. Ambien is rapidly absorbed and should be taken within 30 minutes before bedtime.

Common Side Effects

The most common side effects reported with Ambien are memory disturbance, drowsiness, and sedation. Because of its short half-life, Ambien is unlikely to produce daytime sedation or drowsiness. Other occasional complaints are impaired concentration and memory, a feeling of dissociation ("spacey"), and impaired coordination.

Adverse Reactions and Precautions

Ambien may affect alertness and coordination the next day after taking a single bedtime dose. Patients should exercise caution when driving or performing other tasks requiring alertness while taking this medication. Seniors may be more adversely affected, because it may affect their coordination and reflexes and lead to falls and injury. Taking Ambien with other central nervous system (CNS) depressants such as alcohol, narcotics, and barbiturates may compound these CNS effects.

Prolonged use of Ambien may rarely lead to dependence. Its abuse potential is very low, and it is one of the sedative-hypnotic agents of choice for individuals with a history of alcohol or drug abuse. When Ambien is abruptly withdrawn, mild symptoms of withdrawal may occur. Withdrawal symptoms may include headache, vomiting, impaired concentration, confusion, tremor, and muscle cramps.

Ambien, like other sedative-hypnotics, is a centrally acting depressant and can depress respiration. In healthy adults, Ambien has very little effect on respiratory function, but in patients with compromised respiratory function (such as chronic obstructive pulmonary disease and emphysema), Ambien may depress their "respiratory drive" or their ability to breathe.

Use in Pregnancy and Breastfeeding: Pregnancy Category B

Ambien has not been clinically investigated in pregnant women, so our understanding of the risk in pregnancy is limited. Reproduction studies in animals showed no teratogenic effect (i.e., caused no congenital malformation), but Ambien had some effect on bone development in rats and rabbits. Ambien should not be used during pregnancy, if possible.

Nursing mothers should not take Ambien, because it will pass into breast milk and be ingested by the baby. If stopping the drug is not an alternative, breastfeeding should not be started or should be discontinued.

Possible Drug Interactions

Ambien is one of those few medications that have few or no clinically significant drug interactions. However, patients taking Ambien should not consume alcohol because the combination may increase sedation and drowsiness.

Overdose

Overdoses from oral ingestion of Ambien alone have not proved to be fatal. Reported symptoms of overdose with Ambien include somnolence, dizziness, impaired coordination, and loss of consciousness. More severe symptoms, including fatalities, were reported with overdoses of Ambien in combination with multiple medications, especially with another CNS depressant, including narcotics and barbiturates.

Any suspected overdose should be treated as an emergency. The person should be taken to the emergency room for observation and treatment. The prescription bottle of medication (and any other medication suspected in the overdose) should be brought as well, because the information on the prescription label can be helpful to the treating physician in determining the number of pills ingested.

Special Considerations

- Ambien should be taken only when needed for sleep. Do not take more than the prescribed dose.
- Ambien may cause sedation and drowsiness, especially during initiation of therapy, and impair your alertness. Use caution when driving or performing tasks that require alertness. Avoid alcohol when taking Ambien, because alcohol may intensify these effects.
- Store the medication in its originally labeled, light-resistant container, away from heat and moisture. Heat and moisture may precipitate breakdown of your medication, and the medication may lose its therapeutic effects.
- Keep your medication out of reach of children.

If you have any questions about your medication, consult your physician or pharmacist.

Notes

From Chew RH, Hales RE, Yudofsky SC: *What Your Patients Need to Know About Psychiatric Medications*, Second Edition. Washington, DC, American Psychiatric Publishing, 2009

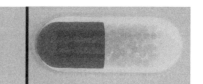

Lunesta (eszopiclone)

Generic name: Eszopiclone
Available strengths: 1 mg, 2 mg, 3 mg tablets
Available in generic: No
Drug class: Nonbenzodiazepine/sedative-hypnotic

General Information

Lunesta (eszopiclone) is used for the treatment of insomnia, which may be due to problems with falling asleep, staying asleep, or early wakening. It is unrelated to other sleep medications such as benzodiazepines and barbiturates. Lunesta is rapidly absorbed after ingestion and has a fast onset of action. It has a short duration of action, and most of the medication is eliminated from the body in about 6 hours. For this reason, Lunesta appears to cause little daytime sedation and drowsiness. When taken at bedtime, Lunesta may decrease the time to fall asleep and may improve sleep maintenance through the night.

Lunesta is a prescription medication, classified as a Schedule IV controlled substance. Although Lunesta's chemical structure is unrelated to the structures of benzodiazepines, it shares many pharmacological properties with benzodiazepines.

Lunesta was evaluated in adults with chronic insomnia in a controlled clinical study of 6 months' duration. The study demonstrated that patients receiving Lunesta over the study period continued to benefit from the medication without developing tolerance. On the basis of the evidence of this study, the U.S. Food and Drug Administration did not limit Lunesta's indication for short-term use as with other sleep medications, and approved Lunesta for long-term treatment of insomnia and sleep maintenance.

Dosing Information

Lunesta comes in 1 mg, 2 mg, and 3 mg tablets. The recommended dose is 2 mg at bedtime, which is usually effective for sleep onset and maintenance. The dose may be increased to 3 mg for those who continue to have difficulty sleeping through the night. For the elderly patient whose primary complaint is difficulty falling asleep, a 1 mg dose is generally effective, and if falling asleep and sleeping through the night is the problem, the dose may be increased to 2 mg.

Common Side Effects

The most common side effects reported with Lunesta are drowsiness, dizziness, lightheadedness, and difficulty with coordination. Because of its short half-life, Lunesta is unlikely to induce daytime sedation or drowsiness. However, some patients, especially the elderly, may experience daytime drowsiness if taking a large dose. Sedation can best be avoided by taking the lowest possible dose that helps you sleep at night and avoiding other sedatives, such as alcohol and antihistamines. Other occasional complaints are impaired concentration and memory, a feeling of dissociation ("spacey"), and incoordination.

Adverse Reactions and Precautions

Lunesta may affect alertness and coordination the next day after taking a single bedtime dose. Patients should exercise caution when driving or performing other tasks requiring alertness. Seniors may be more adversely affected, because it may affect their coordination and reflexes and lead to falls and injury. Taking Lunesta with other central nervous system (CNS) depressants such as alcohol, narcotics, antihistamines, and barbiturates may compound Lunesta's CNS adverse effects.

Sleep medications, especially with short-acting agents like Lunesta, may cause short-term memory loss. When this occurs, you may not remember what has happened for several hours after taking the medication. This short-term memory loss is called **retrograde amnesia.** It is usually not a problem for those who take Lunesta and get a full night's sleep, but for the individual who takes Lunesta while traveling, such as during an airplane flight, and wakes up before the effects of the medication wear off, memory loss can be a problem. Sleep medication is best avoided if you anticipate not being allowed to sleep a full night.

As with other sleep medications, chronic use of Lunesta, especially when the use is regular and at high doses, can lead to dependence. The risk of dependence is very low when Lunesta is prescribed under the care of a physician and taken at the prescribed dosage. When Lunesta is suddenly stopped, symptoms of withdrawal, which are generally mild, may occur and may consist only of jitteriness and unpleasant feelings. Since its introduction, severe withdrawal symptoms have not been reported with Lunesta. Also, when Lunesta is stopped after chronic use, you may experience **rebound insomnia:** you may have more trouble sleeping the first few nights after stopping than before starting the medication. Rebound insomnia is transient and subsides after a few nights. Patients who have been taking Lunesta or other sleep medications for a long time should not suddenly stop the medication without discussing the issue with their physician. The physician may taper the sleep medication gradually to avoid any unpleasant side effects.

Changes in behavior and thinking have been associated with sleep medications. Although the occurrence of such changes is uncommon, patients taking Lunesta should be aware of any changes in their behavior or the emergence of abnormal thinking, including more outgoing or aggressive behavior, confusion, agitation, bizarre behavior, and hallucinations. Worsening of depression, including suicidal thoughts, has also been associated with use of sleep medications in depressed patients. Elderly patients may be more susceptible to changes in behavior and thinking from sleep medications.

Use in Pregnancy and Breastfeeding: Pregnancy Category C

Lunesta has not been clinically investigated in pregnant women, and knowledge of its risk in pregnancy is limited. Lunesta should not be used during pregnancy unless clearly indicated.

It is not known whether Lunesta is excreted in breast milk. It is not recommended that the mother breastfeed her child while taking a sleep medication.

Possible Drug Interactions

Lunesta is metabolized primarily in the liver by hepatic enzymes and thereby eliminated from the body. Some medications when taken together with Lunesta may interfere with the enzymes that metabolize it, and thus slow its elimination. This may elevate the level of Lunesta and increase its pharmacological action and side effects. Patients should be aware of potential drug interactions when the medications in the table below are taken together with Lunesta.

Alcohol	Alcohol has an additive effect on the sedative effects of Lunesta and may make the side effects of incoordination, drowsiness, and dizziness worse.
Antibiotics	The antibiotics erythromycin, Biaxin (clarithromycin), and TAO (troleandomycin) may inhibit the metabolism of Lunesta, elevating drug levels and increasing the potential for side effects.
Antifungal agents	The antifungal agents Nizoral (ketoconazole) and Sporanox (itraconazole) may inhibit the metabolism of Lunesta, elevating drug levels and increasing the potential for side effects.
Antiretroviral agents	The antiretroviral agents Norvir (ritonavir) and Viracept (nelfinavir), used for treatment of HIV, may inhibit the metabolism of Lunesta, elevating drug levels and increasing the potential for side effects.
Prozac (fluoxetine)	Prozac and its active metabolite may inhibit the metabolism of Lunesta, elevating drug levels and increasing the potential for side effects.

Overdose

There is limited clinical experience with overdoses of Lunesta. In one reported case, an individual fully recovered from an overdose with up to 36 mg of Lunesta. The severity of overdose, of course, depends on the total amount of sleep medication ingested and whether it was taken in combination with other medications, especially in combination with other CNS depressants.

Any suspected overdose with Lunesta should be treated as an emergency. The person should be taken to the emergency room for observation and treatment. The prescription bottle of medication (and any other medication suspected in the overdose) should be brought as well, because the information on the prescription label can be helpful to the treating physician in determining the number of pills ingested.

Special Considerations

- Lunesta should be taken only when needed for sleep. Lunesta works quickly and should be taken immediately before going to bed. Do not take more than the prescribed dose.
- Lunesta may cause daytime drowsiness and impair alertness. Use caution when driving or performing tasks that require alertness. Avoid alcohol when taking Lunesta; the combination may increase sedation and drowsiness and impair coordination.

- Store the medication in its originally labeled, light-resistant container, away from heat and moisture. Heat and moisture may precipitate breakdown of your medication, and the medication may lose its therapeutic effects.
- Keep Lunesta out of the reach of children.

If you have any questions about your medication, consult your physician or pharmacist.

Notes

_____

_____

_____

_____

_____

_____

_____

_____

_____

From Chew RH, Hales RE, Yudofsky SC: *What Your Patients Need to Know About Psychiatric Medications*, Second Edition. Washington, DC, American Psychiatric Publishing, 2009

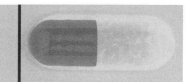

Rozerem (ramelteon)

Generic name: Ramelteon
Available strength: 8 mg tablet
Available in generic: No
Drug class: Nonbenzodiazepine/sedative-hypnotic

General Information

Recently introduced in the United States, **Rozerem (ramelteon)** has been approved by the U.S. Food and Drug Administration for treatment of insomnia. Insomnia may be due to problems with falling asleep, staying asleep, or early wakening. Rozerem is unrelated to other sleep medications, such as benzodiazepines and barbiturates, and it is unique in the way it works: Rozerem mimics the natural hormone melatonin, which is secreted in the brain by the **pineal gland.** Rozerem acts on melatonin receptors, much like the natural hormone that plays a role in regulating sleep and our circadian cycle.

Rapidly absorbed after ingestion, Rozerem has a fast onset of action. It has a short duration of action, and most of the medication is eliminated from the body in 10–12 hours. For this reason Rozerem appears to cause little daytime sedation and drowsiness. When taken at bedtime, Rozerem decreases the time to fall asleep and may improve sleep maintenance through the night.

Rozerem is a prescription medication, but it is not classified as a controlled substance as are most other sedative-hypnotic medications. The long-term use of Rozerem has not been evaluated. There is no addiction potential associated with the medication, nor are withdrawal symptoms or **rebound insomnia** (worsening of insomnia when the medication is discontinued) of any serious consequence.

Dosing Information

Rozerem only comes in an 8 mg tablet. The recommended dose is 8 mg, with the dose taken 30 minutes before bedtime. Rozerem should not be taken with or immediately after meals, especially after a high-fat meal. This may delay the absorption of the medication and diminish its effectiveness.

Common Side Effects

The most common side effects reported with Rozerem are dizziness, headache, nausea, and tiredness. Because of its short half-life, Rozerem is unlikely to induce significant daytime sedation or drowsiness. However, some patients, especially the elderly, may experience some drowsiness during the day.

Adverse Reactions and Precautions

Individuals should be aware that Rozerem may affect their alertness and coordination after taking a single bedtime dose and that, therefore, they should not drive or perform other tasks requiring alertness. Elderly patients whose coordination and reflexes may be affected are susceptible to falling and injuring themselves. Taking Rozerem with other central nervous system (CNS) depressants such as alcohol, narcotics, antihistamines, and barbiturates may compound the CNS effects of those medications.

As with other sleep medications, chronic (especially regular) use of Rozerem may lead to tolerance. The risk of dependence is very low when Rozerem is prescribed under the care of a physician and taken at the prescribed dosage. Withdrawal symptoms and rebound insomnia from discontinuation have not been reported with Rozerem.

Use in Pregnancy and Breastfeeding: Pregnancy Category C

Rozerem has not been clinically investigated in pregnant women, and knowledge of the risk of its use in pregnancy is limited. It is not recommended that Rozerem be used during pregnancy.

It is not known whether Rozerem is excreted in breast milk. It is not recommended that the mother breastfeed her child while taking a sleep medication.

Possible Drug Interactions

Rozerem is metabolized primarily in the liver by hepatic enzymes and thereby eliminated from the body. Some medications when taken together with Rozerem may interfere with the enzymes that metabolize it and thus slow its elimination. This may elevate the level of Rozerem and increase its pharmacological action and side effects. Patients should be aware of potential drug interactions when the medications in the table below are taken together with Rozerem.

Alcohol	Alcohol has an additive effect on the sedative effects of Rozerem and may make the side effects of incoordination, drowsiness, and dizziness worse.
Antifungal agents	The antifungal agents Nizoral (ketoconazole) and Diflucan (fluconazole) may inhibit the metabolism of Rozerem, elevating drug levels and the potential for side effects.
Luvox (fluvoxamine)	The antidepressant Luvox (fluvoxamine) inhibits the metabolism of Rozerem, significantly increasing plasma levels and the potential for side effects.
Rifampin	Rifampin, an antibiotic for treatment of tuberculosis, may affect the levels of Rozerem, decreasing plasma levels and the effectiveness of the sleep medication.

Overdose

There is limited clinical experience with overdoses of Rozerem. The severity of the overdose depends on the total amount of sleep medication ingested and whether the medication was taken in combination with other medications, particularly in combination with other CNS depressants.

Any suspected overdose with Rozerem should be treated as an emergency. The person should be taken to the emergency room for observation and treatment. The prescription bottle of medication (and any other medication suspected in the overdose) should be brought as well, because the information on the prescription label can be helpful to the treating physician in determining the number of pills ingested.

Special Considerations

- Rozerem should be taken only when needed for sleep. Rozerem works quickly and should be taken 30 minutes before going to bed.
- Do not take more than the prescribed dose.
- Rozerem may cause daytime drowsiness and impair alertness. Use caution when driving or performing tasks that require alertness. Avoid alcohol when taking Rozerem; the combination may increase sedation and drowsiness and impair coordination.
- Store the medication in its originally labeled, light-resistant container, away from heat and moisture. Heat and moisture may precipitate the breakdown of your medication, and the medication may lose its therapeutic effects.
- Keep Rozerem out of the reach of children.

If you have any questions about your medication, consult your physician or pharmacist.

Notes

_____

_____

_____

_____

_____

_____

From Chew RH, Hales RE, Yudofsky SC: *What Your Patients Need to Know About Psychiatric Medications*, Second Edition. Washington, DC, American Psychiatric Publishing, 2009

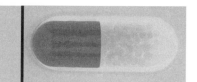

Sonata (zaleplon)

Generic name: Zaleplon
Available strengths: 5 mg, 10 mg tablets
Available in generic: Yes
Drug class: Nonbenzodiazepine/sedative-hypnotic

General Information

Sonata (zaleplon), a sedative-hypnotic medication, is unrelated to the benzodiazepines or barbiturates and was approved for short-term treatment of insomnia. In contrast to the benzodiazepines, Sonata does not appear to have antianxiety or muscle relaxant effects at the recommended hypnotic doses. Sonata has a short duration of action and no active metabolite and appears to cause very little daytime sedation and drowsiness. For this reason Sonata has been favored by international travelers requiring a sleep aid as they cross different time zones. Generally, Sonata should be used for brief treatment of insomnia for no longer than 1 week. However, longer use occasionally may be necessary for some patients; in such cases, careful monitoring is needed to prevent physical or psychological dependence. Like the benzodiazepines, Sonata may be associated with dependence and abuse and is therefore regulated as a controlled substance by federal and state laws.

Dosing Information

The usual starting dose of Sonata is 10 mg at bedtime, and it is rarely necessary to go beyond this amount. Seniors may require only 5 mg at bedtime. Sonata is rapidly absorbed and should be taken within 30 minutes before bedtime.

Common Side Effects

The most common side effects reported with Sonata are memory disturbance, drowsiness, and sedation. Because of its short half-life, Sonata is unlikely to produce daytime sedation or drowsiness. Other occasional complaints are impaired concentration and memory, a feeling of dissociation ("spacey"), and impaired coordination.

Adverse Reactions and Precautions

Sonata may affect alertness and coordination the next day after taking a single bedtime dose. Patients should exercise caution when driving or performing other tasks requiring alertness while taking this medication. Seniors may be more adversely affected, because it may affect their coordination and reflexes and lead to falls and injury. Taking Sonata with other central nervous system (CNS) depressants such as alcohol, narcotics, and barbiturates may compound these CNS effects.

Prolonged use of Sonata may rarely lead to dependence. Its abuse potential is very low, and it is one of the sedative-hypnotic agents of choice for individuals with a history of alcohol or drug abuse. When Sonata is abruptly withdrawn, mild symptoms of withdrawal may occur.

Sonata, like other sedative-hypnotics, is a centrally acting depressant and can depress respiration. In healthy adults, Sonata has very little effect on their respiratory function, but in patients with compromised respiratory function (such as chronic obstructive pulmonary disease and emphysema), Sonata may depress their "respiratory drive" or their ability to breathe.

Use in Pregnancy and Breastfeeding: Pregnancy Category C

Sonata has not been clinically investigated in pregnant women, so our understanding of the risk in pregnancy is limited. Reproduction studies in animals demonstrated that Sonata had an effect on bone development. Sonata should not be used during pregnancy.

Nursing mothers should not take Sonata, because it will pass into breast milk and be ingested by the baby. If stopping the drug is not an alternative, breastfeeding should not be started or should be discontinued.

Possible Drug Interactions

Sonata is one of those few medications that have few or no clinically significant drug interactions. However, patients taking Sonata should not consume alcohol because the combination may increase sedation and drowsiness.

Overdose

Overdoses from oral ingestion of Sonata alone have not proven to be fatal. Reported symptoms of overdose with Sonata include somnolence, dizziness, impaired coordination, and loss of consciousness. More severe symptoms, including fatalities, were reported with overdoses of Sonata in combination with multiple medications, especially with CNS depressants, including narcotics and barbiturates.

Any suspected overdose should be treated as an emergency. The person should be taken to the emergency room for observation and treatment. The prescription bottle of medication (and any other medication suspected in the overdose) should be brought as well, because the information on the prescription label can be helpful to the treating physician in determining the number of pills ingested.

Special Considerations

- Sonata should be taken only when needed for sleep. Do not take more than the prescribed dose.
- Sonata may cause sedation and drowsiness, especially during initiation of therapy, and impair your alertness. Use caution when driving or performing tasks that require alertness. Avoid alcohol when taking Sonata, because alcohol may intensify these effects.
- Store the medication in its originally labeled, light-resistant container, away from heat and moisture. Heat and moisture may precipitate breakdown of your medication, and the medication may lose its therapeutic effects.
- Keep your medication out of reach of children.

If you have any questions about your medication, consult your physician or pharmacist.

Notes

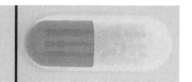

Trazodone (Desyrel)

Generic name: Trazodone
Available strengths: 50 mg, 100 mg, 150 mg, 300 mg tablets;
   150 mg scored tablet (Desyrel Dividose)
Available in generic: Yes (available only in generic)
Drug class: Antidepressant, but prescribed primarily for sleep

General Information

At one time **trazodone**—sold under the brand name Desyrel—was widely prescribed for treatment of depression. However, at the higher doses needed to treat depression, most people could not tolerate its tendency to cause pronounced sedation and drowsiness, especially during the daytime. With the introduction of selective serotonin reuptake inhibitor (SSRI) antidepressants such as Prozac (fluoxetine) and other newer antidepressants, the use of trazodone for depression rapidly declined. SSRIs instead caused insomnia and other sleep difficulties for many people. To counter this side effect, physicians added low doses of trazodone at bedtime for sleep. Today, trazodone is used mostly for treating insomnia and rarely for depression.

Besides its use for treatment of insomnia, trazodone was reported to be effective for reducing agitation and aggression in patients with Alzheimer's disease and other brain disorders. Also, at low doses, trazodone has antianxiety effects and may be effective in treating generalized anxiety disorder. These uses for trazodone, however, are outside their indication; trazodone was approved only for the treatment of depression by the U.S. Food and Drug Administration (FDA). The use of a medication for its approved indications is called its *labeled use*. In clinical practice, however, physicians often prescribe medications for *unlabeled* ("off-label") uses when published clinical studies, case reports, or their own clinical experiences support the efficacy and safety of those treatments.

Dosing Information

When prescribed for insomnia and sleep disturbance, the usual dose of trazodone is 50–100 mg at bedtime, but some patients may need doses as high as 150–200 mg.

For treatment of depression, trazodone is gradually increased to the effective therapeutic dosage of 300–400 mg/day, although some individuals may require dosages up to 600 mg/day. The entire dosage may be taken in one dose at bedtime to prevent daytime somnolence, but some individuals may still have lingering drowsiness the next day.

For treatment of aggression and agitation in Alzheimer's disease patients, 50 mg of trazodone two times a day has been reported to be effective.

Common Side Effects

Common side effects with trazodone are sedation, drowsiness, dizziness, dry mouth, headaches, nausea, indigestion, and visual disturbance. Nausea and indigestion are more frequent at higher dosages and on an empty stomach. Taking trazodone with food may decrease gastrointestinal side effects. Patients may experience visual disturbances—seeing visual trails or afterimages when their eyes move. Generally, these side effects subside over time and are less frequent with lower dosages.

Adverse Reactions and Precautions

Individuals may complain of dizziness from trazodone. Trazodone blocks the body's compensatory response to maintain a stable blood pressure when a person moves from lying down to a sitting position or from sitting to standing, and thus the person becomes dizzy due to a momentary drop in blood pressure. This reaction is known in medical terms as **orthostatic hypotension.** Seniors and those taking other medications to lower blood pressure may be more susceptible to orthostatic hypotension from trazodone.

Some medications can cause a rare condition in males that results in uncontrollable, sustained, painful penile erections, known as **priapism.** In very rare instances, trazodone may induce priapism (in about 1 per 6,000 men taking the medication). Men taking trazodone who experience an uncontrolled erection persisting several hours should seek immediate medical attention. If not treated promptly, priapism may result in permanent impotence due to damage of vascular structures in the penis.

Trazodone is highly sedating and can cause significant drowsiness, especially when starting the medication. Patients should not drive or operate hazardous machinery immediately after taking trazodone.

Use in Pregnancy and Breastfeeding: Pregnancy Category C

Trazodone has not been tested in women to determine its safety in pregnancy. The effects of the drug on the developing fetus in pregnant women are unknown. Women who are pregnant or may become pregnant should discuss this with their physician. If trazodone was prescribed for depression, some women may experience a recurrence of symptoms when they stop trazodone. In these circumstances, the physician may discuss the need to restart the medication or seek an alternative medication or treatment.

Nursing mothers should not take trazodone, because it will pass into breast milk and be ingested by the baby. If stopping the drug is not an alternative, breastfeeding should not be started or should be discontinued.

Possible Drug Interactions

Trazodone, like many other medications, is metabolized in the liver. The combined use of trazodone with certain medications may result in adverse drug interactions because one drug may alter the blood levels of the other. The significant drug interactions reported with trazodone are summarized in the table on the next page.

Other medications, including herbal supplements (such as St. John's wort), that boost serotonin may result in excessive levels of that neurotransmitter when combined with trazodone. This may produce a toxic syndrome known as **serotonin syndrome,** which is caused by excessive serotonin stimulation. The early signs of serotonin syndrome are restlessness, confusion, tremors, flushing, excessive sweating, and involuntary muscle jerks. If the medications are not stopped, the individual may develop more life-threatening complications resulting in muscle disorders, high fever, respiratory problems, clotting problems, and destruction of red blood cells that may lead to acute renal failure. Patients taking SSRIs should be alert to signs of serotonin syndrome, which require immediate medical attention and discontinuation of the serotonin-boosting medications. Anti-

Tegretol (carbamazepine)	When Tegretol is combined with trazodone, Tegretol blood levels may be elevated, with a possible increase in side effects, and trazodone levels may be lowered, with a possible decrease in efficacy.
Tagamet (cimetidine)	Tagamet may inhibit the liver enzyme that metabolizes trazodone and produce elevated blood levels of trazodone, thus increasing the potential for adverse side effects from trazodone.
Prozac (fluoxetine), Paxil (paroxetine), Wellbutrin SR or XL (bupropion)	Prozac, Paxil, and Wellbutrin may inhibit the liver enzyme that metabolizes trazodone and elevate trazodone's blood levels, thus increasing the potential for adverse side effects.
Antiretroviral (anti-HIV) agents Norvir (ritonavir) and Crixivan (indinavir)	Coadministration of Norvir or Crixivan with trazodone may significantly elevate and prolong serum levels of trazodone, which can cause nausea, dizziness, daytime sedation, and tiredness. When these antiretroviral medications are being used, trazodone should be administered in the lowest possible dose.

depressants known as **monoamine oxidase inhibitors** should not be taken with trazodone because the combination may potentially produce a toxic reaction that includes elevated temperature, high blood pressure, and extreme excitation and agitation. Consult your physician or pharmacist before taking any new medications, including over-the-counter medications and herbal supplements, with trazodone.

Patients taking trazodone should avoid alcohol or should consume it in moderation because the combination may increase depression.

Overdose

In contrast to tricyclic and monoamine oxidase inhibitor antidepressants, overdose with trazodone is generally much less dangerous, especially when it is taken alone. Overdoses often involve multiple medications, and the other drugs may increase the risk of more serious complications. The combination of central nervous system depressants, such as alcohol, and trazodone can be lethal, and death is usually from respiratory depression.

Any suspected overdose should be treated as an emergency. The person should be taken to the emergency room for observation and treatment. The prescription bottle of medication (and any other medication suspected in the overdose) should be brought as well, because the information on the prescription label can be helpful to the treating physician in determining the number of pills ingested.

Special Considerations

In short-term studies, antidepressants were found to increase the risk of suicidal thinking and behavior in children and adolescents with major depression and other psychiatric disorders. Because trazodone is an antidepressant, although it is seldom used for treatment of depression, the prescriber must still warn of this risk in children and adolescents taking trazodone for other conditions. According to FDA findings, the risk of suicidal thoughts and behaviors associated with antidepressants is age-related. This phenomenon tends to occur in the younger population and is most likely to occur early in the course of treatment. In adults over 24 years of age, there did not appear to be an increased risk of suicidality with antidepressants compared with placebo. In patients over age 65, the findings showed that antidepressants had a "protective effect" against suicidal thoughts and behavior. Other studies have found that when more people in a community are taking antidepressants, the suicide rate is lower.

The risk of suicide is inherent in depression and may persist until the individual responds to treatment. The family or caregiver should closely observe the patient, especially a child or adolescent, for signs of worsening, suicidal thoughts, and changes in behavior, especially early in the course of therapy and with change in dose; any concerns should be communicated to the physician.

- **Warning:** Always let your physician or a family member know if you have suicidal thoughts. Notify your psychiatrist or family physician whenever your depressive symptoms worsen or whenever you feel unable to control suicidal urges or thoughts.
- Do not discontinue your medication without consulting with your physician. If you miss a dose, take it as soon as possible within 2–3 hours of the scheduled dose. If longer, skip the missed dose and continue on your regular dosing schedule, but do not take double doses.
- If the trazodone is prescribed for sleep, take it about 1 hour before bedtime. Take only the amount prescribed and only when needed.
- Trazodone may be taken with or without food.
- Store the medication in its originally labeled, light-resistant container, away from heat and moisture. Heat and moisture may precipitate breakdown of the medication, and the medication may lose its therapeutic effects.
- Keep your medication out of the reach of children.

If you have any questions about your medication, consult your physician or pharmacist.

Notes

_____

_____

_____

_____

_____

From Chew RH, Hales RE, Yudofsky SC: *What Your Patients Need to Know About Psychiatric Medications*, Second Edition. Washington, DC, American Psychiatric Publishing, 2009

Antidepressants
Selective Serotonin Reuptake Inhibitors and Mixed-Action Antidepressants

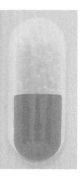

Selective serotonin reuptake inhibitors

Celexa (citalopram)
Lexapro (escitalopram)
Luvox and Luvox CR (fluvoxamine)
Paxil and Paxil CR (paroxetine)
Prozac, Prozac Weekly, and Sarafem (fluoxetine)
Zoloft (sertraline)

Mixed-action antidepressants

Cymbalta (duloxetine)
Effexor and Effexor XR (venlafaxine)
Pristiq (desvenlafaxine)
Remeron (mirtazapine)
Wellbutrin, Wellbutrin SR, and Wellbutrin XL (bupropion)

The antidepressants known as **selective serotonin reuptake inhibitors** (SSRIs) have become widely used to treat major depression and many other psychiatric disorders, including obsessive-compulsive disorder (OCD), panic disorder, generalized anxiety disorder, social anxiety disorder, posttraumatic stress disorder, eating disorders (e.g., bulimia nervosa), and premenstrual dysphoric disorder. The antidepressants in this group are all **serotonin**-specific drugs. They work by boosting the levels of the neurotransmitter serotonin in the central nervous system. The mixed-action antidepressants increase levels of more than one neurotransmitter or have more than one mechanism of action. For instance, Cymbalta, Effexor, and Remeron increase levels of both serotonin and norepinephrine, while Wellbutrin increases levels of dopamine and norepinephrine. All these newer antidepressants are easy to prescribe and take (usually as a single dose in the morning or at bedtime); cause fewer side effects than some of the older antidepressants, such as the **tricyclic antidepressants** (TCAs), and do not require dietary restrictions, such as those required for the **monoamine oxidase inhibitors** (MAOIs). Moreover, the SSRIs and mixed-action antidepressants are usually a good choice for individuals who have medical problems, such as heart disease, hypertension, or seizures.

Neurotransmitters such as serotonin, norepinephrine, and dopamine are chemicals produced by brain cells (called neurons) that enable the neurons to communicate with each other. Serotonin, norepinephrine, and dopamine are released by one neuron into the space between that neuron and the next neuron, allowing an electrical stimulus to continue down the next neuron.

SSRIs work in the brain by inhibiting serotonin from going back to the neuron from which it was originally produced, thereby boosting the levels of serotonin available in the brain. Depression and several other psychiatric disorders, such as OCD, may be the result of abnormally low levels of serotonin in the brain. The low levels of serotonin in turn may produce changes in select areas of the brain, producing psychiatric symptoms such as depression or anxiety. Cymbalta and Effexor block the reuptake of both serotonin and norepinephrine, thereby boosting the levels of both neurotransmitters in the brain. Because of this dual mechanism of action, they are sometimes called **serotonin-norepinephrine reuptake inhibitors** (SNRIs). Wellbutrin blocks the reuptake of norepinephrine and dopamine, and Remeron's principal mechanism of action involves blocking presynaptic α_2-adrenergic receptors and selected serotonin receptors.

When levels of the neurotransmitters are elevated by these antidepressants, those areas of the brain that were previously altered by the low neurotransmitter levels are restored to normal functioning. There is usually a time lag of 3–4 weeks for antidepressants to achieve their optimal effect, which may be the time needed for the brain to make the changes to restore normal functioning.

Common Side Effects

The SSRIs and mixed-action antidepressants are usually well tolerated, and they cause less sedation (except for Remeron) than older antidepressants such as the TCAs. Some individuals, however, complain of "jitters" or restlessness when taking an SSRI, SNRI, or Wellbutrin, especially with those that are more stimulating, such as Prozac, Effexor, or Wellbutrin. Caffeine can also contribute to this "hyper" feeling and should be reduced or avoided by patients taking an SSRI, an SNRI, or Wellbutrin. This side effect may be minimized by starting the antidepressant at a lower dosage and increasing it gradually.

Another frequent complaint is that SSRIs and SNRIs (Cymbalta and Effexor) cause sexual dysfunction, including retarded ejaculation in men and delayed orgasm in women, or intensify a preexisting dysfunction, such as erectile dysfunction. Such side effects may occur in about 50%–60% of individuals taking SSRI antidepressants and in a lower percentage of persons taking SNRIs. Sexual side effects may be minimized with a reduction in dosage or a change to a different SSRI, or they may be eliminated with a change to a different class of antidepressant, such as Wellbutrin (bupropion) or Remeron (mirtazapine).

Other side effects reported with SSRI and SNRI antidepressants include gastrointestinal distress, such as nausea, cramping, heartburn, and diarrhea. Patients may also experience insomnia or daytime sedation from the SSRIs and SNRIs. Taking the antidepressant in the morning may minimize insomnia, or taking it at bedtime may diminish daytime sedation. Headaches may be another bothersome side effect of SSRIs and SNRIs. Generally, patients have fewer complaints of headaches when the dosage is increased gradually.

Adverse Reactions and Precautions

SSRIs and SNRIs can increase the blood levels of other medications metabolized in the liver by inhibiting their metabolism. For example, Paxil has been reported to increase levels of the anticoagulant Coumadin (warfarin), which may increase the risk of bleeding (also refer to the handout for the given medication). Therefore, it is important for physicians to know all of the medications a patient is taking, including over-the-counter medications and herbal supplements. Patients should contact their psychiatrist when any new medications are prescribed by another physician to determine whether caution or closer monitoring is necessary with the psychiatric medications.

Patients taking other drugs that boost serotonin, such as **MAOIs,** in combination with SSRIs or SNRIs may develop a potentially hazardous condition called **serotonin syndrome,** caused by excessive serotonin stimulation in the central nervous system. Rarely, this syndrome may also occur in individuals taking a single SSRI or SNRI agent, especially at higher dosages. Early signs of serotonin syndrome are restlessness, confusion, tremors, flushing, excessive sweating, and involuntary muscle jerks. If the medications are not stopped and unremitting stimulation continues, the individual may develop more life-threatening complications resulting in muscle disorders, high fever, respiratory problems, clotting problems, and destruction of red blood cells that may lead to acute renal failure. Patients taking SSRIs or SNRIs should be alert to signs of serotonin syndrome, which require immediate medical attention and discontinuation of the serotonin-boosting medications.

Overdose

In contrast to the TCAs, overdoses of SSRIs and mixed-action antidepressants are generally much less dangerous, especially when these agents are taken alone. Overdose often involves multiple medications, and the other drugs involved may increase the risk of more serious complications.

Any suspected overdose should be treated as an emergency. The person should be taken to the emergency room for observation and treatment. The prescription bottle of medication (and any other medication suspected in the overdose) should be brought as well, because the information on the prescription label can be helpful to the treating physician in determining the number of pills ingested.

Special Considerations

Most cases of major depression can be treated successfully, usually with medication, psychotherapy, or both. The combination of psychotherapy and antidepressants is very effective in treating moderate to severe depression. The medications improve mood, sleep, energy, and appetite while therapy strengthens coping skills, deals with possible underlying issues, and improves thought patterns and behavior.

In general, antidepressants alone help about 60%–70% of those taking them. Although a few individuals may experience some improvement from antidepressants by the end of the first week, most people do not see significant benefits from their antidepressants until after 3–4 weeks, and it can sometimes take as long as 8 weeks for the medication to achieve its full effects. Thus it is critical that patients continue to take their antidepressant long enough for the medication to be beneficial and that patients not get discouraged and stop their medication prematurely.

We do not fully understand the exact mechanisms by which antidepressants work. They appear to disrupt the chain of events that produce abnormalities in how the brain deals with emotions or stress and result in the symptoms of depression. When an individual does not respond to an SSRI or mixed-action antidepressant, does it make sense for the physician to switch the patient's medication to another medication in the same class if they all have similar modes of action? In practice, patients who do not respond fully to one antidepressant often may respond to another one in the same class. This may not adequately explain the paradox. The molecular structure of an antidepressant may be effective for one individual but not for another. Sometimes it takes trial and error to find the right antidepressant, or combination, for a given individual.

In short-term studies, antidepressants were found to increase the risk of suicidal thinking and behavior in children and adolescents with major depression and other psychiatric disorders. The FDA requires the prescriber to warn of this risk in children and adolescents when starting antidepressant therapy. According to the FDA findings, the risk of suicidal thoughts and behaviors associated with antidepressants is age-related. This phenomenon tends to occur in the younger population and is most likely to occur early in the course of treatment. In adults over 24 years of age, there did not appear to be an increased risk of suicidality with antidepressants compared with placebo. In patients over age 65, the findings showed that antidepressants had a "protective effect" against suicidal thoughts and behavior. Other studies have found that when more people in a community are taking antidepressants, the suicide rate is lower.

The risk of suicide is inherent in depression and may persist until the individual responds to treatment. Closely observe children and adolescents taking antidepressants for signs of worsening, suicidal thoughts, and changes in behavior, especially early in the course of therapy and with change in dosages. Similarly, adults with depressive disorder taking antidepressants should be closely observed for any signs of clinical worsening and suicidal thoughts and behaviors, especially during the first few months of therapy.

Warning: Always let your physician or family member know if you have suicidal thoughts. Notify your psychiatrist or family physician whenever your depressive symptoms worsen or whenever you feel unable to control suicidal urges or thoughts.

For more information, refer to the handout for the antidepressant that was prescribed for you.

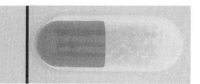

Celexa (citalopram)

Generic name: Citalopram
Available strengths: 10 mg, 20 mg, 40 mg tablets;
   10 mg/5 mL oral solution
Available in generic: Yes
Drug class: Selective serotonin reuptake inhibitor
   antidepressant

General Information

Celexa (citalopram) was approved by the U.S. Food and Drug Administration (FDA) for the treatment of major depressive disorders. The use of a medication for its approved indications is called its *labeled use.* In clinical practice, however, physicians often prescribe medications for *unlabeled* ("off-label") uses when published clinical studies, case reports, or their own clinical experiences support the efficacy and safety of those treatments. Unlabeled uses of Celexa include treatment of other psychiatric disorders, including obsessive-compulsive disorder (OCD), panic disorder, generalized anxiety disorder, social anxiety disorder, posttraumatic stress disorder, and premenstrual dysphoric disorder.

Celexa is a **serotonin**-specific medication that works by blocking the reuptake of the neurotransmitter serotonin back into brain cells, thereby increasing its levels in the brain. Depression and other mental disorders may be caused by abnormally low levels of serotonin. This abnormality may in turn produce changes in affected areas of the brain, resulting in psychiatric symptoms such as depression or anxiety. The presumed action of Celexa and other selective serotonin reuptake inhibitors (SSRIs) is to increase serotonin levels, which may help to restore those areas of the brain to normal functioning.

Dosing Information

For depression, the usual starting dosage of Celexa is 20 mg once a day in the morning or evening. Seniors and people with chronic medical illness may require a lower starting dosage of 10 mg once a day. If no improvement is seen after 3–4 weeks, the dosage may be increased in increments of 10 mg to a usual maximum dosage of 40 mg/day, although it is not uncommon for some patients with severe depression to require up to 80 mg/day. Treatment of other psychiatric disorders, such as OCD, may require higher dosages than those used to treat depression. For patients who cannot take a tablet, Celexa also comes in a liquid form.

For most people, it may take as long as 3–4 weeks to experience the optimal effects of the medication. The duration of medication treatment depends on the individual's personal psychiatric history and family history.

For instance, the length of medication treatment will be longer for those who have had two or more previous episodes of major depressive disorder. For most people, the medication may be tapered 6–9 months after their depression responds to treatment. However, a small percentage of patients will continue to have depressive symptoms after their antidepressant is reduced or stopped. These individuals may benefit from continuing to take Celexa for 1 year or longer.

Common Side Effects

The most frequently reported side effects with Celexa are gastrointestinal disturbance, principally nausea, vomiting, indigestion, diarrhea, or loose stools. Nervousness, jitteriness, and trouble sleeping are other commonly reported side effects. Occasionally, individuals may experience headaches, sleepiness, and excessive sweating. Celexa has very little influence on appetite and weight changes, unlike some of the other SSRIs such as Paxil.

Celexa may induce sexual dysfunction in both men and women. The sexual side effects reported are delayed orgasm in women and retarded ejaculation in men. Some people may experience decreased desire or lack of interest in sexual activity. However, the adverse effects on sexual function with Celexa are generally less frequent than with Prozac or Paxil.

Patients should discuss these side effects with their physician, especially if they continue to be bothersome 3–4 weeks after the medication is started. If a rash or any other severe symptoms develop, patients should contact their physician immediately.

Adverse Reactions and Precautions

Celexa may cause drowsiness in some people. Patients should not drive or operate machinery until they are certain that their alertness or coordination is not affected by the medication. Patients with a known allergy to Celexa or who have experienced a severe reaction after taking it should not take Celexa.

Use in Pregnancy and Breastfeeding: Pregnancy Category C

Celexa has not been tested in women to determine its safety in pregnancy. The effects of the medication on the developing fetus in pregnant women are unknown. However, newborn babies exposed to antidepressants such as SSRIs late in the third trimester developed complications requiring prolonged hospitalization, respiratory support, and tube feeding. Women who are pregnant or may become pregnant should discuss this with their physician. Some women may experience a recurrence of their depression when they stop their antidepressant. In these circumstances it may be necessary to restart the medication or seek an alternative medication or treatment.

Nursing mothers should not take Celexa, because small amounts will pass into breast milk and be ingested by the baby. If stopping the drug is not an alternative, breastfeeding should not be started or should be discontinued.

Possible Drug Interactions

The combined use of Celexa with certain other medications may result in adverse drug interactions, because one medication may alter the blood levels of the other. Fortunately, Celexa has a lower incidence of reported drug interactions than some of the other SSRIs, such as Prozac, Paxil, or Zoloft. The possible drug interactions with Celexa are summarized in the table on the next page.

Coumadin (warfarin)	Celexa may increase Coumadin levels and its anticoagulant effects, resulting in bleeding. This interaction is less likely than with other SSRIs, but Coumadin therapy should be monitored closely when starting any SSRI.
Erythromycin	Antibiotics in the erythromycin family may increase Celexa blood levels and increase the potential for adverse side effects.
Tagamet (cimetidine)	Tagamet may increase Celexa blood levels and increase the potential for adverse side effects.
Antifungal agents such as Nizoral (ketoconazole), Sporanox (itraconazole), and Diflucan (fluconazole)	Antifungals may elevate blood levels of Celexa and increase the potential for adverse side effects.

Other medications, including herbal supplements (such as St. John's wort), that boost serotonin may result in excessive levels of that neurotransmitter when combined with Celexa and produce a toxic syndrome known as **serotonin syndrome.** The early signs of serotonin syndrome are restlessness, confusion, tremors, flushing, and involuntary muscle jerks. If the medications are not stopped, the individual may develop more life-threatening complications resulting in muscle disorders, high fever, respiratory problems, clotting problems, and destruction of red blood cells that may lead to acute renal failure. Patients taking Celexa should be alert to the possible signs of serotonin syndrome, which require immediate medical attention and discontinuation of the serotonin-boosting medications.

Antidepressants known as **monoamine oxidase inhibitors** (MAOIs) should not be taken together with Celexa, because the combination may potentially produce a toxic reaction that includes elevated temperature, high blood pressure, and extreme excitation and agitation. Patients should consult their physician or pharmacist before taking any new medications, including over-the-counter medications and herbal supplements, with Celexa.

Patients taking Celexa should avoid alcohol or should consume it in moderation because the combination may worsen depression.

Overdose

Like other SSRIs, Celexa is much safer in overdose than the older tricyclic antidepressants and some of the newer antidepressants. In the reported overdoses with Celexa, the majority of fatalities were in combination with other medications and/or alcohol. However, fatalities were reported in several cases when Celexa alone was taken in very high doses.

Any suspected overdose should be treated as an emergency. The person should be taken to the emergency room for observation and treatment. The prescription bottle of medication (and any other medication suspected in the overdose) should be brought as well, because the information on the prescription label can be helpful to the treating physician in determining the number of pills ingested.

Special Considerations

Most cases of major depression can be treated successfully, usually with medication, psychotherapy, or both. The combination of psychotherapy and antidepressants is very effective in treating moderate to severe depression. The medications improve mood, sleep, energy, and appetite while therapy strengthens coping skills, deals with possible underlying issues, and improves thought patterns and behavior.

In general, antidepressants alone help about 60%–70% of those taking them. Although a few individuals may experience some improvement from antidepressants by the end of the first week, most people do not see significant benefits from their antidepressants until after 3–4 weeks, and it can sometimes take as long as 8 weeks for the medication to produce its full effects. Thus it is critical that patients continue to take their antidepressant long enough for the medication to be beneficial and that patients not get discouraged and stop their medication prematurely if they do not feel better immediately.

In short-term studies, antidepressants were found to increase the risk of suicidal thinking and behavior in children and adolescents with major depression and other psychiatric disorders. The U.S. Food and Drug Administration (FDA) requires the prescriber to warn of this risk in children and adolescents when starting antidepressant therapy. According to the FDA findings, the risk of suicidal thoughts and behaviors associated with antidepressants is age-related. This phenomenon tends to occur in the younger population and is most likely to occur early in the course of treatment. In adults over 24 years of age, there did not appear to be an increased risk of suicidality with antidepressants compared with placebo. In patients over age 65, the findings showed that antidepressants had a "protective effect" against suicidal thoughts and behavior. Other studies have found that when more people in a community are taking antidepressants, the suicide rate is lower.

The risk of suicide is inherent in depression and may persist until the individual responds to treatment. After antidepressant therapy is being started or changed, the person, especially a child or adolescent, should be closely observed for worsening signs of depression, and the family or caregiver should communicate any concerns to the physician.

- **Warning:** Always let your physician or a family member know if you have suicidal thoughts. Notify your psychiatrist or your family physician whenever your depressive symptoms worsen or whenever you feel unable to control suicidal urges or thoughts.
- Do not discontinue Celexa abruptly. Your dosage should be tapered gradually to prevent any discontinuation symptoms.
- If you miss a dose, take it as soon as possible, within 2–3 hours of the scheduled dose. If it is close to the next scheduled dose, skip the missed dose and continue on your regular dosing schedule. Do not take double doses.
- Celexa may be taken with or without food.
- Store the medication in its originally labeled, light-resistant container, away from heat and moisture. Heat and moisture may precipitate breakdown of your medication, and the medication may lose its therapeutic effects.
- Keep your medication out of reach of children.

If you have any questions about your medication, consult your physician or pharmacist.

Notes

_____

_____

_____

From Chew RH, Hales RE, Yudofsky SC: *What Your Patients Need to Know About Psychiatric Medications,* Second Edition. Washington, DC, American Psychiatric Publishing, 2009

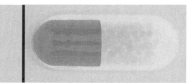

Lexapro (escitalopram)

Generic name: Escitalopram
Available strengths: 5 mg, 10 mg, 20 mg tablets;
   5 mg/5 mL oral solution
Available in generic: No
Drug class: Selective serotonin reuptake inhibitor antidepressant

General Information

Lexapro (escitalopram) is a purified molecule of Celexa (citalopram), a selective serotonin reuptake inhibitor (SSRI) antidepressant. Celexa has two mirror-image forms (designated as *S* and *R* forms), much like our left and right hands, which are mirror images but opposite. Lexapro is made up of only the *S* form. What is the advantage of Lexapro over Celexa? It is thought that the primarily antidepressant action is from the *S* form and that the *R* form has little or no antidepressant activity and may interfere with the active molecule and contribute to side effects. Lexapro, containing only the purified *S* form, is presumed to provide better antidepressant activity than Celexa and, as reported in clinical trials, produce fewer side effects.

Lexapro is approved by the U.S. Food and Drug Administration (FDA) to treat major depressive disorder and general anxiety disorder. The use of a medication for its approved indications is called its *labeled use*. In clinical practice, however, physicians often prescribe medications for *unlabeled* ("off-label") uses when published clinical studies, case reports, or their own clinical experiences support the efficacy and safety for those treatments. Unlabeled uses of Lexapro include treatment of other psychiatric disorders, including obsessive-compulsive disorder, panic disorder, social anxiety disorder, posttraumatic stress disorder, and premenstrual dysphoric disorder.

Lexapro is a **serotonin**-specific medication that works by blocking the reuptake of the neurotransmitter serotonin back into brain cells, thereby increasing its levels in the brain. Depression and other mental disorders may be caused by abnormally low levels of serotonin. This abnormality may in turn produce changes in affected areas of the brain, resulting in psychiatric symptoms such as depression or anxiety. The presumed action of Lexapro and other SSRIs is to increase serotonin levels, which may help to restore those areas of the brain to normal functioning.

Dosing Information

For depression and generalized anxiety disorder, the usual starting dosage of Lexapro is 10 mg once a day in the morning or evening. If improvement is not seen after 3–4 weeks, the dosage may be increased to 20 mg once a day. Generally, for treatment of depression, most people need a dosage of 10–20 mg/day, but some patients with more severe depression may require higher dosages. Treatment of other mental disorders may also require higher dosages than those used for depression. Seniors and people with severe or chronic medical illnesses may require a lower starting dosage of 5 mg/day as well as a lower maintenance dosage of 10 mg/day. For patients who cannot take a tablet, Lexapro also comes in a liquid form.

For most people, it may take as long as 3–4 weeks to experience the optimal effects of the medication. The duration of medication treatment depends on the individual's personal psychiatric history and family history. For instance, the length of medication treatment will be longer for those who have had two or more previous episodes of major depressive disorder. For most people, the medication may be tapered 6 months after their depression responds to treatment. However, a small percentage of patients will continue to have depressive symptoms after their antidepressant is reduced or stopped. These individuals may benefit from continuing to take Lexapro for 1 year or longer.

Common Side Effects

The most frequently reported side effects with Lexapro are gastrointestinal disturbance, principally nausea, vomiting, indigestion, diarrhea, or loose stools. Nervousness, jitteriness, and trouble sleeping are other commonly reported side effects. Occasionally, individuals may experience headaches, sleepiness, and excessive sweating. Lexapro has very little influence on appetite and weight changes, unlike some of the other SSRIs such as Paxil.

Lexapro may induce sexual dysfunction in both men and women. The sexual side effects reported are delayed orgasm in women and retarded ejaculation in men. Some people may experience decreased desire or lack of interest in sexual activity. However, the adverse effects on sexual function with Lexapro are generally less frequent than with Prozac or Paxil.

Patients should discuss these side effects with their physician, especially if they continue to be bothersome 3–4 weeks after the medication is started. If a rash or any other severe symptoms develop, patients should contact their physician immediately.

Adverse Reactions and Precautions

Lexapro may cause drowsiness in some people. Patients should not drive or operate machinery until they are certain that their alertness or coordination is not affected by the medication. Patients with a known allergy to Lexapro or who have experienced a severe reaction after taking it should not take Lexapro.

Use in Pregnancy and Breastfeeding: Pregnancy Category C

Lexapro has not been tested in women to determine its safety in pregnancy. The effects of the medication on the developing fetus in pregnant women are unknown. However, newborn babies exposed to antidepressants such as SSRIs late in the third trimester developed complications requiring prolonged hospitalization, respiratory support, and tube feeding. Women who are pregnant or may become pregnant should discuss this with their physician. Some women may experience a recurrence of their depression when they stop their antidepressant. In these circumstances it may be necessary to restart the medication or seek an alternative medication or treatment.

Nursing mothers should not take Lexapro because small amounts will pass into breast milk and be ingested by the baby. If stopping the drug is not an alternative, breastfeeding should not be started or should be discontinued.

Possible Drug Interactions

The combined use of Lexapro with certain other medications may result in adverse drug interactions, because one medication may alter the blood levels of the other. Fortunately, Lexapro has a very low incidence of reported drug interactions than with some of the other SSRIs, such as Prozac, Paxil, or Zoloft. The possible drug interactions with Lexapro are summarized in the table on the next page.

Coumadin (warfarin)	Lexapro may increase Coumadin levels and its anticoagulant effects, resulting in bleeding. This interaction is less likely than with other SSRIs, but Coumadin therapy should be monitored closely when starting any SSRI.
Erythromycin	Antibiotics in the erythromycin family may increase Lexapro blood levels and increase the potential for adverse side effects.
Tagamet (cimetidine)	Tagamet may increase Lexapro blood levels and increase the potential for adverse side effects.
Antifungal agents such as Nizoral (ketoconazole), Sporanox (itraconazole), and Diflucan (fluconazole)	Antifungals may elevate blood levels of Lexapro and increase the potential for adverse side effects.

Other medications, including herbal supplements (such as St. John's wort), that boost serotonin may result in excessive levels of that neurotransmitter when combined with Lexapro and produce a toxic syndrome known as **scrotonin syndrome.** The early signs of serotonin syndrome are restlessness, confusion, tremors, flushing, and involuntary muscle jerks. If the medications are not stopped, the individual may develop more life-threatening complications resulting in muscle disorders, high fever, respiratory problems, clotting problems, and destruction of red blood cells that may lead to acute renal failure. Patients taking Lexapro should be alert to the possible signs of serotonin syndrome, which require immediate medical attention and discontinuation of the serotonin-boosting medications.

Antidepressants known as **monoamine oxidase inhibitors** (MAOIs) should not be taken together with Lexapro, because the combination may potentially produce a toxic reaction that includes elevated temperature, high blood pressure, and extreme excitation and agitation. Patients should consult their physician or pharmacist before taking any new medications, including over-the-counter medications and herbal supplements, with Lexapro.

Patients taking Lexapro should avoid alcohol or should consume it in moderation because the combination may worsen depression.

Overdose

Like other SSRIs, Lexapro is much safer in overdose than the older tricyclic antidepressants and some of the newer antidepressants. In the reported overdoses with Lexapro, the majority of fatalities were in combination with other medications and/or alcohol. However, fatalities were reported in several cases when Lexapro alone was taken in very high doses.

Any suspected overdose should be treated as an emergency. The person should be taken to the emergency room for observation and treatment. The prescription bottle of medication (and any other medication suspected in the overdose) should be brought as well, because the information on the prescription label can be helpful to the treating physician in determining the number of pills ingested.

Special Considerations

Most cases of major depression can be treated successfully, usually with medication, psychotherapy, or both. The combination of psychotherapy and antidepressants is very effective in treating moderate to severe depression. The medications improve mood, sleep, energy, and appetite while therapy strengthens coping skills, deals with possible underlying issues, and improves thought patterns and behavior.

In general, antidepressants alone help about 60%–70% of those taking them. Although a few individuals may experience some improvement from antidepressants by the end of the first week, most people do not see significant benefits from their antidepressants until after 3–4 weeks, and it can sometimes take as long as 8 weeks for the medication to produce its full effects. Thus it is critical that patients continue to take their antidepressant long enough for the medication to be beneficial and that patients not get discouraged and stop their medication prematurely if they do not feel better immediately.

In short-term studies, antidepressants were found to increase the risk of suicidal thinking and behavior in children and adolescents with major depression and other psychiatric disorders. The FDA requires the prescriber to warn of this risk in children and adolescents when starting antidepressant therapy. According to the FDA findings, the risk of suicidal thoughts and behaviors associated with antidepressants is age-related. This phenomenon tends to occur in the younger population and is most likely to occur early in the course of treatment. In adults over 24 years of age, there did not appear to be an increased risk of suicidality with antidepressants compared with placebo. In patients over age 65, the findings showed that antidepressants had a "protective effect" against suicidal thoughts and behavior. Other studies have found that when more people in a community are taking antidepressants, the suicide rate is lower.

The risk of suicide is inherent in depression and may persist until the individual responds to treatment. After starting or changing antidepressant therapy, the person, especially a child or adolescent, should be closely observed for worsening signs of depression, and the family or caregiver should communicate any concerns to the physician.

- **Warning:** Always let your physician or a family member know if you have suicidal thoughts. Notify your psychiatrist or your family physician whenever your depressive symptoms worsen or whenever you feel unable to control suicidal urges or thoughts.
- Do not discontinue Lexapro abruptly. Your dosage should be tapered gradually to prevent discontinuation symptoms.
- If you miss a dose, take it as soon as possible, within 2–3 hours of the scheduled dose. If it is close to the next scheduled dose, skip the missed dose and continue on your regular dosing schedule. Do not take double doses.
- Lexapro may be taken with or without food.
- Store the medication in its originally labeled, light-resistant container, away from heat and moisture. Heat and moisture may precipitate breakdown of your medication, and the medication may lose its therapeutic effects.
- Keep your medication out of reach of children.

If you have any questions about your medication, consult your physician or pharmacist.

Notes

_____

_____

_____

From Chew RH, Hales RE, Yudofsky SC: *What Your Patients Need to Know About Psychiatric Medications*, Second Edition. Washington, DC, American Psychiatric Publishing, 2009

Luvox and Luvox CR
(fluvoxamine)

Generic name: Fluvoxamine
Available strengths: 25 mg, 50 mg, 100 mg tablets;
   100 mg, 150 mg sustained-release capsules (Luvox CR)
Available in generic: Yes
Drug class: Selective serotonin reuptake inhibitor antidepressant

General Information

Luvox (fluvoxamine) was approved by the U.S. Food and Drug Administration (FDA) for the treatment of obsessive-compulsive disorder (OCD) and social aniety disorder, but not depression. The use of a medication for its approved indications is called its *labeled use*. In clinical practice, however, physicians often prescribe medications for *unlabeled* ("off-label") uses when published clinical studies, case reports, or their own clinical experiences support the efficacy and safety of those treatments. Physicians may use Luvox for treatment of major depression, panic disorder, posttraumatic stress disorder, premenstrual dysphoric disorder, nocturnal enuresis (incontinence of urine) in children, and bulimia nervosa.

Luvox is a **serotonin**-specific medication that works by blocking the reuptake of the neurotransmitter serotonin back into brain cells, thereby increasing its levels in the brain. OCD, depression, and other mental disorders may be caused by abnormally low levels of serotonin. This abnormality may in turn produce changes in affected areas of the brain, resulting in psychiatric symptoms such as depression or anxiety. The presumed action of Luvox and other selective serotonin reuptake inhibitors (SSRIs) is to increase serotonin levels, which may help to restore those areas of the brain to normal functioning. OCD may also be successfully treated with other SSRIs as well as the tricyclic antidepressant (TCA) Anafranil (clomipramine).

Dosing Information

The recommended starting dose of Luvox is 50 mg as a single bedtime dose. The dose is increased weekly in increments of 25–50 mg. The maximum dosage should not exceed 300 mg/day. When dosages are greater than 100 mg/day, Luvox should be taken twice a day, in either equally divided doses or with the larger dose at bedtime. The inconvenience of twice-daily dosing may be circumvented by switching to Luvox CR, which can be administered as a single dose at bedtime. Seniors and people with severe and chronic illness may require lower dosages (50–100 mg/day) than the average person.

In treating children (ages 8–17 years) with OCD, the recommended starting dose is 25 mg administered as a single bedtime dose. The dose is increased by 25 mg every 4–7 days until clinical response is achieved. Generally, the dosage for children up to 11 years old should not exceed 200 mg/day, whereas adolescents may require a maximum dosage of 300 mg/day, similar to the average adult. Girls, in general, may require lower dosages.

Common Side Effects

The most frequently reported side effects with Luvox are gastrointestinal disturbance, principally nausea, vomiting, indigestion, diarrhea, or loose stools. Nervousness, jitteriness, and trouble sleeping are other commonly reported side effects. Occasionally, individuals may experience headaches, sleepiness, and excessive sweating.

Luvox may induce sexual dysfunction in both men and women. The sexual side effects reported are delayed orgasm in women and retarded ejaculation in men. Some people may experience decreased desire or lack of interest in sexual activity. However, the adverse effects on sexual function with Luvox are generally less frequent than with Prozac or Paxil.

Patients should discuss these side effects with their physician, especially if they continue to be bothersome 3–4 weeks after the medication is started. If a rash or any other severe symptoms develop, patients should contact their physician immediately.

Adverse Reactions and Precautions

Luvox may cause drowsiness in some people. Patients should not drive or operate machinery until they are certain that their alertness or coordination is not affected by the medication. Patients with a known allergy to Luvox or who have experienced a severe reaction after taking it should not take Luvox.

Use in Pregnancy and Breastfeeding: Pregnancy Category C

Luvox has not been tested in women to determine its safety in pregnancy. The effects of the medication on the developing fetus in pregnant women are unknown. However, newborn babies exposed to antidepressants such as SSRIs late in the third trimester developed complications requiring prolonged hospitalization, respiratory support, and tube feeding. Women who are pregnant or may become pregnant should discuss this with their physician. Some women may experience a recurrence of their depression when they stop their antidepressant. In these circumstances it may be necessary to restart the medication or seek an alternative medication or treatment.

Nursing mothers should not take Luvox because small amounts will pass into breast milk and be ingested by the baby. If stopping the drug is not an alternative, breastfeeding should not be started or should be discontinued.

Possible Drug Interactions

The combined use of Luvox with certain other medications may result in adverse drug interactions, because one medication may alter the blood levels of the other. The clinically significant drug interactions reported with Luvox are summarized in the table on the next page.

Coumadin (warfarin)	Luvox may increase Coumadin levels and its anticoagulant effects, resulting in bleeding; Coumadin therapy should be monitored closely when starting any SSRI.
Tricyclic antidepressants (TCAs)	Luvox may increase the levels of TCAs and the potential for toxicity.
Clozaril (clozapine)	Luvox may increase the levels of Clozaril and increase its potential for adverse side effects.
Theophylline	Luvox may elevate levels of theophylline and cause toxicity; consequently, theophylline levels should be monitored closely.
Tegretol (carbamazepine)	Luvox may increase levels of Tegretol, possibly resulting in toxicity.
Smoking	Smoking may lower blood levels and decrease the effectiveness of Luvox. Smokers may require higher doses than nonsmokers.

Other medications, including herbal supplements (such as St. John's wort), that boost serotonin may result in excessive levels of that neurotransmitter when combined with Luvox and produce a toxic syndrome known as **serotonin syndrome.** The early signs of serotonin syndrome are restlessness, confusion, tremors, flushing, and involuntary muscle jerks. If the medications are not stopped, the individual may develop more life-threatening complications resulting in muscle disorders, high fever, respiratory problems, clotting problems, and destruction of red blood cells that may lead to acute renal failure. Hence, patients taking Luvox should be alert to the possible signs of serotonin syndrome, which require immediate medical attention and discontinuation of the serotonin-boosting medications.

Antidepressants known as **monoamine oxidase inhibitors** (MAOIs) should not be taken together with Luvox, because the combination may potentially produce a toxic reaction that includes elevated temperature, high blood pressure, and extreme excitation and agitation. Patients should consult their physician or pharmacist before taking any new medications, including over-the-counter medications and herbal supplements, with Luvox.

Patients taking Luvox should avoid alcohol or should consume it in moderation because the combination may worsen depression.

Overdose

Like other SSRIs, Luvox is much safer in overdose than the older TCAs and some of the newer antidepressants. However, fatal outcomes have been reported when Luvox was taken in combination with other medications.

Any suspected overdose should be treated as an emergency. The person should be taken to the emergency room for observation and treatment. The prescription bottle of medication (and any other medication suspected in the overdose) should be brought as well, because the information on the prescription label can be helpful to the treating physician in determining the number of pills ingested.

Special Considerations

Most cases of major depression can be treated successfully, usually with medication, psychotherapy, or both. The combination of psychotherapy and antidepressants is very effective in treating moderate to severe depression. The medications improve mood, sleep, energy, and appetite while therapy strengthens coping skills, deals with possible underlying issues, and improves thought patterns and behavior.

In general, antidepressants alone help about 60%–70% of those taking them. Although a few individuals may experience some improvement from antidepressants by the end of the first week, most people do not see significant benefits from their antidepressants until after 3–4 weeks, and it can sometimes take as long as 8 weeks for the medication to produce its full effects. Thus it is critical that patients continue to take their antidepressant long enough for the medication to be beneficial and that patients not get discouraged and stop their medication prematurely if they do not feel better immediately.

In short-term studies, antidepressants were found to increase the risk of suicidal thinking and behavior in children and adolescents with major depression and other psychiatric disorders. The FDA requires the prescriber to warn of this risk in children and adolescents when starting antidepressant therapy. According to the FDA findings, the risk of suicidal thoughts and behaviors associated with antidepressants is age-related. This phenomenon tends to occur in the younger population and is most likely to occur early in the course of treatment. In adults over 24 years of age, there did not appear to be an increased risk of suicidality with antidepressants compared with placebo. In patients over age 65, the findings showed that antidepressants had a "protective effect" against suicidal thoughts and behavior. Other studies have found that when more people in a community are taking antidepressants, the suicide rate is lower.

The risk of suicide is inherent in depression and may persist until the individual responds to treatment. After starting or changing antidepressant therapy, the person, especially a child or adolescent, should be closely observed for worsening signs of depression, and the family or caregiver should communicate any concerns to the physician.

- **Warning:** Always let your physician or a family member know if you have suicidal thoughts. Notify your psychiatrist or your family physician whenever your depressive symptoms worsen or whenever you feel unable to control suicidal urges or thoughts.
- Do not discontinue Luvox abruptly. Your dosage should be tapered gradually to prevent discontinuation symptoms.
- If you miss a dose, take it as soon as possible, within 1–2 hours of the scheduled dose. If it is close to the next scheduled dose, skip the missed dose and continue on your regular dosing schedule. Do not take double doses.
- Luvox may be taken with or without food.
- Store the medication in its originally labeled, light-resistant container, away from heat and moisture. Heat and moisture may precipitate breakdown of your medication, and the medication may lose its therapeutic effects.
- Keep your medication out of reach of children.

If you have any questions about your medication, consult your physician or pharmacist.

Notes

_____

_____

_____

From Chew RH, Hales RE, Yudofsky SC: *What Your Patients Need to Know About Psychiatric Medications*, Second Edition. Washington, DC, American Psychiatric Publishing, 2009

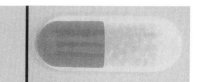

Paxil and Paxil CR
(paroxetine)

Generic name: Paroxetine
Available strengths: 10 mg, 20 mg, 30 mg, 40 mg tablets;
   10 mg/5 mL oral suspension; 12.5 mg, 25 mg,
   37.5 mg controlled-release tablets (Paxil CR)
Available in generic: Yes, except Paxil CR
Drug class: Selective serotonin reuptake inhibitor antidepressant

General Information

Paxil (paroxetine) was approved by the U.S. Food and Drug Administration (FDA) for treatment of major depressive disorder, panic disorder, obsessive-compulsive disorder (OCD), social anxiety disorder, generalized anxiety disorder, and posttraumatic stress disorder. The use of a medication for its approved indications is called its *labeled use*. In clinical practice, however, physicians often prescribe medications for *unlabeled* ("off-label") uses when published clinical studies, case reports, or their own clinical experiences support the efficacy and safety of those treatments. Paxil may be used to treat other psychiatric disorders, including premenstrual dysphoric disorder and eating disorders such as bulimia nervosa, which is characterized by symptoms of binge eating and vomiting.

Paxil is a **serotonin**-specific medication that works by blocking the reuptake of the neurotransmitter serotonin back into brain cells, thereby increasing its levels in the brain. Depression and other mental disorders may be caused by abnormally low levels of serotonin. This abnormality may in turn produce changes in affected areas of the brain, resulting in psychiatric symptoms such as depression or anxiety. The presumed action of Paxil and other selective serotonin reuptake inhibitors (SSRIs) is to increase serotonin levels, which may help to restore those areas of the brain to normal functioning.

Dosing Information

For depression, the usual starting dose of Paxil is 20 mg, taken once a day, usually in the morning. With the controlled-release tablet, Paxil CR, the starting dose is 25 mg, taken once a day in the morning. If no improvement is seen after 3–4 weeks, the dosage is incrementally increased to a maximum daily dosage of 50 mg for Paxil and 62.5 mg for Paxil CR. Seniors and people with severe or chronic medical illnesses may require lower starting dosages. Treatment of other psychiatric disorders such as OCD or panic disorder may require initially lower starting dosages of Paxil or Paxil CR but require higher ending dosages. For example, in the treatment of panic disorder, the starting dosage is 10 mg/day of Paxil and 12.5 mg/day of Paxil CR, but the maximum dosage for Paxil and Paxil CR is 60 mg/day and 75 mg/day, respectively. For patients who cannot take a tablet, Paxil also comes in a liquid form.

Paxil CR is a controlled-release, and not a sustained-release, formulation. The controlled-release tablet does not provide a longer duration of action over Paxil but offers a smoother rate of absorption with fewer gastrointestinal side effects, such as nausea. The enteric-coated tablets of Paxil CR should not be chewed, crushed, or cut but swallowed whole, because the tablet structure is what makes the medication controlled-release.

For most people, it may take as long as 3–4 weeks to experience the optimal effects of the medication. The duration of medication treatment depends on the individual's personal psychiatric history and family history. For instance, the length of medication treatment will be longer for those who have had two or more previous episodes of major depressive disorder. For most people, the medication may be tapered 6–9 months after their depression responds to treatment. However, a small percentage of patients will continue to have depressive symptoms after their antidepressant is reduced or stopped. These individuals may benefit from continuing to take Paxil for 1 year or longer.

Common Side Effects

The most frequent complaints reported with Paxil are gastrointestinal side effects, including nausea, vomiting, cramping, diarrhea, and heartburn. These side effects may be dramatically reduced by switching to the controlled-release tablet, Paxil CR. Drowsiness and daytime sedation may be other frequent side effects experienced by individuals taking Paxil. However, a significant number of people taking SSRIs, including Paxil, may experience jitteriness, nervousness, and insomnia, which is common with this class of antidepressants because of its activating properties in the central nervous system.

Paxil is associated with a significant rate of sexual dysfunction in men and women taking the antidepressant. The sexual side effects reported are delayed orgasm in women and retarded ejaculation in men. Some people may experience decreased desire or lack of interest in sexual activity. Occasionally, individuals report headaches, sleepiness, excessive sweating, stomach cramps, diarrhea, and constipation.

People taking Paxil may also experience weight gain.

Patients should discuss these side effects with their physician, especially if they continue to be bothersome 3–4 weeks after the medication is started. If a rash or any other severe symptoms develop, patients should contact their physician immediately.

Adverse Reactions and Precautions

Paxil may cause drowsiness in some people. Patients should not drive or operate machinery until they are certain that their alertness or coordination is not affected by the medication. Patients with a known allergy to Paxil or who have experienced a severe reaction after taking it should not take Paxil.

Use in Pregnancy and Breastfeeding: Pregnancy Category C

Paxil has not been tested in women to determine its safety in pregnancy. The effects of the medication on the developing fetus in pregnant women are unknown. However, newborn babies exposed to antidepressants such as

SSRIs late in the third trimester developed complications requiring prolonged hospitalization, respiratory support, and tube feeding. Women who are pregnant or may become pregnant should discuss this with their physician. Some women may experience a recurrence of their depression when they stop their antidepressant. In these circumstances it may be necessary to restart the medication or seek an alternative medication or treatment.

Nursing mothers should not take Paxil because small amounts will pass into breast milk and be ingested by the baby. If stopping the drug is not an alternative, breastfeeding should not be started or should be discontinued.

Possible Drug Interactions

The combined use of Paxil with certain other medications may result in adverse drug interactions, because one medication may alter the blood levels of the other. The clinically significant drug interactions reported with Paxil are summarized in the table below.

Coumadin (warfarin)	Paxil may increase Coumadin levels and its anticoagulant effects, resulting in bleeding; Coumadin therapy should be monitored closely when starting any SSRI.
Tricyclic antidepressants (TCAs)	Paxil may increase the levels of TCAs and the potential for toxicity.
Thioridazine	Paxil may increase the level of thioridazine, an antipsychotic medication, and increase the risk of cardiac arrhythmias.
Phenobarbital	Phenobarbital may decrease the level of Paxil and make it less effective.
Dilantin (phenytoin)	Dilantin may decrease the level of Paxil and make it less effective.
Tagamet (cimetidine)	Tagamet may increase the level of Paxil and increase the potential for side effects.
Imitrex (sumatriptan)	When Imitrex, a medication for treatment of migraine headaches, was combined with Paxil, some patients reported weakness, jerkiness, and loss of coordination.

Other medications, including herbal supplements (such as St. John's wort), that boost serotonin may result in excessive levels of that neurotransmitter when combined with Paxil and produce a toxic syndrome known as **serotonin syndrome.** The early signs of serotonin syndrome are restlessness, confusion, tremors, flushing, and involuntary muscle jerks. If the medications are not stopped, the individual may develop more life-threatening complications resulting in muscle disorders, high fever, respiratory problems, clotting problems, and destruction of red blood cells that may lead to acute renal failure. Patients taking Paxil should be alert to the possible signs of serotonin syndrome, which require immediate medical attention and discontinuation of the serotonin-boosting medications.

Antidepressants known as **monoamine oxidase inhibitors** (MAOIs) should not be taken together with Paxil, because the combination may potentially produce a toxic reaction that includes elevated temperature, high blood pressure, and extreme excitation and agitation. Patients should consult their physician or pharmacist before taking any new medications, including over-the-counter medications and herbal supplements, with Paxil.

Patients taking Paxil should avoid alcohol or should consume it in moderation because the combination may worsen depression.

Overdose

Like other SSRIs, Paxil is much safer in overdose than the older TCAs and some of the newer antidepressants. There are no reports of fatality following overdose with Paxil alone. However, fatal outcomes have been reported when Paxil was taken in combination with other medications.

Any suspected overdose should be treated as an emergency. The person should be taken to the emergency room for observation and treatment. The prescription bottle of medication (and any other medication suspected in the overdose) should be brought as well, because the information on the prescription label can be helpful to the treating physician in determining the number of pills ingested.

Special Considerations

Most cases of major depression can be treated successfully, usually with medication, psychotherapy, or both. The combination of psychotherapy and antidepressants is very effective in treating moderate to severe depression. The medications improve mood, sleep, energy, and appetite while therapy strengthens coping skills, deals with possible underlying issues, and improves thought patterns and behavior.

In general, antidepressants alone help about 60%–70% of those taking them. Although a few individuals may experience some improvement from antidepressants by the end of the first week, most people do not see significant benefits from their antidepressants until after 3–4 weeks, and it can sometimes take as long as 8 weeks for the medication to produce its full effects. Thus it is critical that patients continue to take their antidepressant long enough for the medication to be beneficial and that patients not get discouraged and stop their medication prematurely if they do not feel better immediately.

In short-term studies, antidepressants were found to increase the risk of suicidal thinking and behavior in children and adolescents with major depression and other psychiatric disorders. The FDA requires the prescriber to warn of this risk in children and adolescents when starting antidepressant therapy. According to the FDA findings, the risk of suicidal thoughts and behaviors associated with antidepressants is age-related. This phenomenon tends to occur in the younger population and is most likely to occur early in the course of treatment. In adults over 24 years of age, there did not appear to be an increased risk of suicidality with antidepressants compared with placebo. In patients over age 65, the findings showed that antidepressants had a "protective effect" against suicidal thoughts and behavior. Other studies have found that when more people in a community are taking antidepressants, the suicide rate is lower.

The risk of suicide is inherent in depression and may persist until the individual responds to treatment. After starting or changing antidepressant therapy, the person, especially a child or adolescent, should be closely observed for worsening signs of depression, and the family or caregiver should communicate any concerns to the physician.

- **Warning:** Always let your physician or a family member know if you have suicidal thoughts. Notify your psychiatrist or your family physician whenever your depressive symptoms worsen or whenever you feel unable to control suicidal urges or thoughts.
- Do not discontinue Paxil abruptly. Your dosage should be tapered gradually to prevent discontinuation symptoms.
- If you miss a dose, take it as soon as possible, within 2–3 hours of the scheduled dose. If it is close to the next scheduled dose, skip the missed dose and continue on your regular dosing schedule. Do not take double doses.
- Paxil may be taken with or without food.
- Swallow tablets of Paxil CR whole, and do not crush or chew the tablet.
- Store the medication in its originally labeled, light-resistant container, away from heat and moisture. Heat and moisture may precipitate breakdown of your medication, and the medication may lose its therapeutic effects.
- Keep your medication out of reach of children.

If you have any questions about your medication, consult your physician or pharmacist.

Notes

From Chew RH, Hales RE, Yudofsky SC: *What Your Patients Need to Know About Psychiatric Medications,* Second Edition. Washington, DC, American Psychiatric Publishing, 2009

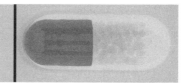

Prozac, Prozac Weekly, and Sarafem (fluoxetine)

Generic name: Fluoxetine

Available strengths: 10 mg, 15 mg, 20 mg, 40 mg capsules or tablets;
   90 mg delayed-release capsule (Prozac Weekly);
   20 mg/5 mL oral solution

Available in generic: Yes, except Prozac Weekly

Drug class: Selective serotonin reuptake inhibitor
   antidepressant

General Information

Prozac (fluoxetine) was approved by the U.S. Food and Drug Administration (FDA) for the treatment of major depressive disorder, obsessive-compulsive disorder (OCD), bulimia nervosa (a binge eating and vomiting disorder), and premenstrual dysphoric disorder (PMDD). In clinical studies, the use of fluoxetine in children and adolescents (ages 7–17) was found to be safe and effective for treating OCD and major depression. Fluoxetine was recently approved by the FDA in this population for treatment of OCD and major depression. The use of a medication for its approved indications is called its *labeled use*. In clinical practice, however, physicians often prescribe medications for *unlabeled* ("off-label") uses when published clinical studies, case reports, or their own clinical experiences support the efficacy and safety of those treatments. Prozac may be used to treat other psychiatric disorders, including panic disorder, generalized anxiety disorder, social anxiety disorder, and posttraumatic stress disorder.

Prozac was the first selective serotonin reuptake inhibitor (SSRI) approved by the FDA for the treatment of PMDD. The symptoms occur during a specific phase of the menstrual cycle just prior to menstrual bleeding, and the woman typically presents with labile mood, anger, irritability, and depression. Fluoxetine is marketed under the brand name Sarafem specifically for PMDD.

Prozac is a **serotonin**-specific medication that works by blocking the reuptake of the neurotransmitter serotonin back into brain cells, thereby increasing its levels in the brain. Depression and other mental disorders may be caused by abnormally low levels of serotonin. This abnormality may in turn produce changes in affected areas of the brain, resulting in psychiatric symptoms such as depression or anxiety. The presumed action of Prozac and other SSRIs is to increase serotonin levels, which may help to restore those areas of the brain to normal functioning.

Dosing Information

The usual starting dose of Prozac in depression is 20 mg (capsule or tablet), taken once a day in the morning. In treating young and lower-weight children, the recommended starting dosage is 10 mg/day. If no improvement is seen after 3–4 weeks, the dosage may be increased in increments of 10 mg to a maximum dosage of 60 mg/day. If the patient's symptoms are stable with a 20 mg/day dosage, the dosage may be switched to 90 mg of the delayed-release Prozac Weekly once a week for dosing convenience, with similar therapeutic effect. Seniors and people with severe or chronic medical conditions may require a lower starting dosage. Generally, higher dosages of Prozac are required for treatment of other psychiatric disorders. Treatment of OCD, for example, may require a dosage of 80–100 mg/day for the average adult and 20–60 mg/day for children and adolescents. For treatment of PMDD, Prozac is marketed under the brand name Sarafem, which merely contains Prozac. For patients who cannot take a tablet or capsule, Prozac also comes in liquid form.

For most people, it may take as long as 3–4 weeks to experience the optimal effects of the medication. The duration of medication treatment depends on the individual's personal psychiatric history and family history. For instance, the length of medication treatment will be longer for those who have had two or more previous episodes of major depressive disorder. For most people, the medication may be tapered 6 months after their depression responds to treatment. However, a small percentage of patients will continue to have depressive symptoms after their antidepressant is reduced or stopped. These individuals may benefit from continuing to take Prozac for 1 year or longer.

Common Side Effects

The most common side effects reported with Prozac are nervousness, jitteriness, nausea, and insomnia. There is a high rate of sexual dysfunction in individuals taking Prozac. The most frequent sexual side effects reported were delayed or lack of orgasm in women and retarded ejaculation in men. Some people may experience decreased desire or lack of interest in sexual drive. Occasionally, individuals report headaches, sleepiness, changes in appetite, excessive sweating, stomach cramps, diarrhea, and constipation with Prozac.

Patients should discuss these side effects with their physician, especially if they continue to be bothersome 3–4 weeks after the medication is started. If a rash or any other severe symptoms develop, patients should contact their physician immediately.

Adverse Reactions and Precautions

Prozac may cause drowsiness in some people. Patients should not drive or operate machinery until they are certain that their alertness or coordination is not affected by the medication. Patients with a known allergy to Prozac or who have experienced a severe reaction after taking it should not take Prozac.

Use in Pregnancy and Breastfeeding: Pregnancy Category C

Prozac has not been tested in women to determine its safety in pregnancy. The effects of the medication on the developing fetus in pregnant women are unknown. However, newborn babies exposed to antidepressants such as SSRIs late in the third trimester developed complications requiring prolonged hospitalization, respiratory support, and tube feeding. Women who are pregnant or may become pregnant should discuss this with their physician. Some women may experience a recurrence of their depression when they stop their antidepressant. In these circumstances it may be necessary to restart the medication or seek an alternative medication or treatment.

Nursing mothers should not take Prozac because small amounts will pass into breast milk and be ingested by the baby. If stopping the drug is not an alternative, breastfeeding should not be started or should be discontinued.

Possible Drug Interactions

Prozac may increase the levels of other medications by inhibiting their metabolism in the liver. This interaction may result in higher levels of the inhibited medication and thus increase its potential for toxicity. The clinically significant drug interactions with Prozac are summarized in the table below.

Coumadin (warfarin)	Prozac may increase Coumadin levels and its anticoagulant effects, resulting in bleeding. This interaction is less likely than with other SSRIs, but Coumadin therapy should be monitored closely when starting any SSRI.
Tricyclic antidepressants (TCAs)	Prozac may increase the levels of TCAs and the potential for toxicity.
Valium (diazepam)	Prozac may elevate levels of diazepam and diazepam-like medications, enhancing sedation and impairment of coordination.
Anticonvulsants	Prozac may elevate levels of anticonvulsants such as Dilantin (phenytoin), Tegretol (carbamazepine), and Depakote (divalproex sodium), increasing the potential for toxicity.
Antipsychotics	Prozac may elevate levels of antipsychotic medications, including Haldol (haloperidol), Clozaril (clozapine), thioridazine, and Risperdal (risperidone), possibly increasing their side effects.

Other medications, including herbal supplements (such as St. John's wort), that boost serotonin may result in excessive levels of that neurotransmitter when combined with Prozac and produce a toxic syndrome known as **serotonin syndrome.** The early signs of serotonin syndrome are restlessness, confusion, tremors, flushing, and involuntary muscle jerks. If the medications are not stopped, the individual may develop more life-threatening complications resulting in muscle disorders, high fever, respiratory problems, clotting problems, and destruction of red blood cells that may lead to acute renal failure. Patients taking Prozac should be alert to the possible signs of serotonin syndrome, which require immediate medical attention and discontinuation of the serotonin-boosting medications.

Antidepressants known as **monoamine oxidase inhibitors** (MAOIs) should not be taken together with Prozac, because the combination may potentially produce a toxic reaction that includes elevated temperature, high blood pressure, and extreme excitation and agitation. Patients should consult their physician or pharmacist before taking any new medications, including over-the-counter medications and herbal supplements, with Prozac.

Patients taking Prozac should avoid alcohol or should consume it in moderation because the combination may worsen depression.

Overdose

Like other SSRIs, Prozac is much safer in overdose than the older TCAs and some of the newer antidepressants. However, unlike the other SSRIs, Prozac has a very long duration of action, and therefore it takes much longer to eliminate Prozac from the body. Deaths from massive overdoses of Prozac have been reported. Usually, Prozac was combined with other medications in cases of fatal outcomes. The most common symptoms associated with Prozac overdose include somnolence, confusion, nausea, vomiting, rapid heart rate, and seizures.

Any suspected overdose should be treated as an emergency. The person should be taken to the emergency room for observation and treatment. The prescription bottle of medication (and any other medication suspected in the overdose) should be brought as well, because the information on the prescription label can be helpful to the treating physician in determining the number of pills ingested.

Special Considerations

Most cases of major depression can be treated successfully, usually with medication, psychotherapy, or both. The combination of psychotherapy and antidepressants is very effective in treating moderate to severe depression. The medications improve mood, sleep, energy, and appetite while therapy strengthens coping skills, deals with possible underlying issues, and improves thought patterns and behavior.

In general, antidepressants alone help about 60%–70% of those taking them. Although a few individuals may experience some improvement from antidepressants by the end of the first week, most people do not see significant benefits from their antidepressants until after 3–4 weeks, and it can sometimes take as long as 8 weeks for the medication to produce its full effects. Thus it is critical that patients continue to take their antidepressant long enough for the medication to be beneficial and that patients not get discouraged and stop their medication prematurely if they do not feel better immediately.

In short-term studies, antidepressants were found to increase the risk of suicidal thinking and behavior in children and adolescents with major depression and other psychiatric disorders. The FDA requires the prescriber to warn of this risk in children and adolescents when starting antidepressant therapy. According to the FDA findings, the risk of suicidal thoughts and behaviors associated with antidepressants is age-related. This phenomenon tends to occur in the younger population and is most likely to occur early in the course of treatment. In adults over 24 years of age, there did not appear to be an increased risk of suicidality with antidepressants compared with placebo. In patients over age 65, the findings showed that antidepressants had a "protective effect" against suicidal thoughts and behavior. Other studies have found that when more people in a community are taking antidepressants, the suicide rate is lower.

The risk of suicide is inherent in depression and may persist until the individual responds to treatment. After starting or changing antidepressant therapy, the person, especially a child or adolescent, should be closely observed for worsening signs of depression, and the family or caregiver should communicate any concerns to the physician.

- **Warning:** Always let your physician or a family member know if you have suicidal thoughts. Notify your psychiatrist or your family physician whenever your depressive symptoms worsen or whenever you feel unable to control suicidal urges or thoughts.
- Do not discontinue Prozac abruptly. Your dosage should be tapered gradually to prevent discontinuation symptoms.
- If you miss a dose, take it as soon as possible, within 2–3 hours of the scheduled dose. If it is close to the next scheduled dose, skip the missed dose and continue on your regular dosing schedule. Do not take double doses.
- Prozac may be taken with or without food.
- Store the medication in its originally labeled, light-resistant container, away from heat and moisture. Heat and moisture may precipitate breakdown of your medication, and the medication may lose its therapeutic effects.
- Keep your medication out of reach of children.

If you have any questions about your medication, consult your physician or pharmacist.

Notes

From Chew RH, Hales RE, Yudofsky SC: *What Your Patients Need to Know About Psychiatric Medications*, Second Edition. Washington, DC, American Psychiatric Publishing, 2009

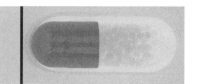

Zoloft (sertraline)

Generic name: Sertraline
Available strengths: 25 mg, 50 mg, 100 mg tablets;
   20 mg/mL oral concentrate
Available in generic: Yes
Drug class: Selective serotonin reuptake inhibitor
   antidepressant

General Information

Zoloft (sertraline) was approved by the U.S. Food and Drug Administration (FDA) for treatment of major depressive disorder, panic disorder, obsessive-compulsive disorder, social anxiety disorder, premenstrual dysphoric disorder, and posttraumatic stress disorder. The use of a medication for its approved indications is called its *labeled use*. In clinical practice, however, physicians often prescribe medications for *unlabeled* ("off-label") uses when published clinical studies, case reports, or their own clinical experiences support the efficacy and safety of those treatments. Zoloft may be used to treat other psychiatric disorders, including generalized anxiety disorder.

Zoloft is a **serotonin**-specific medication that works by blocking the reuptake of the neurotransmitter serotonin back into brain cells, thereby increasing its levels in the brain. Depression and other mental disorders may be caused by abnormally low levels of serotonin. This abnormality may in turn produce changes in affected areas of the brain, resulting in psychiatric symptoms such as depression or anxiety. The presumed action of Zoloft and other selective serotonin reuptake inhibitors (SSRIs) is to increase serotonin levels, which may help to restore those areas of the brain to normal functioning.

Dosing Information

For depression, the usual starting dose of Zoloft is 50 mg, once a day, which is best taken in the morning. Seniors and people with chronic or severe medical illnesses may require a lower starting dose of 25 mg, taken once a day. For patients with an anxiety disorder, such as panic disorder, the usual starting daily dose is also 25 mg. If no improvement is seen after 3–4 weeks, the dosage of Zoloft may be increased in increments of 50 mg/day to a maximum of 200 mg/day. Treatment of other psychiatric disorders usually requires higher dosages than those used in treating depression. For patients who cannot take a tablet, Zoloft also comes in a liquid form.

For most people, it may take as long as 3–4 weeks to experience the optimal effects of the medication. The duration of medication treatment depends on the individual's personal psychiatric history and family history.

For instance, the length of medication treatment will be longer for those who have had two or more previous episodes of major depressive disorder. For most people, the medication may be tapered 6 months after their depression responds to treatment. However, a small percentage of patients will continue to have depressive symptoms after their antidepressant is reduced or stopped. These individuals may benefit from continuing to take Zoloft for 1 year or longer.

Common Side Effects

The most frequently reported side effects with Zoloft are gastrointestinal disturbance, principally nausea, vomiting, indigestion, diarrhea, or loose stools. Nervousness, jitteriness, and trouble sleeping are other commonly reported side effects. Occasionally, individuals may experience headaches, sleepiness, and excessive sweating.

Zoloft may induce sexual dysfunction in both men and women. The sexual side effects reported are delayed orgasm in women and retarded ejaculation in men. Some people may experience decreased desire or lack of interest in sexual activity. However, the adverse effects on sexual function with Zoloft are generally less frequent than with Prozac or Paxil.

Patients should discuss these side effects with their physician, especially if they continue to be bothersome 3–4 weeks after the medication is started. If a rash or any other severe symptoms develop, patients should contact their physician immediately.

Adverse Reactions and Precautions

Zoloft may cause drowsiness in some people. Patients should not drive or operate machinery until they are certain that their alertness or coordination is not affected by the medication. Patients with a known allergy to Zoloft or who have experienced a severe reaction after taking it should not take Zoloft.

Use in Pregnancy and Breastfeeding: Pregnancy Category C

Zoloft has not been tested in women to determine its safety in pregnancy. The effects of the medication on the developing fetus in pregnant women are unknown. However, newborn babies exposed to antidepressants such as SSRIs late in the third trimester developed complications requiring prolonged hospitalization, respiratory support, and tube feeding. Women who are pregnant or may become pregnant should discuss this with their physician. Some women may experience a recurrence of their depression when they stop their antidepressant. In these circumstances it may be necessary to restart the medication or seek an alternative medication or treatment.

Nursing mothers should not take Zoloft, because small amounts will pass into breast milk and be ingested by the baby. If stopping the antidepressant is not an alternative, breastfeeding should not be started or should be discontinued.

Possible Drug Interactions

The combined use of Zoloft with certain other medications may result in adverse drug interactions, because one medication may alter the blood levels of the other. The clinically significant drug interactions reported with Zoloft are summarized in the table on the next page.

Coumadin (warfarin)	Zoloft may increase the anticoagulant action of Coumadin and increase risk of bleeding.
Tricyclic antidepressants (TCAs)	Zoloft may increase the levels of TCAs, primarily desipramine (Norpramin) and imipramine (Tofranil), and the potential for toxicity.
Tagamet (cimetidine)	Tagamet may increase the level of Zoloft and increase the potential for side effects.

Other medications, including herbal supplements (such as St. John's wort), that boost serotonin may result in excessive levels of that neurotransmitter when combined with Zoloft and produce a toxic syndrome known as **serotonin syndrome.** The early signs of serotonin syndrome are restlessness, confusion, tremors, flushing, and involuntary muscle jerks. If the medications are not stopped, the individual may develop more life-threatening complications resulting in muscle disorders, high fever, respiratory problems, clotting problems, and destruction of red blood cells that may lead to acute renal failure. Patients taking Zoloft should be alert to the possible signs of serotonin syndrome, which require immediate medical attention and discontinuation of the serotonin-boosting medications.

Antidepressants known as **monoamine oxidase inhibitors** (MAOIs) should not be taken together with Zoloft, because the combination may potentially produce a toxic reaction that includes elevated temperature, high blood pressure, and extreme excitation and agitation. Patients should consult their physician or pharmacist before taking any new medications, including over-the-counter medications and herbal supplements, with Zoloft.

Patients taking Zoloft should avoid alcohol or should consume it in moderation because the combination may worsen depression.

Overdose

Like other SSRIs, Zoloft is much safer in overdose than the older TCAs and some of the newer antidepressants. There are no reports of fatality after overdose with Zoloft alone. However, fatal outcomes have been reported when Zoloft was taken in combination with other medications.

Any suspected overdose should be treated as an emergency. The person should be taken to the emergency room for observation and treatment. The prescription bottle of medication (and any other medication suspected in the overdose) should be brought as well, because the information on the prescription label can be helpful to the treating physician in determining the number of pills ingested.

Special Considerations

Most cases of major depression can be treated successfully, usually with medication, psychotherapy, or both. The combination of psychotherapy and antidepressants is very effective in treating moderate to severe depression. The medications improve mood, sleep, energy, and appetite while therapy strengthens coping skills, deals with possible underlying issues, and improves thought patterns and behavior.

In general, antidepressants alone help about 60%–70% of those taking them. Although a few individuals may experience some improvement from antidepressants by the end of the first week, most people do not see significant benefits from their antidepressants until after 3–4 weeks, and it can sometimes take as long as 8 weeks for the medication to produce its full effects. Thus it is critical that patients continue to take their antidepressant long enough for the medication to be beneficial and that patients not get discouraged and stop their medication prematurely if they do not feel better immediately.

In short-term studies, antidepressants were found to increase the risk of suicidal thinking and behavior in children and adolescents with major depression and other psychiatric disorders. The FDA requires the prescriber to warn of this risk in children and adolescents when starting antidepressant therapy. According to the FDA findings, the risk of suicidal thoughts and behaviors associated with antidepressants is age-related. This phenomenon tends to occur in the younger population and is most likely to occur early in the course of treatment. In adults over 24 years of age, there did not appear to be an increased risk of suicidality with antidepressants compared with placebo. In patients over age 65, the findings showed that antidepressants had a "protective effect" against suicidal thoughts and behavior. Other studies have found that when more people in a community are taking antidepressants, the suicide rate is lower.

The risk of suicide is inherent in depression and may persist until the individual responds to treatment. After starting or changing antidepressant therapy, the person, especially a child or adolescent, should be closely observed for worsening signs of depression, and the family or caregiver should communicate any concerns to the physician.

- **Warning:** Always let your physician or a family member know if you have suicidal thoughts. Notify your psychiatrist or your family physician whenever your depressive symptoms worsen or whenever you feel unable to control suicidal urges or thoughts.
- Do not discontinue Zoloft abruptly. Your dosage should be tapered gradually to prevent discontinuation symptoms.
- If you miss a dose, take it as soon as possible, within 2–3 hours of the scheduled dose. If it is close to the next scheduled dose, skip the missed dose and continue on your regular dosing schedule. Do not take double doses.
- Zoloft may be taken with or without food.
- Store the medication in its originally labeled, light-resistant container, away from heat and moisture. Heat and moisture may precipitate breakdown of your medication, and the medication may lose its therapeutic effects.
- Keep your medication out of reach of children.

If you have any questions about your medication, consult your physician or pharmacist.

Notes

_____

_____

_____

_____

_____

_____

From Chew RH, Hales RE, Yudofsky SC: *What Your Patients Need to Know About Psychiatric Medications*, Second Edition. Washington, DC, American Psychiatric Publishing, 2009

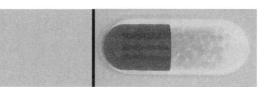

Cymbalta (duloxetine)

Generic name: Duloxetine
Available strengths: 20 mg, 30 mg, 60 mg capsules
Available in generic: No
Drug class: Serotonin-norepinephrine reuptake
    inhibitor antidepressant

General Information

Cymbalta (duloxetine) is unlike the selective serotonin reuptake inhibitor (SSRI) antidepressants such as Prozac (fluoxetine), which are relatively serotonin-specific in action. Cymbalta has a dual mechanism of action. Presumably, it works by altering the neurotransmission of both **serotonin** and **norepinephrine,** two important neurotransmitters in the brain.

During neurotransmission, *neurotransmitters* are released by one neuron into the space between that neuron and the next neuron. The neurotransmitters come into contact with specific sites on the surface membrane of neurons called *receptors*. From there, the chemical signal is transformed into an electrical impulse that travels down the neuron, causing further release of neurotransmitters. This process of neurotransmission is repeated along a chain of neurons. During neurotransmission, after neurotransmitters are released and the chemical signal is transferred to neurons, the neurotransmitters are recaptured back into brain cells by a process known as *reuptake*. By blocking the neurotransmitters from going back into the neurons from where they were released, the antidepressant can amplify the effects of the neurotransmitter.

Cymbalta exerts its antidepressant effect principally by blocking the reuptake of serotonin and norepinephrine. This action is similar to that of the SSRIs, but notably different in that Cymbalta also inhibits the reuptake of norepinephrine. Through reuptake inhibition, Cymbalta boosts serotonin and norepinephrine neurotransmission. For this reason, Cymbalta is called a *serotonin-norepinephrine reuptake inhibitor* (SNRI). Depression and other mental disorders may be caused by abnormally low levels (or abnormal neurotransmission) of serotonin, norepinephrine, or both. This abnormality may in turn produce changes in affected areas of the brain, resulting in psychiatric symptoms such as depression or anxiety. When neurotransmission is improved by the antidepressant, the affected areas of the brain are restored to normal functioning, reducing the symptoms of the illness.

Cymbalta was originally approved by the U.S. Food and Drug Administration (FDA) for the treatment of major depression and management of pain and abnormal sensations caused by complications of diabetes mellitus, known as *diabetic peripheral neuropathy* (DPN). It is now approved also for treatment of generalized anxiety disorder and for fibromyalgia, a condition defined by symptoms of fatigue, chronic generalized pain, and sensitivity to touch. The use of a medication for its approved indications is called its *labeled use*. In clinical practice, however, physicians often prescribe medications for *unlabeled* ("off-label") uses when published clinical studies, case reports, or their own clinical experiences support the efficacy and safety of those treatments. Physicians may use Cymbalta "off-label" to treat other pain conditions, panic disorder, posttraumatic stress disorder, social phobia, and urinary difficulties (incontinence).

Dosing Information

For major depression, Cymbalta is usually initiated at a total daily dose of 40–60 mg, administered in divided doses (20–30 mg two times a day). Generally, 60 mg/day was found to be the optimal dosage. For treating pain symptoms, some patients may need higher dosages (90–120 mg/day in divided doses). The safety and effectiveness of dosages higher than 120 mg/day have not been adequately evaluated, and, therefore, use of the medication at dosages higher than 120 mg/day is not recommended.

Common Side Effects

The most common side effects reported with Cymbalta are nausea, vomiting, constipation, dry mouth, dizziness, increased sweating (e.g., night sweats), fatigue, and insomnia. Side effects generally occur soon after starting the medication or when increasing the dosage. If side effects become intolerable, the physician may decrease the dosage to allow the individual to adjust to the medication before increasing it again slowly.

Sexual side effects, including delayed orgasm in women and retarded ejaculation in men, occur with Cymbalta at about the same rate as with the SNRI antidepressant Effexor (venlafaxine), but at a rate lower than the 50%–60% rate reported with the SSRIs.

Cymbalta does not appear to induce weight gain. In clinical trials, patients taking Cymbalta gained less weight than those taking placebo (sugar tablets).

Adverse Reactions and Precautions

Patients taking normal dosages of Cymbalta may develop mild elevation of blood pressure (hypertension). The increase in blood pressure is usually modest, and very few patients have to discontinue Cymbalta because of hypertension. Generally, lowering the dosage will normalize blood pressure. For this reason, the patient's blood pressure should be checked before starting Cymbalta and routinely during therapy as a precautionary measure, especially for individuals with preexisting hypertension or those with a history of heart disease.

Cymbalta may worsen uncontrolled narrow-angle glaucoma, an eye disorder caused by increased intraocular pressure. Therefore, Cymbalta should be avoided in patients with poorly controlled narrow-angle glaucoma.

Abrupt discontinuation of Cymbalta may precipitate withdrawal symptoms, including dizziness, nausea, headache, vomiting, irritability, and nightmare. Withdrawal symptoms may be avoided by tapering the dosage gradually before discontinuation.

Cymbalta's pharmacological action may cause urinary difficulty and hesitancy. Men with an enlarged prostate may be particularly prone to this adverse effect.

Use in Pregnancy and Breastfeeding: Pregnancy Category C

Cymbalta has not been tested in women to determine its safety in pregnancy. The effects of the medication on the developing fetus are unknown. However, newborn babies exposed to antidepressants such as Cymbalta and

SSRIs late in the third trimester developed complications requiring prolonged hospitalization, respiratory support, and tube feeding. Women who are pregnant or may become pregnant should discuss this with their physician. Some women may experience a recurrence of their depression when they stop their antidepressant. In these circumstances it may be necessary to restart the medication or seek an alternative medication or treatment.

Nursing mothers should not take Cymbalta, because small amounts will pass into breast milk and be ingested by the baby. If stopping the antidepressant is not an alternative, breastfeeding should not be started or should be discontinued.

Possible Drug Interactions

Cymbalta, like many other medications, is metabolized in the liver. The combined use with certain medications may result in adverse drug interactions, because one medication may alter the blood levels of the other. Fortunately, the number of reported drug interactions with Cymbalta are few. The significant drug interactions that have been reported with Cymbalta are summarized in the table below.

Luvox (fluvoxamine)	Luvox, a selective serotonin reuptake inhibitor (SSRI), may inhibit the metabolism of Cymbalta. This may result in significantly elevated levels of Cymbalta, potentially increasing adverse side effects. When a patient's medication is switched to Cymbalta after discontinuation of Luvox, the treatment should begin with a smaller-than-normal dosage of Cymbalta, because significant levels of Luvox may still be present in the body.
Paxil (paroxetine) and Prozac (fluoxetine)	Paxil and Prozac, two SSRIs, are potent inhibitors of the enzyme that metabolizes Cymbalta. This may result in significantly elevated levels of Cymbalta, potentially increasing adverse effects. When a patient's medication is switched to Cymbalta after discontinuation of Paxil or Prozac, treatment should begin with a smaller-than-normal dosage of Cymbalta, because significant levels of the SSRI may still be present in the body.
Tagamet (cimetidine)	Tagamet may inhibit the metabolism of Cymbalta and elevate its levels, potentially increasing adverse side effects.
Cipro (ciprofloxacin)	Cipro and antibiotics in this family may inhibit the metabolism of Cymbalta and elevate its levels, potentially increasing the likelihood of adverse side effects.

Other medications, including herbal supplements (such as St. John's wort), that boost serotonin may result in excessive levels of that neurotransmitter when combined with Cymbalta and produce a toxic syndrome known as **serotonin syndrome.** The early signs of serotonin syndrome are restlessness, confusion, tremors, flushing, and involuntary muscle jerks. If the medications are not stopped, the individual may develop more life-threatening complications resulting in muscle disorders, high fever, respiratory problems, clotting problems, and destruction of red blood cells that may lead to acute renal failure. Patients taking Cymbalta should be alert to the possible signs of serotonin syndrome, which require immediate medical attention and discontinuation of the serotonin-boosting medications.

Antidepressants known as **monoamine oxidase inhibitors** (MAOIs) should not be taken together with Cymbalta, because the combination may potentially produce a toxic reaction that includes elevated temperature, high blood pressure, and extreme excitation and agitation. Patients should consult their physician or pharmacist before taking any new medications, including over-the-counter medications and herbal supplements, with Cymbalta.

Patients taking Cymbalta should avoid alcohol or should consume it in moderation because the combination may worsen depression. Smoking may significantly reduce the serum levels of Cymbalta by as much as one-third. Individuals who smoke while taking Cymbalta may require higher dosages to achieve therapeutic levels.

Overdose

There is limited clinical experience with Cymbalta overdose, and no cases of fatal acute overdose have been reported. In contrast with overdoses involving tricyclic and MAOI antidepressants, overdose with Cymbalta should be much less dangerous, especially when it is taken alone. However, overdoses often involve multiple medications, and the combination of medications may present more serious complications. The combination of central nervous system depressants (e.g., alcohol, narcotics, benzodiazepines) and Cymbalta can be lethal, and death is usually from respiratory depression.

Any suspected overdose should be treated as an emergency. The person should be taken to the emergency room for observation and treatment. The prescription bottle of medication (and any other medication suspected in the overdose) should be brought as well, because the information on the prescription label can be helpful to the treating physician in determining the number of pills ingested.

Special Considerations

Most cases of major depression can be treated successfully, usually with medication, psychotherapy, or both. The combination of psychotherapy and antidepressants is very effective in treating moderate to severe depression. The medications improve mood, sleep, energy, and appetite, while therapy strengthens coping skills, deals with possible underlying issues, and improves thought patterns and behavior. Cymbalta may also be very beneficial for treating anxiety.

In general, antidepressants alone help about 60%–70% of those taking them. Although a few individuals may experience some improvement from antidepressants by the end of the first week, most people do not see significant benefits from their antidepressants until after 3–4 weeks, and it can sometimes take as long as 8 weeks for the medication to produce its full effects. Thus it is critical that patients continue to take their antidepressant long enough for the medication to be beneficial and that patients not get discouraged and stop their medication prematurely if they do not feel better immediately.

In short-term studies, antidepressants were found to increase the risk of suicidal thinking and behavior in children and adolescents with major depression and other psychiatric disorders. The FDA requires the prescriber to warn of this risk in children and adolescents when starting antidepressant therapy. According to the FDA findings, the risk of suicidal thoughts and behaviors associated with antidepressants is age-related. This phenomenon tends to occur in the younger population and is most likely to occur early in the course of treatment. In adults over 24 years of age, there did not appear to be an increased risk of suicidality with antidepressants compared with placebo. In patients over age 65, the findings showed that antidepressants had a "protective effect" against suicidal thoughts and behavior. Other studies have found that when more people in a community are taking antidepressants, the suicide rate is lower.

The risk of suicide is inherent in depression and may persist until the individual responds to treatment. After starting or changing antidepressant therapy, the person, especially a child or adolescent, should be closely observed for worsening signs of depression, and the family or caregiver should communicate any concerns to the physician.

- **Warning:** Always let your physician or a family member know if you have suicidal thoughts. Notify your psychiatrist or your family physician whenever your depressive symptoms worsen or whenever you feel unable to control suicidal urges or thoughts.
- Do not discontinue Cymbalta abruptly. Your dosage should be tapered gradually to prevent discontinuation symptoms.
- If you miss a dose, take it as soon as possible, within 2–3 hours of the scheduled dose. If it is close to the next scheduled dose, skip the missed dose and continue on your regular dosing schedule. Do not take double doses.
- Cymbalta should be swallowed whole and not crushed or chewed, nor should the capsule be opened and sprinkled in food.
- Cymbalta may be taken with or without food.
- Store the medication in its originally labeled, light-resistant container, away from heat and moisture. Heat and moisture may precipitate breakdown of your medication, and the medication may lose its therapeutic effects.
- Keep your medication out of reach of children.

If you have any questions about your medication, consult your physician or pharmacist.

Notes

_____

_____

_____

_____

_____

_____

_____

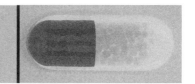

Effexor and Effexor XR
(venlafaxine)

Generic name: Venlafaxine
Available strengths: 25 mg, 37.5 mg, 50 mg, 75 mg,
    100 mg immediate-release tablets; 37.5 mg, 75 mg,
    150 mg controlled-release capsules (Effexor XR)
Available in generic: No
Drug class: Serotonin-norepinephrine reuptake
    inhibitor antidepressant

General Information

Effexor (venlafaxine) is unlike the selective serotonin reuptake inhibitors (SSRI) antidepressants such as Prozac (fluoxetine), which are relatively serotonin-specific in action. Effexor has a dual mechanism of action. Presumably, it works by altering the neurotransmission of both **serotonin** and **norepinephrine,** two important neurotransmitters in the brain.

During neurotransmission, *neurotransmitters* are released by one neuron into the space between that neuron and the next neuron. The neurotransmitters come into contact with specific sites on the surface membrane of neurons called *receptors.* From there, the chemical signal is transformed into an electrical impulse that travels down the neuron, causing further release of neurotransmitters. This process of neurotransmission is repeated along a chain of neurons. During neurotransmission, after neurotransmitters are released and the chemical signal is transferred to neurons, the neurotransmitters are recaptured back into brain cells by a process known as *reuptake.* By blocking the neurotransmitters from going back into the neurons from where they were released, the antidepressant can amplify the effects of the neurotransmitter.

Effexor exerts its antidepressant effect principally by blocking the reuptake of serotonin and norepinephrine. This action is similar to that of the SSRIs, but notably different in that Effexor also inhibits the reuptake of norepinephrine. Through reuptake inhibition, Effexor boosts serotonin and norepinephrine neurotransmission. For this reason, Effexor is called a *serotonin-norepinephrine reuptake inhibitor* (SNRI). Depression and other mental disorders may be caused by abnormally low levels (or abnormal neurotransmission) of serotonin, norepinephrine, or both. This abnormality may in turn produce changes in affected areas of the brain, resulting in psychiatric symptoms such as depression or anxiety. When neurotransmission is improved by the antidepressant, the affected areas of the brain are restored to normal functioning, reducing the symptoms of the illness.

The U.S. Food and Drug Administration (FDA) approved Effexor and Effexor XR for treatment of depression, but only Effexor XR for treatment of generalized anxiety disorder, social phobia, and panic disorder. The use of a medication for its approved indications is called its *labeled use*. In clinical practice, however, physicians often prescribe medications for *unlabeled* ("off-label") uses when published clinical studies, case reports, or their own clinical experiences support the efficacy and safety of those treatments. Physicians may also prescribe Effexor and Effexor XR to treat posttraumatic stress disorder, premenstrual syndrome, and attention-deficit/hyperactivity disorder. Effexor has also proved useful in treating more seriously depressed patients with melancholic depression, which may not respond as well to other antidepressants.

Dosing Information

Effexor comes in two formulations: immediate-release tablets (Effexor) and extended-release capsules (Effexor XR). In general, physicians prefer to prescribe Effexor in the extended-release form because it offers the convenience of once-daily dosing and because the slow-release form may be better tolerated over the immediate-release tablet.

The recommended starting dosage is 75 mg/day, taken in two or three divided doses in the immediate-release tablets or once a day in the extended-release capsule. For some patients, especially for seniors and those with chronic medical problems, a starting dosage of 37.5 mg/day of Effexor XR may be better tolerated, with subsequent increases in dosage to 75 mg/day. The dosage then may be increased after another week or two, depending on tolerability and clinical response, to 150 mg/day. If needed, further dosage increases are made gradually. For outpatient treatment of moderate depression, the dosage range for Effexor XR is usually between 75 mg/day and 225 mg/day. For more severe depression and depression refractory to other treatments, higher dosages may be needed. The usual maximum dosage for Effexor is 375 mg/day and for Effexor XR is 225 mg/day.

Common Side Effects

The most common side effects from taking Effexor are nausea, vomiting, dry mouth, nervousness, anxiety, dizziness, headaches, and insomnia. Side effects generally occur after starting the medication or when increasing the dosage. If side effects become intolerable, the physician may decrease the dosage to allow the individual to adjust to the medication before increasing it again slowly.

Sexual side effects, including delayed orgasm in women and retarded ejaculation in men, occur with Effexor at about the same rate as with the SNRI antidepressant Cymbalta (duloxetine), but at a rate lower than the 50%–60% rate reported with the SSRIs.

Adverse Reactions and Precautions

In about 5% of patients taking normal dosages of Effexor, mild elevation of blood pressure (hypertension) may occur. At higher dosages, the incidence of Effexor-induced hypertension may be higher. The increase in blood pressure is usually modest, and very few patients have to discontinue Effexor because of hypertension. Generally, lowering the dosage will normalize blood pressure. For this reason, patients' blood pressure should be checked before starting Effexor and routinely during therapy as a precautionary measure, especially for individuals with preexisting hypertension or those with a history of heart disease.

Effexor may cause drowsiness in some people. Patients should not drive or operate machinery until they are certain that their alertness or coordination is not affected by the medication. Patients with a known allergy to Effexor or who have experienced a severe reaction after taking it should not take Effexor.

Use in Pregnancy and Breastfeeding: Pregnancy Category C

Effexor has not been tested in women to determine its safety in pregnancy. The effects of the medication on the developing fetus are unknown. Women who are pregnant or may become pregnant should discuss this with their physician. Some women may experience a recurrence of their depression when they stop their antidepressant. In these circumstances it may be necessary to restart the medication or seek an alternative medication or treatment.

Nursing mothers should not take Effexor, because small amounts will pass into breast milk and be ingested by the baby. If stopping the antidepressant is not an alternative, breastfeeding should not be started or should be discontinued.

Possible Drug Interactions

Effexor, like many other medications, is metabolized in the liver. The combined use with certain medications may result in adverse drug interactions because one medication may alter the blood levels of the other. Fortunately, the number of reported drug interactions with Effexor is few. The significant drug interactions that have been reported with Effexor are summarized in the table below.

Tagamet (cimetidine)	Tagamet may inhibit the metabolism of Effexor. This may result in elevated levels of Effexor, potentially increasing adverse side effects. Blood pressure should be monitored closely with this combination.
Selective serotonin reuptake inhibitors (SSRIs)	SSRIs, particularly Paxil, may inhibit the metabolism of Effexor and elevate blood levels. When this combination is used for treatment of refractory depression, blood pressure should be monitored closely. Patients should also be monitored for signs of serotonin syndrome.
Tricyclic antidepressants (TCAs)	Effexor may increase levels of TCAs when this combination is used, potentially increasing adverse side effects from the TCA. Patients should also be monitored for signs and symptoms of serotonin syndrome.
Haldol (haloperidol)	Effexor may decrease the clearance of Haldol and increase its blood levels, potentially increasing adverse side effects of the antipsychotic medication.

Other medications, including herbal supplements (such as St. John's wort), that boost serotonin may result in excessive levels of that neurotransmitter when combined with Effexor and produce a toxic syndrome known as **serotonin syndrome.** The early signs of serotonin syndrome are restlessness, confusion, tremors, flushing, and involuntary muscle jerks. If the medications are not stopped, the individual may develop more life-threatening complications resulting in muscle disorders, high fever, respiratory problems, clotting problems, and destruction of red blood cells that may lead to acute renal failure. Patients taking Effexor should be alert to the possible signs of serotonin syndrome, which require immediate medical attention and discontinuation of the serotonin-boosting medications.

Antidepressants known as **monoamine oxidase inhibitors** (MAOIs) should not be taken together with Effexor, because the combination may potentially produce a toxic reaction that includes elevated temperature, high blood pressure, and extreme excitation and agitation. Patients should consult their physician or pharmacist before taking any new medications, including over-the-counter medications and herbal supplements, with Effexor.

Patients taking Effexor should avoid alcohol or should consume it in moderation because the combination may worsen depression.

Overdose

In contrast to tricyclic and MAOI antidepressants, overdose with Effexor is generally much less dangerous, especially when taken alone. Patients more often overdose with multiple medications, and other medications may increase the risk of more serious complications. The combination of central nervous system depressants (e.g., alcohol, narcotics, benzodiazepines) and Effexor can be lethal, and death is usually from respiratory depression.

Depending on the amount ingested and whether the medication was combined with alcohol or other drugs, reported reactions with Effexor overdose include changes in consciousness (from somnolence to coma), rapid heart rate, seizures, vomiting, arrhythmia, low blood pressure, liver damage, serotonin syndrome, and death.

Any suspected overdose should be treated as an emergency. The person should be taken to the emergency room for observation and treatment. The prescription bottle of medication (and any other medication suspected in the overdose) should be brought as well, because the information on the prescription label can be helpful to the treating physician in determining the number of pills ingested.

Special Considerations

Most cases of major depression can be treated successfully, usually with medication, psychotherapy, or both. The combination of psychotherapy and antidepressants is very effective in treating moderate to severe depression. The medications improve mood, sleep, energy, and appetite, while therapy strengthens coping skills, deals with possible underlying issues, and improves thought patterns and behavior. Effexor may also be very beneficial for treating anxiety.

In general, antidepressants alone help about 60%–70% of those taking them. Although a few individuals may experience some improvement from antidepressants by the end of the first week, most people do not see significant benefits from their antidepressants until after 3–4 weeks, and it can sometimes take as long as 8 weeks for the medication to produce its full effects. Thus it is critical that patients continue to take their antidepressant long enough for the medication to be beneficial and that patients not get discouraged and stop their medication prematurely if they do not feel better immediately.

In short-term studies, antidepressants were found to increase the risk of suicidal thinking and behavior in children and adolescents with major depression and other psychiatric disorders. The FDA requires the prescriber to warn of this risk in children and adolescents when starting antidepressant therapy. According to the FDA findings, the risk of suicidal thoughts and behaviors associated with antidepressants is age-related. This phenomenon tends to occur in the younger population and is most likely to occur early in the course of treatment. In adults over 24 years of age, there did not appear to be an increased risk of suicidality with antidepressants compared with placebo. In patients over age 65, the findings showed that antidepressants had a "protective effect" against suicidal thoughts and behavior. Other studies have found that when more people in a community are taking antidepressants, the suicide rate is lower. The risk of suicide is inherent in depression and may persist until the individual responds to treatment. After starting or changing antidepressant therapy, the person, especially a child or adolescent, should be closely observed for worsening signs of depression, and the family or caregiver should communicate any concerns to the physician.

- **Warning:** Always let your physician or a family member know if you have suicidal thoughts. Notify your psychiatrist or your family physicians whenever your depressive symptoms worsen or whenever you feel unable to control suicidal urges or thoughts.
- Do not discontinue Effexor abruptly. Your dosage should be tapered gradually to prevent discontinuation symptoms.
- If you miss a dose, take it as soon as possible, within 2–3 hours of the scheduled dose. If it is close to the next scheduled dose, skip the missed dose and continue on your regular dosing schedule. Do not take double doses.
- Effexor should be taken with food to decrease gastrointestinal side effects.
- Store the medication in its originally labeled, light-resistant container, away from heat and moisture. Heat and moisture may precipitate breakdown of your medication, and the medication may lose its therapeutic effects.
- Keep your medication out of reach of children.

If you have any questions about your medication, consult your physician or pharmacist.

Notes

From Chew RH, Hales RE, Yudofsky SC: *What Your Patients Need to Know About Psychiatric Medications,* Second Edition. Washington, DC, American Psychiatric Publishing, 2009

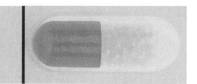

Pristiq (desvenlafaxine)

Generic name: desvenlafaxine
Available strengths: 50 mg, 100 mg extended-release capsules
Available in generic: No
Drug class: Serotonin-norepinephrine reuptake inhibitor
antidepressant

General Information

Introduced in February 2008, Pristiq (desvenlafaxine) is the latest addition to the family of antidepressants. Currently, it has only received U.S. Food and Drug Administration (FDA) approval for the treatment of major depressive disorder in adults, but use for other disorders, such as anxiety disorders, may be granted by the FDA in the future. Pristiq comes in 50 mg and 100 mg extended-release capsules and can be dosed once a day. Desvenlafaxine is the major metabolite of Effexor (venlafaxine) and is very similar to the parent compound. In the liver, venlafaxine is converted to desvenlafaxine by an enzyme that removes a component (a methyl group) from venlafaxine's structure. Both venlafaxine and desvenlafaxine are effective antidepressants.

What are the advantages of Pristiq over Effexor? According to the manufacturer, Pristiq may be started at the therapeutic dose of 50 mg (once a day), without having to be started at lower doses and increased slowly to reach therapeutic doses, as with Effexor. Another advantage, according to the manufacturer, is that Pristiq bypasses a metabolic step and therefore may have fewer drug interactions with other medications than does Effexor.

Like Effexor, Pristiq achieves its principal antidepressant action by blocking reuptake of the neurotransmitters **serotonin** and **norepinephrine** and thereby preventing the breakdown of these neurotransmitters within neurons. Hence, Pristiq is a *serotonin-norepinephrine reuptake inhibitor* (SNRI), whose actions are similar to those of Effexor and Cymbalta (duloxetine) in this group of antidepressants. Through reuptake inhibition, Pristiq augments serotonin and norepinephrine neurotransmission. Depression and other mental disorders may be caused by abnormally low levels (or abnormal neurotransmission) of serotonin, norepinephrine, or both. This abnormality may in turn produce changes in affected areas of the brain, resulting in psychiatric symptoms such as depression or anxiety. When neurotransmission is improved by the antidepressant, the affected areas of the brain are restored to normal functioning, reducing the symptoms of the illness.

Dosing Information

The starting dose for Pristiq is usually 50 mg once daily, preferably taken in the morning with or without food, but at higher dosages the medication may be given in divided doses (twice daily). If the patient has taken the medication at the initial dose for an adequate time and an optimal effect has not been achieved, the dose may be increased. Across the treatment spectrum, doses of 50–400 mg were shown to be effective, but more side effects occur with higher doses. Until more experience is gained with Pristiq, clinicians will generally start with lower doses and increase the dose slowly as needed.

Common Side Effects

Frequent complaints after starting Pristiq include nausea, constipation, sweating, fatigue, dizziness, and headaches. Patients may also experience jitteriness, decreased appetite, insomnia, and sleepiness during the day. Men may experience sexual dysfunction when taking Pristiq. When Pristiq is taken at higher doses, these side effects are more frequent. If the side effect can be tolerated, the medication is often continued and the bothersome side effect typically subsides. When the side effect is intolerable, the patient should consult his or her physician but should not stop taking the antidepressant abruptly.

Adverse Reactions and Precautions

As with Effexor, mild elevation of blood pressure has been reported with Pristiq. Typically, blood pressure normalizes when the patient becomes adjusted to the new medication. Those with preexisting high blood pressure or some other underlying medical condition should check their blood pressure regularly while taking Pristiq. Patients should consult their physician if they experience sustained elevation of blood pressure and should seek immediate medical attention if their blood pressure is abnormally high.

Combining Pristiq with other medications that boost serotonin may precipitate a potentially hazardous condition called the **serotonin syndrome,** a reaction due to excessive serotonin stimulation in the brain. Serotonergic medications include tricyclic antidepressants (TCAs), selective serotonin reuptake inhibitor (SSRI) antidepressants, and triptan anti-migraine agents, such as Imitrex (sumatriptan). The early signs of serotonin syndrome are restlessness, confusion, tremors, flushing, excessive sweating, and involuntary muscle jerks. If the medications are not stopped, the individual may develop more life-threatening complications resulting in severe muscle contractions, high fever, respiratory problems, clotting problems, destruction of red blood cells (that may lead to acute renal failure), coma, and death.

Pristiq should *not* be combined with **monoamine oxidase inhibitors** (MAOIs), such as Nardil (phenelzine), Parnate (tranylcypromine), and Emsam (selegiline). When a switch between treatments is being made, at least 14 days must elapse after discontinuation of the MAOI before Pristiq is started, and 7 days after discontinuation of Pristiq before an MAOI is started. The drug interaction may precipitate symptoms that include abnormal elevation of blood pressure, sweating, rapid heartbeat, elevated body temperature, flushing, nausea, vomiting, and tremors, which may lead to seizures, coma, and death if medical intervention is not immediate.

Pristiq should not be abruptly discontinued without consulting a physician. To avoid unpleasant symptoms associated with abrupt discontinuation, the dose should be tapered slowly before the medication is stopped. Withdrawal symptoms may include irritability, anxiety, insomnia, headaches, and nausea.

Use in Pregnancy and Breastfeeding: Pregnancy Category C

The safety of taking Pristiq during pregnancy has not been established. The risk to the mother or fetus cannot be ruled out, because there are no adequate studies of or information on women taking Pristiq during pregnancy. Women who are pregnant or may become pregnant should discuss this with their physician.

Nursing mothers should not take Pristiq, because small amounts will pass into breast milk and be ingested by the baby. If stopping the antidepressant is not an alternative, breastfeeding should not be started or should be discontinued.

Possible Drug Interactions

Nizoral (ketoconazole)	Ketoconazole, an antifungal agent, may inhibit the metabolism of Pristiq and increase the blood levels of the antidepressant, which can lead to higher incidence of side effects.
Selective serotonin reuptake inhibitors (SSRIs), serotonin-norepinephrine reuptake inhibitors (SNRIs), other antidepressants, triptans (e.g., Imitrex)	Combining Pristiq with other serotonin-enhancing agents, including anti-migraine medications such as Imitrex, or other serotonergic antidepressants may trigger life-threatening symptoms associated with serotonin syndrome.
Monoamine oxidase inhibitors (MAOIs) (e.g., Nardil, Parnate, Emsam)	Concomitant use of Pristiq with an MAOI is contraindicated.
Coumadin (warfarin)	Pristiq may alter the anticoagulant effect of warfarin and lead to an increased risk of bleeding. Monitor anticoagulation when starting, changing the dose of, or discontinuing Pristiq.
Aspirin and NSAIDs (nonsteroidal anti-inflammatory drugs) such as Motrin and Naprosyn	Pristiq and other SNRIs may increase the risk of gastrointestinal bleeding when combined with aspirin or NSAIDs.

Overdose

There is limited information on overdose of Pristiq, since it is a rather new medication. However, the knowledge of overdose with Pristiq can be gleaned from overdoses with Effexor, because Pristiq is the major active metabolite of Effexor.

Depending on the amount ingested and whether the medication was combined with alcohol or other drugs, reported reactions with Effexor overdose (these reactions would also be expected with Pristiq) include changes in consciousness (from somnolence to coma), rapid heart rate, seizures, vomiting, arrhythmia, low blood pressure, liver damage, serotonin syndrome, and death.

Any suspected overdose should be treated as an emergency. The person should be taken to the emergency room for observation and treatment. The prescription bottle of medication (and any other medication suspected in the overdose) should be brought as well, because the information on the prescription label can be helpful to the treating physician in determining the number of pills ingested.

Special Considerations

In short-term studies, antidepressants were found to increase the risk of suicidal thinking and behavior in children and adolescents with major depression and other psychiatric disorders. The FDA requires the prescriber to warn of this risk in children and adolescents when starting or changing antidepressant therapy. According to the FDA findings, the risk of suicidal thoughts and behaviors associated with antidepressants is age-related. This phenomenon tends to occur in the younger population and is most likely to occur early in the course of treatment. In adults over 24 years of age, there did not appear to be an increased risk of suicidality with antidepressants compared with placebo. In patients over age 65, the findings showed that antidepressants had a "protective effect" against suicidal thoughts and behavior. Other studies have found that when more people in a community are taking antidepressants, the suicide rate is lower. The risk of suicide is inherent in depression and may persist until the individual responds to treatment.

The risk of suicide is inherent in depression and may persist until the individual responds to treatment. After starting or changing antidepressant therapy, the person, especially a child or adolescent, should be closely observed for worsening signs of depression, and the family or caregiver should communicate any concerns to the physician.

- **Warning:** Always let your physician or a family member know if you have suicidal thoughts. Notify your psychiatrist or your family physicians whenever your depressive symptoms worsen or whenever you feel unable to control suicidal urges or thoughts.
- Pristiq can be taken with or without food, but if it causes nausea or upsets your stomach, take it with food.
- Do not discontinue Pristiq abruptly. Your dosage should be tapered gradually to prevent discontinuation symptoms.
- Pristiq may induce drowsiness. Know how it affects you before operating a motor vehicle or hazardous machinery. Avoid alcohol while taking Pristiq.
- Have your blood pressure checked on a routine basis when taking Pristiq.
- Store the medication in its originally labeled, light-resistant container, away from heat and moisture. Heat or moisture may precipitate breakdown of your medication, and the medication may lose its therapeutic effects.
- Keep your medication out of reach of children.

If you have any questions about your medication, consult your physician or pharmacist.

Notes

_____

_____

_____

_____

_____

_____

_____

From Chew RH, Hales RE, Yudofsky SC: *What Your Patients Need to Know About Psychiatric Medications*, Second Edition. Washington, DC, American Psychiatric Publishing, 2009

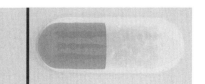

Remeron (mirtazapine)

Generic name: Mirtazapine
Available strengths: 7.5 mg, 15 mg, 30 mg, 45 mg tablets;
   15 mg, 30 mg, 45 mg quick-dissolving tablets
   (Remeron SolTab)
Available in generic: Yes
Drug class: Norepinephrine-serotonin modulator
   antidepressant

General Information

Remeron (mirtazapine) exerts its antidepressant action principally through antagonism of certain types of receptors, thereby altering neurotransmission of **serotonin** and **norepinephrine** in the brain. *Neurotransmitters*, such as serotonin and norepinephrine, are chemicals produced by brain cells called neurons that enable them to communicate with each other. The neurotransmitters are released by one neuron into the space between that neuron and the next neuron. The neurotransmitters come into contact with specific sites on the surface membrane of neurons called *receptors*. From there, the chemical signal is transformed into an electrical impulse that travels down the neuron, causing further release of neurotransmitters. This process of neurotransmission is repeated along a chain of neurons.

Depression and other mental disorders may be caused by abnormally low levels (or abnormal transmission) of serotonin, norepinephrine, or both. This abnormality may in turn produce changes in affected areas of the brain, resulting in psychiatric symptoms such as depression or anxiety. When neurotransmission is improved by the antidepressant, the affected areas of the brain are restored to normal functioning, reducing the symptoms of the illness. There is usually a time lag of 3–4 weeks for antidepressants to achieve their optimal effect, which may be the time needed for the brain to make the changes to restore previously affected areas to normal functioning, hence reducing or eliminating the symptoms of the illness.

Remeron was approved by the U.S. Food and Drug Administration (FDA) for the treatment of major depressive disorder. The use of a medication for its approved indications is called its *labeled use*. In clinical practice, however, physicians often prescribe medications for *unlabeled* ("off-label") uses when published clinical studies, case reports, or their own clinical experiences support the efficacy and safety of those treatments. Unlabeled uses of Remeron include treatment of anxiety disorders with or without depression, posttraumatic stress disorder, and insomnia.

Physicians may use Remeron in combination with a selective serotonin reuptake inhibitor (SSRI) such as Zoloft (sertraline) or Lexapro (escitalopram) to augment the antidepressant effect. This augmentation strategy may be successful in treating refractory depression for which the response to a single antidepressant was inadequate.

Dosing Information

The recommended starting dose is 15 mg, taken once a day, preferably in the evening prior to bedtime. After 1–2 weeks, the dosage may be increased in increments of 15 mg/day at intervals of 1–2 weeks up to a maximum of 45 mg/day. Remeron also comes in quick-dissolving tablets (Remeron SolTab) for ease of swallowing.

Common Side Effects

Remeron is usually well tolerated, and only infrequently is the medication stopped because of intolerable side effects. The most common side effects are dry mouth, drowsiness, sedation, and weight gain. Daytime sleepiness may be managed by taking a single dose close to bedtime.

For some patients taking Remeron, increased appetite and weight gain may be problematic. About 20% of patients taking Remeron gain weight with long-term use. In addition, Remeron may have effects on cholesterol and triglycerides. Cholesterol may significantly increase in about 15%, and triglycerides in about 6%, of the patients taking Remeron. Management of weight gain is usually accomplished by controlling appetite and diet and through exercise. Cholesterol and triglyceride levels should be checked before and periodically (at least annually) during treatment with Remeron. Any patient with Remeron-induced weight gain should be monitored closely, especially if at risk for diabetes and heart disease.

Unlike SSRIs, Remeron rarely induces sexual dysfunction. It is a useful alternative to other antidepressants that produce sexual dysfunction.

Adverse Reactions and Precautions

Remeron may cause drowsiness in some people. Patients should not drive or operate machinery until they are certain that their alertness or coordination is not affected by the medication. Patients with a known allergy to Remeron or who have experienced a severe reaction after taking it should not take Remeron.

Use in Pregnancy and Breastfeeding: Pregnancy Category C

Remeron has not been tested in women to determine its safety in pregnancy. The effects of the medication on the developing fetus in pregnant women are unknown. Women who are pregnant or may become pregnant should discuss this with their physician. Some women may experience a recurrence of their depression when they stop their antidepressant. In these circumstances it may be necessary to restart the medication or seek an alternative medication or treatment.

Nursing mothers should not take Remeron, because small amounts will pass into breast milk and be ingested by the baby. If stopping the drug is not an alternative, breastfeeding should not be started or should be discontinued.

Possible Drug Interactions

Remeron, like many other medications, is metabolized in the liver. The combined use with certain medications may result in adverse drug interactions because one medication may alter the blood levels of the other.

Fortunately, the number of reported drug interactions with Remeron is few. The significant drug interactions that have been reported with Remeron are summarized in the table below.

Tagamet (cimetidine)	Tagamet may increase the blood levels of Remeron, potentially causing side effects.
Tegretol (carbamazepine)	Tegretol reduces the blood levels of Remeron, possibly decreasing its antidepressant effects.
Luvox (fluvoxamine)	Luvox may significantly increase the blood levels of Remeron to toxic levels.

Other medications, including herbal supplements (such as St. John's wort), that boost serotonin may result in excessive levels of that neurotransmitter when combined with Remeron and produce a toxic syndrome known as **serotonin syndrome.** The early signs of serotonin syndrome are restlessness, confusion, tremors, flushing, and involuntary muscle jerks. If the medications are not stopped, the individual may develop more life-threatening complications resulting in muscle disorders, high fever, respiratory problems, clotting problems, and destruction of red blood cells that may lead to acute renal failure. Patients taking Remeron should be alert to the possible signs of serotonin syndrome, which require immediate medical attention and discontinuation of the serotonin-boosting medications.

Antidepressants known as **monoamine oxidase inhibitors** (MAOIs) should not be taken together with Remeron, because the combination may potentially produce a toxic reaction that includes elevated temperature, high blood pressure, and extreme excitation and agitation. Patients should consult their physician or pharmacist before taking any new medications, including over-the-counter medications and herbal supplements, with Remeron.

Patients taking Remeron should avoid alcohol or should consume it in moderation because the combination may worsen depression.

Overdose

Compared with some other antidepressants, such as tricyclic antidepressants, Remeron is relatively safe in overdose. However, when multiple medications are involved in overdose, the other medications may increase the risk of more serious complications.

Any suspected overdose should be treated as an emergency. The person should be taken to the emergency room for observation and treatment. The prescription bottle of medication (and any other medication suspected in the overdose) should be brought as well, because the information on the prescription label can be helpful to the treating physician in determining the number of pills ingested.

Special Considerations

Most cases of major depression can be treated successfully, usually with medication, psychotherapy, or both. The combination of psychotherapy and antidepressants is very effective in treating moderate to severe depression. The medications improve mood, sleep, energy, and appetite, while therapy strengthens coping skills, deals with possible underlying issues, and improves thought patterns and behavior.

In general, antidepressants alone help about 60%–70% of those taking them. Although a few individuals may experience some improvement from antidepressants by the end of the first week, most people do not see significant benefits from their antidepressants until after 3–4 weeks, and it can sometimes take as long as

8 weeks for the medication to produce its full effects. Thus it is critical that patients continue to take their antidepressant long enough for the medication to be beneficial and that patients not get discouraged and stop their medication prematurely if they do not feel better immediately.

In short-term studies, antidepressants were found to increase the risk of suicidal thinking and behavior in children and adolescents with major depression and other psychiatric disorders. The FDA requires the prescriber to warn of this risk in children and adolescents when starting antidepressant therapy. According to the FDA findings, the risk of suicidal thoughts and behaviors associated with antidepressants is age-related. This phenomenon tends to occur in the younger population and is most likely to occur early in the course of treatment. In adults over 24 years of age, there did not appear to be an increased risk of suicidality with antidepressants compared with placebo. In patients over age 65, the findings showed that antidepressants had a "protective effect" against suicidal thoughts and behavior. Other studies have found that when more people in a community are taking antidepressants, the suicide rate is lower.

The risk of suicide is inherent in depression and may persist until the individual responds to treatment. After starting or changing antidepressant therapy, the person, especially a child or adolescent, should be closely observed for worsening signs of depression, and the family or caregiver should communicate any concerns to the physician.

- **Warning:** Always let your physician or a family member know if you have suicidal thoughts. Notify your psychiatrist or your family physician whenever your depressive symptoms worsen or whenever you feel unable to control suicidal urges or thoughts.
- Do not discontinue Remeron without consulting your physician.
- If you miss a dose, take it as soon as possible. If it is close to the next scheduled dose, skip the missed dose and continue on your regular dosing schedule. Do not take double doses.
- Remeron may be taken with or without food.
- Store the medication in its originally labeled, light-resistant container, away from heat and moisture. Heat and moisture may precipitate breakdown of your medication, and the medication may lose its therapeutic effects.
- Keep your medication out of reach of children.

If you have any questions about your medication, consult your physician or pharmacist.

Notes

_____

_____

_____

_____

From Chew RH, Hales RE, Yudofsky SC: *What Your Patients Need to Know About Psychiatric Medications*, Second Edition. Washington, DC, American Psychiatric Publishing, 2009

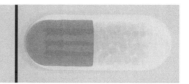

Wellbutrin, Wellbutrin SR, and Wellbutrin XL (bupropion)

Generic name: Bupropion

Available strengths: 75 mg, 100 mg immediate-release tablets;
100 mg, 150 mg, 200 mg sustained-release tablets
(Wellbutrin SR); 150 mg, 300 mg extended-release tablets
(Wellbutrin XL)

Available in generic: Yes

Drug class: Dopamine-norepinephrine reuptake inhibitor
antidepressant

General Information

Unlike the **selective serotonin reuptake inhibitors** (SSRIs) such as Prozac (fluoxetine), **Wellbutrin (bupropion)** has more than one mechanism of action. Presumably, it works primarily by altering the neurotransmission of **dopamine** and **norepinephrine** in the brain. *Neurotransmitters*, such as dopamine and norepinephrine, are chemicals produced by brain cells called neurons that enable them to communicate with each other. The neurotransmitters are released by one neuron into the space between that neuron and the next neuron. The neurotransmitters come into contact on specific sites on the surface membrane of the neuron called receptors. From there, the chemical signal is transformed into an electrical impulse that travels down the neuron, causing further release of neurotransmitters. This process of neurotransmission is repeated along a chain of neurons. Wellbutrin works in the brain by inhibiting dopamine and norepinephrine from going back into the neurons where they were originally produced; therefore the antidepressant increases levels of the neurotransmitters. Consequently, Wellbutrin is classified as a *dopamine-norepinephrine reuptake inhibitor* (DNRI).

Depression and other mental disorders may be caused by abnormally low levels of certain neurotransmitters in the brain. This abnormality may in turn produce changes in affected areas of the brain, resulting in psychiatric symptoms such as depression or anxiety. When levels of the neurotransmitter are elevated by the antidepressant, the affected areas of the brain that were previously altered by the low neurotransmitter levels are restored to normal functioning. There is usually a time lag of 3–4 weeks for antidepressants to achieve their optimal effect, which may be the time needed for the brain to make the changes to restore previously affected areas to normal functioning, hence reducing or eliminating the symptoms of the illness.

Wellbutrin was approved by the U.S. Food and Drug Administration (FDA) for the treatment of major depressive disorder and smoking cessation (with the sustained-release tablet, which is marketed under the brand **Zyban**). The use of a medication for its approved indications is called its *labeled use*. In clinical practice, however, physicians often prescribe medications for *unlabeled* ("off-label") uses when published clinical studies, case reports, or their own clinical experiences support the efficacy and safety of those treatments. A common unlabeled use of Wellbutrin is for the treatment of attention-deficit/hyperactivity disorder in both children and adults. It is a safe alternative to stimulants such as Ritalin (methylphenidate) or Dexedrine (dextroamphetamine).

Physicians may use Wellbutrin in combination with another antidepressant, such as an SSRI (e.g., Zoloft, Lexapro, Paxil) to augment the antidepressant effect. This augmentation strategy may be successful in treating refractory depression for which response to a single antidepressant was inadequate. Because Wellbutrin is associated with few or no sexual side effects, it is a good alternative for individuals who have had sexual dysfunction from other antidepressants such as SSRIs or Effexor. Wellbutrin generally has not been effective in the treatment of anxiety disorders, such as panic disorder, in part because Wellbutrin is activating and anxious patients prefer other agents, such as an SSRI, over Wellbutrin.

Dosing Information

Wellbutrin is available in three formulations: immediate-release (Wellbutrin), sustained-release (Wellbutrin SR), and extended-release (Wellbutrin XL) tablets. All three contain the same active ingredient, but the rate in which they are absorbed from the stomach and intestines into the bloodstream varies. Immediate-release Wellbutrin is more quickly absorbed and eliminated and usually needs to be taken three times a day. Wellbutrin SR tablets have a slower release and can be taken twice daily. Wellbutrin XL requires only once-daily dosing. Because of the convenience of the sustained- and extended-release tablets, they have largely replaced the earlier immediate-release formulation; they also are associated with fewer side effects.

The usual starting dose of Wellbutrin SR or Wellbutrin XL is 150 mg, taken once a day, for 1 week. Generally, the target dosage for treatment of depression is 300 mg/day. The dosage may be increased after 1 week, to 150 mg twice a day with Wellbutrin SR or 300 mg once a day with Wellbutrin XL. The maximum recommended dosage is 400 mg/day for the sustained-release (in divided doses) and 450 mg/day (in a single dose) for the extended-release formulation.

Common Side Effects

Wellbutrin SR and Wellbutrin XL are usually well tolerated, and only infrequently is the medication stopped because of intolerable side effects. The most common side effects of Wellbutrin SR and Wellbutrin XL are dry mouth, nervousness, tremors, and insomnia. Insomnia may be managed by taking the daily dose of Wellbutrin XL early in the morning or by taking the second dose of Wellbutrin SR early in the evening, with a separation of 6–8 hours between the morning and evening doses.

Other antidepressants, such as **monoamine oxidase inhibitors** (MAOIs), **tricyclic antidepressants** (TCAs), and SSRIs frequently induce sexual dysfunction. In contrast, patients taking Wellbutrin generally do not encounter this problem. Moreover, Wellbutrin does not induce weight gain and is a useful alternative for patients who experience excessive weight gain from other antidepressants.

Adverse Reactions and Precautions

A concern with Wellbutrin is the potential for developing seizures at higher dosages. Seizures occurred mainly with the immediate-release form of Wellbutrin, and the risk of seizures has significantly decreased with the introduction of the sustained-release and extended-release formulations. To reduce the risk of seizures, the manufacturer recommends limiting a single dose to a maximum of 200 mg for Wellbutrin SR and 150 mg for Wellbutrin; the maximum total daily dosage of either formulation should not exceed 400 mg/day. With the recent advance formulation of Wellbutrin XL, a single daily dose is safe up to 300 mg, but the maximum total dosage should not exceed 450 mg/day. The concurrent use of stimulants, alcohol, and cocaine with Wellbutrin may increase the risk of seizures. In patients with head injury or an eating disorder such as bulimia nervosa and anorexia nervosa, the risk of seizures is apparently increased when taking Wellbutrin. In patients with a seizure disorder, Wellbutrin should be avoided.

Wellbutrin must be used with caution in patients with liver impairment, and the dosage may need to be reduced.

Use in Pregnancy and Breastfeeding: Pregnancy Category B

Wellbutrin has not been tested in women to determine its safety in pregnancy. The effects of the medication on the developing fetus in pregnant women are unknown. In animal studies, there was no evidence of harm to the fetus when exposed to Wellbutrin. Animal studies, however, are not always predictive of effects in humans. Women who are pregnant or may become pregnant should discuss this with their physician. Some women may experience a recurrence of their depression when they stop their antidepressant. In these circumstances it may be necessary to restart the medication or seek an alternative medication or treatment.

Nursing mothers should not take Wellbutrin, because small amounts will pass into breast milk and be ingested by the baby. If stopping the antidepressant is not an alternative, breastfeeding should not be started or should be discontinued.

Possible Drug Interactions

Wellbutrin, like many other medications, is metabolized in the liver. The combined use with certain medications may result in adverse drug interactions because one medication may alter the blood levels of the other. Fortunately, the number of reported drug interactions with Wellbutrin is few. The significant drug interactions that have been reported with Wellbutrin are summarized in the table below.

Tegretol (carbamazepine)	Tegretol reduces the blood levels of Wellbutrin, possibly decreasing its antidepressant effects.
Antiparkinsonian agents (e.g., levodopa, Sinemet)	If Wellbutrin is combined with antiparkinsonian medications to treat Parkinson's disease, dopamine levels in the brain may be elevated, increasing the probability of side effects such as hallucinations.
Norvir (ritonavir)	The AIDS medication Norvir may increase blood levels of Wellbutrin, increasing the risk of Wellbutrin toxicity and adverse effects, especially seizures in high-risk individuals.
Antiarrhythmic medications Rythmol (propafenone) and Tambocor (flecainide)	These medications are used to regulate heart rhythm and prevent arrhythmias (antiarrhythmic). The metabolism of these drugs may be inhibited by Wellbutrin, which may hazardously affect their therapeutic action and toxicity.

Antidepressants known as monoamine oxidase inhibitors, or MAOIs, should not be taken together with Wellbutrin, because the combination may potentially produce a toxic reaction that includes elevated temperature, high blood pressure, and extreme excitation and agitation. Patients should consult their physician or pharmacist before taking any new medications, including over-the-counter medications and herbal supplements, with Wellbutrin.

Patients taking Wellbutrin should avoid alcohol or should consume it in moderation because the combination may worsen depression.

Overdose

Compared with some other antidepressants, such as TCAs, Wellbutrin is safe in overdose. In most cases of Wellbutrin overdose, the most serious reaction was seizures, but patients generally recovered without significant aftereffects. However, when multiple medications are involved in overdose, the other medications may increase the risk of more serious complications.

Any suspected overdose should be treated as an emergency. The person should be taken to the emergency room for observation and treatment. The prescription bottle of medication (and any other medication suspected in the overdose) should be brought as well, because the information on the prescription label can be helpful to the treating physician in determining the number of pills ingested.

Special Considerations

Most cases of major depression can be treated successfully, usually with medication, psychotherapy, or both. The combination of psychotherapy and antidepressants is very effective in treating moderate to severe depression. The medications improve mood, sleep, energy, and appetite, while therapy strengthens coping skills, deals with possible underlying issues, and improves thought patterns and behavior.

In general, antidepressants alone help about 60%–70% of those taking them. Although a few individuals may experience some improvement from antidepressants by the end of the first week, most people do not see significant benefits from their antidepressants until after 3–4 weeks, and it can sometimes take as long as 8 weeks for the medication to produce its full effects. Thus it is critical that patients continue to take their antidepressant long enough for the medication to be beneficial and that patients not get discouraged and stop their medication prematurely if they do not feel better immediately.

In short-term studies, antidepressants were found to increase the risk of suicidal thinking and behavior in children and adolescents with major depression and other psychiatric disorders. The FDA requires the prescriber to warn of this risk in children and adolescents when starting antidepressant therapy. According to the FDA findings, the risk of suicidal thoughts and behaviors associated with antidepressants is age-related. This phenomenon tends to occur in the younger population and is most likely to occur early in the course of treatment. In adults over 24 years of age, there did not appear to be an increased risk of suicidality with antidepressants compared with placebo. In patients over age 65, the findings showed that antidepressants had a "protective effect" against suicidal thoughts and behavior. Other studies have found that when more people in a community are taking antidepressants, the suicide rate is lower.

The risk of suicide is inherent in depression and may persist until the individual responds to treatment. After starting or changing antidepressant therapy, the person, especially a child or adolescent, should be closely observed for worsening signs of depression, and the family or caregiver should communicate any concerns to the physician.

- **Warning:** Always let your physician or a family member know if you have suicidal thoughts. Notify your psychiatrist or your family physician whenever your depressive symptoms worsen or whenever you feel unable to control suicidal urges or thoughts.

- Do not discontinue Wellbutrin without consulting with your physician.
- If you miss a dose, take it as soon as possible. If it is close to the next scheduled dose, skip the missed dose and continue on your regular dosing schedule. Do not take double doses.
- Do not crush or cut the sustained-release or extended-release tablets; swallow them whole.
- Wellbutrin may be taken with or without food.
- Be aware that Wellbutrin is also prescribed for smoking cessation under the brand name Zyban, which contains sustained-release Wellbutrin. To prevent the co-administration of Wellbutrin and Zyban, inform your physician if you are taking a Wellbutrin medication.
- Store the medication in its originally labeled, light-resistant container, away from heat and moisture. Heat and moisture may precipitate breakdown of your medication, and the medication may lose its therapeutic effects.
- Keep your medication out of reach of children.

If you have any questions about your medication, consult your physician or pharmacist.

Notes

From Chew RH, Hales RE, Yudofsky SC: *What Your Patients Need to Know About Psychiatric Medications*, Second Edition. Washington, DC, American Psychiatric Publishing, 2009

Tricyclic Antidepressants

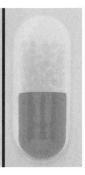

Amitriptyline
Anafranil (clomipramine)
Norpramin (desipramine)
Pamelor (nortriptyline)
Sinequan (doxepin)
Surmontil (trimipramine)*[1]
Vivactil (protriptyline)*
Tofranil and Tofranil-PM (imipramine)

The **tricyclic antidepressants** represent an older class of antidepressants that were once widely used in the treatment of depression. The word *tricyclic* refers to their three-ring chemical structures. For convenience, this handout shall refer to the tricyclic antidepressants as **TCAs.** These agents have been supplanted by newer antidepressants that are as effective but are much safer and have fewer side effects. They are still used to treat depression, but more frequently these agents are used to treat conditions outside of their approved indications, such as insomnia, chronic pain syndromes, generalized anxiety disorder, panic disorder, eating disorders (e.g., bulimia nervosa), and premenstrual dysphoric disorder. The use of a medication for its approved indication is called its *labeled use.* In clinical practice, however, physicians often prescribe medications for *unlabeled* ("off-label") uses when published clinical studies, case reports, or their own clinical experiences support the efficacy and safety of those treatments.

The TCAs are similar not only in structure but also in pharmacological effects. Presumably, these agents work by inhibiting the reuptake of **serotonin** and **norepinephrine,** two important neurotransmitters in the central nervous system, back into brain cells. *Neurotransmitters,* such as serotonin and norepinephrine, are chemicals produced by brain cells called neurons that enable them to communicate with one another. The neurotransmitters are released by one neuron into the space between that neuron and the next neuron. The neurotransmitters come into contact with specific sites on the surface membrane of neurons called *receptors.* From there, the chemical signal is transformed into an electrical impulse that travels down the neuron, causing further release of neurotransmitters. This process of neurotransmission is repeated along a chain of neurons. During neurotransmission, after neurotransmitters are released and the chemical signal is transferred to adjacent neurons, the neurotransmitters are recaptured back into brain cells by a process known as **reuptake.** By blocking the neurotransmitters from going back into the neurons from where they were released, the antidepressant can amplify the effects of the neurotransmitter.

The TCAs vary in their reuptake action depending on their chemical structure. One drug may have relatively greater norepinephrine reuptake blocking action, whereas another may have predominantly serotonin reuptake blocking properties. Most TCAs, however, block both serotonin and norepinephrine reuptake to varying degrees.

---

[1]*No separate handouts for Surmontil and Vivactil are included because these TCAs are not widely used.

Depression and other mental disorders may be due to abnormally low levels of certain neurotransmitters in the brain. This abnormality may in turn produce changes in affected areas of the brain, resulting in psychiatric symptoms such as depression or anxiety. When neurotransmission is improved by the antidepressant, the affected areas of the brain are restored to normal functioning, reducing the symptoms of the illness.

Common Side Effects

The TCAs are associated with numerous side effects and may not be tolerated by some individuals. Side effects often limit the usefulness of these agents, especially at higher dosages. Side effects can be managed sometimes by increasing the dosage slowly or by reducing the dosage. Monitoring blood drug levels for a selected TCA can also ensure the greatest benefit with the fewest side effects, because drug blood levels may identify patients with excessively high levels when toxic effects are suspected or those with low levels of drug in whom lack of absorption or rapid metabolism is suspected.

Most of the side effects from taking antidepressants usually subside greatly within 3–4 weeks, although this does not always occur. In the meantime, practical strategies may help minimize some of the side effects. Because TCAs are generally sedating, taking the prescribed medication before bedtime often results in a reduction of daytime side effects, especially drowsiness. When a medication is prescribed in divided doses, taking the larger dose at bedtime often helps. Other common side effects include feeling "spacey," a sense of being "slowed down," and forgetfulness.

Because the TCAs inhibit **cholinergic neurons** in the nervous system, they frequently produce a cluster of symptoms called **anticholinergic** side effects, which include dry mouth and skin, blurred vision, constipation, and difficulty urinating. Usually, individuals become tolerant to these side effects, but excessive anticholinergic effects may lead to confusion and a psychiatric disorder called delirium if not monitored closely. Sometimes the physician may prescribe another medication to counteract the anticholinergic action of the antidepressant. For example, a physician may prescribe a 1% pilocarpine eyedrop to treat blurred vision and bethanechol (e.g., Urecholine), a cholinergic agent, to treat urinary difficulties. For constipation, an over-the-counter stool softener such as Colace (docusate) is usually helpful.

Individuals may experience dizziness from TCAs. Dizziness may be caused by the drugs' effect in momentarily dropping blood pressure; they block the body's compensatory response to maintain a stable blood pressure when a person moves from lying down to a sitting position or from sitting to standing. This reaction is known in medical terms as **orthostatic hypotension.** Seniors and those taking medications to lower blood pressure may be more susceptible to orthostatic hypotension from these antidepressants.

Weight gain is another common problem, particularly with amitriptyline, Pamelor (nortriptyline), and Sinequan (doxepin). Most individuals gain several pounds while taking TCAs. If the individual's weight does not stabilize, the physician may switch the patient's medication to one of the newer, weight-neutral antidepressants, such as the **selective serotonin reuptake inhibitors** (SSRIs).

TCAs may also produce sexual difficulties, including impotence and ejaculatory difficulty in men and decreased sexual drive in both men and women. If this is a problem, the physician may switch the patient's medication to another antidepressant, such as bupropion (Wellbutrin SR or Wellbutrin XL), that does not interfere with sexual functioning.

Adverse Reactions and Precautions

As previously stated, seniors and individuals taking medications to lower blood pressure may be particularly susceptible to orthostatic hypotension from the TCAs. Patients taking these antidepressants should be cautious when rising suddenly to their feet. If lying down, patients should rise gradually to a sitting position before standing to avoid a sudden change in blood pressure. If lightheaded or dizzy, they should sit and wait for a minute or two to allow the blood pressure to adjust before standing up.

TCAs also may aggravate a potentially serious eye condition called **narrow-angle glaucoma.** Individuals should inform their psychiatrist if they have this condition.

In patients with a history of seizure disorder, use of the TCAs must be monitored closely because these antidepressants may lower the threshold for, and trigger, seizures. They may also slow cardiac conduction, which may result in a disturbance in heart rhythms called an arrhythmia. This side effect is more common in seniors and in people with a history of cardiac arrhythmias. For these individuals an electrocardiogram is recommended prior to and periodically (at least annually) during antidepressant treatment.

Overdose

TCAs are extremely lethal in acute overdoses, particularly in children. Overdoses often result in death, especially when TCAs are combined with other drugs or alcohol. Disturbance of cardiac rhythm is usually the leading cause of death in fatal TCA overdoses.

Any suspected overdose should be treated as an emergency. The person should be taken to the emergency room for observation and treatment. The prescription bottle of medication (and any other medication suspected in the overdose) should be brought as well, because the information on the prescription label can be helpful to the treating physician in determining the number of pills ingested.

Special Considerations

Most cases of major depression can be treated successfully, usually with medication, psychotherapy, or both. The combination of psychotherapy and antidepressants is very effective in treating moderate to severe depression. The medications improve mood, sleep, energy, and appetite, while therapy strengthens coping skills, deals with possible underlying issues, and improves thought patterns and behavior.

In general, antidepressants alone help about 60%–70% of those taking them. Although a few individuals may experience some improvement from antidepressants by the end of the first week, most people do not see significant benefits from their antidepressants until after 3–4 weeks, and it can sometimes take as long as 8 weeks for the medication to produce its full effects. Thus it is critical that patients continue to take their antidepressant long enough for the medication to be beneficial and that patients not get discouraged and stop their medication prematurely if they do not feel better immediately.

Researchers do not fully understand the exact mechanisms by which antidepressants work, but they appear to disrupt the chain of events that produce abnormalities in how the brain deals with emotions or stress, resulting in the symptoms of depression. When an individual does not respond to a tricyclic, does it make sense for the physician to switch the patient's medication to another TCA, since TCAs all have similar modes of action? In practice, patients who do not respond fully to one antidepressant often may respond to another one in the same class. This may not adequately explain the paradox. The molecular structure of one agent may be effective for one person but not for another. Sometimes it takes trial and error to find the right antidepressant, or combination of antidepressants, to successfully treat the person.

In short-term studies, antidepressants were found to increase the risk of suicidal thinking and behavior in children and adolescents with major depression and other psychiatric disorders. The FDA requires the prescriber to warn of this risk in children and adolescents when starting antidepressant therapy. According to the FDA findings, the risk of suicidal thoughts and behaviors associated with antidepressants is age-related. This phenomenon tends to occur in the younger population and is most likely to occur early in the course of treatment. In adults over 24 years of age, there did not appear to be an increased risk of suicidality with antidepressants compared with placebo. In patients over age 65, the findings showed that antidepressants had a "protective effect" against suicidal thoughts and behavior. Other studies have found that when more people in a community are taking antidepressants, the suicide rate is lower.

The risk of suicide is inherent in depression and may persist until the individual responds to treatment. Closely observe children and adolescents taking antidepressants for signs of worsening, suicidal thoughts, and changes in behavior, especially early in the course of therapy and with change in dosages. Similarly, adults with depressive disorder taking antidepressants should be closely observed for any signs of clinical worsening and suicidal thoughts and behaviors, especially during the first few months of therapy.

Warning: Always let your physician or a family member know if you have suicidal thoughts. Notify your psychiatrist or your family physician whenever your depressive symptoms worsen or whenever you feel unable to control suicidal urges or thoughts.

For more information, refer to the handout for the antidepressant that was prescribed for you.

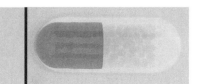

Amitriptyline

Generic name: Amitriptyline
Available strengths: 10 mg, 25 mg, 50 mg, 75 mg, 100 mg,
    150 mg tablets
Available in generic: Yes
Drug class: Tricyclic antidepressant

General Information

Amitriptyline is commonly known by the former brand name Elavil. The brand Elavil has been discontinued, and currently amitriptyline is only available generically in the United States from various manufacturers. Amitriptyline exerts its antidepressant action principally by inhibiting the reuptake of the neurotransmitters **serotonin** and, to a lesser extent, **norepinephrine,** thereby boosting neurotransmission in the central nervous system. Amitriptyline also has other pharmacological effects, which are associated with its side effects. Depression and other mental disorders may be due to abnormally low levels of certain neurotransmitters in the brain. This abnormality may in turn produce changes in affected areas of the brain, resulting in psychiatric symptoms such as depression or anxiety. Amitriptyline exerts its antidepressant action presumably by boosting the levels of serotonin and norepinephrine. There is usually a time lag of 3–4 weeks for antidepressants to achieve their optimal effect, which may be the time needed for the brain to restore normal functioning before reducing the symptoms of the illness.

Amitriptyline was approved by the U.S. Food and Drug Administration (FDA) for the treatment of depression. The use of a medication for its approved indications is called its *labeled use*. In clinical practice, however, physicians often prescribe medications for *unlabeled* ("off-label") uses when published clinical studies, case reports, or their own clinical experiences support the efficacy and safety of those treatments. Unlabeled uses of amitriptyline include treatment of chronic pain syndromes (e.g., migraine headaches, diabetic neuropathy, peripheral neuropathy, arthritic pain, and fibromyalgia). For fibromyalgia, a disorder causing aching muscles, fatigue, and other symptoms, there is some evidence, albeit limited, that low-dose amitriptyline in combination with fluoxetine (Prozac) may be more effective than any of these agents alone. Physicians may also use amitriptyline in combination with another antidepressant, such as fluoxetine for example, to augment the antidepressant action. This strategy is often successful in treating depression that is not fully responsive to a single antidepressant.

Dosing Information

The recommended starting dosage is 50–75 mg/day, preferably taken at bedtime. The dosage is increased by 25–50 mg weekly, depending on tolerability, to 150–200 mg/day. This dosage may be taken in divided doses, but a large portion of the total dosage may be taken at bedtime to minimize daytime sedation. If depressive symptoms persist after 8 weeks, the physician may further increase the dosage up to maximum of 300 mg/day or switch the patient's medication to another antidepressant.

Common Side Effects

Because the tricyclic antidepressants (TCAs) inhibit **cholinergic neurons** in the nervous system, they frequently produce a cluster of symptoms called **anticholinergic** side effects, which include dry mouth and skin, blurred vision, constipation, and difficulty urinating. Usually, individuals become tolerant to these side effects, but excessive anticholinergic effects may lead to confusion and a psychiatric disorder called delirium if not monitored closely. Sometimes the physician may prescribe another medication to counteract the anticholinergic action of the antidepressant. For example, a physician may prescribe a 1% pilocarpine eyedrop to treat blurred vision and bethanechol (e.g., Urecholine), a cholinergic agent, to treat urinary difficulties. For constipation, an over-the-counter stool softener such as Colace (docusate) is usually helpful.

Individuals may experience dizziness from TCAs. Dizziness may be caused by the drugs' effect in momentarily dropping blood pressure; they block the body's compensatory response to maintain a stable blood pressure when a person moves from lying down to a sitting position or from sitting to standing. This reaction is known in medical terms as **orthostatic hypotension.** Seniors and those taking medications to lower blood pressure may be more susceptible to orthostatic hypotension from these antidepressants.

Weight gain is another common problem. Most individuals gain several pounds while taking TCAs, including amitriptyline. If the individual's weight does not stabilize, the physician may switch the patient's medication to one of the newer, weight-neutral antidepressants, such as the selective serotonin reuptake inhibitors (SSRIs).

Amitriptyline may also produce sexual difficulties, including impotence and ejaculatory difficulty in men and decreased sexual drive in both men and women. If this is a problem, the physician may switch the patient's medication to another antidepressant, such as bupropion (Wellbutrin SR or Wellbutrin XL), that does not interfere with sexual functioning.

Adverse Reactions and Precautions

Amitriptyline may cause significant drowsiness and blurred vision in some people. Patients should not drive, operate machinery, or perform other potentially hazardous tasks until they are certain that their vision, alertness, or coordination is not affected by the medication. Patients with a known allergy to amitriptyline or who have experienced a severe reaction after taking it should not take amitriptyline.

Amitriptyline may affect cardiac conduction by slowing the electrical impulses that travel across cardiac tissues, leading to a disturbance in heart rhythms called an arrhythmia. This side effect is common in seniors and in people with a history of arrhythmias or cardiovascular disease. Therefore, patients over 65 years of age and those with a history of heart disease should obtain a pretreatment electrocardiogram and periodic checks (at least annually).

As previously stated, seniors and individuals taking medications to lower blood pressure may be susceptible to amitriptyline-induced orthostatic hypotension. In such susceptible individuals, the sudden drop in blood pressure from rising too rapidly may cause fainting. To prevent this from occurring, the individual should rise slowly, allowing blood pressure to adjust gradually.

136

Use in Pregnancy and Breastfeeding: Pregnancy Category D

TCAs are *not* recommended during pregnancy, especially during the first 3 months. The anticholinergic side effects induced by TCAs may also affect the baby (these effects are known as **fetal anticholinergic syndrome**).

Amitriptyline has not been tested in women to determine its safety in pregnancy. However, amitriptyline is placed in a higher-risk pregnancy category because there have been reported cases of babies born with reduced limbs from mothers who took amitriptyline during pregnancy. The exposure of amitriptyline during pregnancy in these women did not confirm a definite association between amitriptyline and this defect. Amitriptyline is known to cross the placenta, and its use during pregnancy must be clearly weighed against the potential risk of the medication to the developing fetus. Women who are pregnant or may become pregnant should discuss this with their physician. Some women may experience a recurrence of their depression when they stop their antidepressant. In these circumstances it may be necessary to restart the medication or seek an alternative medication or treatment.

Nursing mothers should not take amitriptyline, because small amounts will pass into breast milk and be ingested by the baby. If stopping the drug is not an alternative, breastfeeding should not be started or should be discontinued.

Possible Drug Interactions

The combined use of amitriptyline with certain other medications may result in adverse drug interactions, because one medication may alter the blood levels of the other. The significant drug interactions with amitriptyline are summarized in the table below.

Tagamet (cimetidine)	The combination of amitriptyline and Tagamet may increase the levels of amitriptyline and increase the frequency and severity of side effects.
Tegretol (carbamazepine)	This combination may result in decreased levels of amitriptyline and lower its positive pharmacological effects; the combination may also increase Tegretol levels, resulting in more side effects and increased toxicity.
Coumadin (warfarin)	Amitriptyline may increase Coumadin levels and its anticoagulant effect, resulting in bleeding.
Catapres (clonidine)	This combination may result in dangerous elevation of blood pressure and should be avoided.
Quinidine	The combination of amitriptyline and quinidine, an antiarrhythmia medication, may increase the risk of arrhythmias and should be avoided.
Depakote, Depakote ER, or Depakene	The combination of Depakote, Depakote ER, or Depakene and amitriptyline may elevate amitriptyline levels, thus increasing the likelihood of side effects.
Anticholinergic agents (e.g., Cogentin, Benadryl)	Anticholinergic side effects may increase when amitriptyline is combined with an anticholinergic agent or another medication with anticholinergic side effects.
Antabuse (disulfiram)	The combination of Antabuse and TCAs has been reported to cause a rare but potentially serious reaction called *organic brain syndrome*, which affects mental function.

Antidepressants known as **monoamine oxidase inhibitors** (MAOIs) should not be taken together with amitriptyline, because the combination may potentially produce a toxic reaction that includes elevated temperature, high blood pressure, and extreme excitation and agitation. Patients should consult their physician or pharmacist before taking any new medications, including over-the-counter medications and herbal supplements, with amitriptyline.

Patients taking amitriptyline should avoid alcohol or should consume it in moderation because the combination may worsen depression.

Overdose

Amitriptyline, like other TCAs, is extremely lethal in acute overdose, especially in children. Overdoses may result in death, especially when the antidepressant is combined with other medications or alcohol. Disturbance of cardiac rhythm is usually the leading cause of death.

Any suspected overdose should be treated as an emergency. The person should be taken to the emergency room for observation and treatment. The prescription bottle of medication (and any other medication suspected in the overdose) should be brought as well, because the information on the prescription label can be helpful to the treating physician in determining the number of pills ingested.

Special Considerations

Most cases of major depression can be treated successfully, usually with medication, psychotherapy, or both. The combination of psychotherapy and antidepressants is very effective in treating moderate to severe depression. The medications improve mood, sleep, energy, and appetite, while therapy strengthens coping skills, deals with possible underlying issues, and improves thought patterns and behavior.

In general, antidepressants alone help about 60%–70% of those taking them. Although a few individuals may experience some improvement from antidepressants by the end of the first week, most people do not see significant benefits from their antidepressants until after 3–4 weeks, and it can sometimes take as long as 8 weeks for the medication to produce its full effects. Thus it is critical that patients continue to take their antidepressant long enough for the medication to be beneficial and that patients not get discouraged and stop their medication prematurely if they do not feel better immediately.

In short-term studies, antidepressants were found to increase the risk of suicidal thinking and behavior in children and adolescents with major depression and other psychiatric disorders. The FDA requires the prescriber to warn of this risk in children and adolescents when starting antidepressant therapy. According to the FDA findings, the risk of suicidal thoughts and behaviors associated with antidepressants is age-related. This phenomenon tends to occur in the younger population and is most likely to occur early in the course of treatment. In adults over 24 years of age, there did not appear to be an increased risk of suicidality with antidepressants compared with placebo. In patients over age 65, the findings showed that antidepressants had a "protective effect" against suicidal thoughts and behavior. Other studies have found that when more people in a community are taking antidepressants, the suicide rate is lower.

The risk of suicide is inherent in depression and may persist until the individual responds to treatment. After starting or changing antidepressant therapy, the person, especially a child or adolescent, should be closely observed for worsening signs of depression, and the family or caregiver should communicate any concerns to the physician.

- **Warning:** Always let your physician or a family member know if you have suicidal thoughts. Notify your psychiatrist or your family physician whenever your depressive symptoms worsen or whenever you feel unable to control suicidal urges or thoughts.

- Do not discontinue amitriptyline without consulting your physician. Amitriptyline should not be stopped abruptly, but gradually tapered down before discontinuation. Abrupt discontinuation of amitriptyline may cause nausea, headache, and malaise.
- If you miss a dose, take it as soon as possible. If it is close to the next scheduled dose, skip the missed dose and continue on your regular dosing schedule. Do not take double doses.
- Amitriptyline may cause significant drowsiness. Until you are certain that your alertness and coordination are not affected by your medication, you should avoid driving and operating machinery.
- If you experience blurred vision, you should avoid driving, operating machinery, or performing potentially hazardous tasks. Consult your physician if you experience blurred vision.
- Do not take amitriptyline if you have a known allergy to amitriptyline or have experienced a severe reaction to it.
- Store the medication in its originally labeled, light-resistant container, away from heat and moisture. Heat and moisture may precipitate breakdown of your medication, and the medication may lose its therapeutic effects.
- Keep your medication out of reach of children. TCAs are extremely dangerous in acute overdose in young children.

If you have any questions about your medication, consult your physician or pharmacist.

Notes

From Chew RH, Hales RE, Yudofsky SC: *What Your Patients Need to Know About Psychiatric Medications*, Second Edition. Washington, DC, American Psychiatric Publishing, 2009

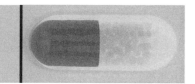

Anafranil (clomipramine)

Generic name: Clomipramine
Available strengths: 25 mg, 50 mg, 75 mg capsules
Available in generic: Yes
Drug class: Tricyclic antidepressant

General Information

Anafranil (clomipramine) exerts its antidepressant action principally by inhibiting the reuptake of the neurotransmitters **serotonin** and, to a lesser extent, **norepinephrine,** thereby boosting neurotransmission in the central nervous system. Anafranil has a broad range of pharmacological effects, some of which are associated with its side effects. Depression and other mental disorders may be due to abnormally low levels of certain neurotransmitters in the brain. This abnormality may in turn produce changes in affected areas of the brain, resulting in psychiatric symptoms such as depression, anxiety, or obsessive-compulsive behavior. It has been postulated, for example, that obsessive-compulsive disorder (OCD) is linked to dysfunction of serotonin neurotransmission, because agents such as Anafranil and selective serotonin reuptake inhibitors (SSRIs) such as Prozac (fluoxetine), Paxil (paroxetine), or Zoloft (sertraline) are effective in reducing OCD symptoms.

Anafranil exerts its antidepressant and anti-OCD actions presumably by boosting the levels of serotonin and norepinephrine. There is usually a time lag of 3–4 weeks for antidepressants to achieve their optimal effect, which may be the time needed for the brain to restore normal functioning before reducing the symptoms of the illness. For patients with OCD, the lag time for a positive response may be as long as 8 weeks. Anafranil was approved by the U.S. Food and Drug Administration (FDA) only for the treatment of OCD. The use of a medication for its approved indications is called its *labeled use*. In clinical practice, however, physicians often prescribe medications for *unlabeled* ("off-label") uses when published clinical studies, case reports, or their own clinical experiences support the efficacy and safety of those treatments. Unlabeled uses of Anafranil include treatment of depression, generalized anxiety disorder, panic disorder, eating disorder (bulimia nervosa), and posttraumatic stress disorder.

Dosing Information

The recommended starting dose of Anafranil is 25–50 mg, taken once daily, preferably at bedtime. The dosage is gradually increased, as tolerated, by 25–50 mg in the first 2 weeks, up to 100 mg/day. At higher dosages, Anafranil may be administered in divided doses to minimize side effects, but a large portion of the total dosage may be taken at bedtime to prevent daytime sedation. Depending on response and tolerability, the dosage may be increased gradually over the course of several weeks or more to a maximum of 250 mg/day.

Common Side Effects

Because the tricyclic antidepressants (TCAs) inhibit **cholinergic neurons** in the nervous system, they frequently produce a cluster of symptoms called **anticholinergic** side effects, which include dry mouth and skin, blurred vision, constipation, and difficulty urinating. Usually, individuals become tolerant to these side effects, but excessive anticholinergic effects may lead to confusion and a psychiatric disorder called delirium if not monitored closely. Sometimes the physician may prescribe another medication to counteract the anticholinergic action of the antidepressant. For example, a physician may prescribe a 1% pilocarpine eyedrop to treat blurred vision and bethanechol (e.g., Urecholine), a cholinergic agent, to treat urinary difficulties. For constipation, an over-the-counter stool softener such as Colace (docusate) is usually helpful.

Individuals may experience dizziness from TCAs. Dizziness may be caused by the drugs' effect in momentarily dropping blood pressure; they block the body's compensatory response to maintain a stable blood pressure when a person moves from lying down to a sitting position or from sitting to standing. This reaction is known in medical terms as **orthostatic hypotension.** Seniors and those taking medications to lower blood pressure may be more susceptible to orthostatic hypotension from these antidepressants.

Weight gain is another common problem. Most individuals gain several pounds while taking TCAs, including Anafranil. If the individual's weight does not stabilize, the physician may switch the patient's medication to one of the newer, weight-neutral antidepressants, such as the selective serotonin reuptake inhibitors (SSRIs).

Anafranil may also produce sexual difficulties, including impotence and ejaculatory difficulty in men and decreased sexual drive in both men and women. If this is a problem, the physician may switch the patient's medication to another antidepressant, such as bupropion (Wellbutrin SR or Wellbutrin XL), that does not interfere with sexual functioning.

Adverse Reactions and Precautions

Anafranil may cause significant drowsiness and blurred vision in some people. Patients should not drive, operate machinery, or perform other potentially hazardous tasks until they are certain that their vision, alertness, or coordination is not affected by the medication. Patients with a known allergy to Anafranil or who have experienced a severe reaction after taking it should not take Anafranil.

Anafranil may affect cardiac conduction by slowing the electrical impulses that travel across cardiac tissues, leading to a disturbance in heart rhythms called an arrhythmia. This side effect is common in seniors and in people with a history of arrhythmias or cardiovascular disease. Therefore, patients over 65 years of age and those with a history of heart disease should obtain a pretreatment electrocardiogram and periodic checks (at least annually).

As previously stated, seniors and individuals taking medications to lower blood pressure may be susceptible to Anafranil-induced orthostatic hypotension. In such susceptible individuals, the sudden drop in blood pressure from rising too rapidly may cause fainting. To prevent this from occurring, the individual should rise slowly, allowing blood pressure to adjust gradually.

There is a small risk that clomipramine can cause seizures, especially at higher dosages (up to 250 mg/day). Individuals who have a history of seizures or have some type of risk for seizures (from, e.g., brain injury, alcoholism, or other predisposing factors) should consult with their physician, because their physician may need to limit the maximum daily dosage.

142

Use in Pregnancy and Breastfeeding: Pregnancy Category C

Anafranil has not been tested in women to determine its safety in pregnancy, and it is not known whether it increases birth defects or spontaneous miscarriages because clinical experience is limited. In general, TCAs are *not* recommended during pregnancy, especially during the first 3 months. The anticholinergic side effects induced by TCAs may also affect the baby (these effects are known as **fetal anticholinergic syndrome**). Thus, use during pregnancy must be clearly weighed against the potential risk of the medication to the developing fetus. Women who are pregnant or may become pregnant should discuss this with their physician. Some women may experience recurrence of OCD or depression when they stop taking Anafranil. In these circumstances it may be necessary to restart the medication or seek an alternative medication or treatment.

Nursing mothers should not take Anafranil, because small amounts will pass into breast milk and be ingested by the baby. If stopping the drug is not an alternative, breastfeeding should not be started or should be discontinued.

Possible Drug Interactions

The combined use of Anafranil with certain other medications may result in adverse drug interactions, because one medication may alter the blood levels of the other. The significant drug interactions with Anafranil are summarized in the table below.

Selective serotonin reuptake inhibitors (SSRIs)	The combination of Anafranil and an SSRI may significantly increase the level of Anafranil, resulting in adverse or toxic reactions.
Tegretol (carbamazepine)	This combination may result in decreased levels of Anafranil and may lower its positive pharmacological effects; the combination may also increase Tegretol levels, resulting in more side effects and increased toxicity.
Coumadin (warfarin)	Anafranil may increase Coumadin levels and its anticoagulant effect, resulting in bleeding.
Catapres (clonidine)	This combination may result in dangerous elevation of blood pressure and should be avoided.
Quinidine	The combination of Anafranil and quinidine, an antiarrhythmia medication, may increase the risk of arrhythmias and should be avoided.
Depakote, Depakote ER, or Depakene	The combination of Depakote, Depakote ER, or Depakene and Anafranil may elevate Anafranil levels, which may increase the likelihood of side effects.
Anticholinergic agents (e.g., Cogentin, Benadryl)	Anticholinergic side effects may increase when Anafranil is combined with an anticholinergic agent or another medication with anticholinergic side effects.
Antabuse (disulfiram)	The combination of Antabuse and TCAs has been reported to cause a rare but potentially serious reaction called *organic brain syndrome*, which affects mental function.

Antidepressants known as **monoamine oxidase inhibitors** (MAOIs) should not be taken together with Anafranil, because the combination may potentially produce a toxic reaction that includes elevated temperature, high blood pressure, and extreme excitation and agitation. Patients should consult their physician or pharmacist before taking any new medications, including over-the-counter medications and herbal supplements, with Anafranil.

Patients taking Anafranil should avoid alcohol or should consume it in moderation because the combination may worsen depression.

Overdose

Anafranil, like other TCAs, is extremely lethal in acute overdose, especially in children. Overdoses may result in death, especially when the antidepressant is combined with other medications or alcohol. Disturbance of cardiac rhythm is usually the leading cause of death.

Any suspected overdose should be treated as an emergency. The person should be taken to the emergency room for observation and treatment. The prescription bottle of medication (and any other medication suspected in the overdose) should be brought as well, because the information on the prescription label can be helpful to the treating physician in determining the number of pills ingested.

Special Considerations

Most cases of major depression can be treated successfully, usually with medication, psychotherapy, or both. The combination of psychotherapy and antidepressants is very effective in treating moderate to severe depression. The medications improve mood, sleep, energy, and appetite, while therapy strengthens coping skills, deals with possible underlying issues, and improves thought patterns and behavior.

In general, antidepressants alone help about 60%–70% of those taking them. Although a few individuals may experience some improvement from antidepressants by the end of the first week, most people do not see significant benefits from their antidepressants until after 3–4 weeks, and it can sometimes take as long as 8 weeks for the medication to produce its full effects. Thus it is critical that patients continue to take their antidepressant long enough for the medication to be beneficial and that patients not get discouraged and stop their medication prematurely if they do not feel better immediately.

In short-term studies, antidepressants were found to increase the risk of suicidal thinking and behavior in children and adolescents with major depression and other psychiatric disorders. The FDA requires the prescriber to warn of this risk in children and adolescents when starting antidepressant therapy. According to the FDA findings, the risk of suicidal thoughts and behaviors associated with antidepressants is age-related. This phenomenon tends to occur in the younger population and is most likely to occur early in the course of treatment. In adults over 24 years of age, there did not appear to be an increased risk of suicidality with antidepressants compared with placebo. In patients over age 65, the findings showed that antidepressants had a "protective effect" against suicidal thoughts and behavior. Other studies have found that when more people in a community are taking antidepressants, the suicide rate is lower.

The risk of suicide is inherent in depression and may persist until the individual responds to treatment. After starting or changing antidepressant therapy, the person, especially a child or adolescent, should be closely observed for worsening signs of depression, and the family or caregiver should communicate any concerns to the physician.

- **Warning:** Always let your physician or a family member know if you have suicidal thoughts. Notify your psychiatrist or your family physician whenever your depressive symptoms worsen or whenever you feel unable to control suicidal urges or thoughts.

- Do not discontinue Anafranil without consulting your physician. Anafranil should not be stopped abruptly, but gradually tapered down before discontinuation. Abrupt discontinuation of Anafranil may cause nausea, headache, and malaise.
- If you miss a dose, take it as soon as possible. If it is close to the next scheduled dose, skip the missed dose and continue on your regular dosing schedule. Do not take double doses.
- Anafranil may cause significant drowsiness. Until you are certain that your alertness and coordination are not affected by your medication, you should avoid driving and operating machinery.
- If you experience blurred vision, you should you should avoid driving, operating machinery, or performing potentially hazardous tasks. Consult your physician if you experience blurred vision.
- Do not take Anafranil if you have a known allergy to Anafranil or have experienced a severe reaction to it.
- Store the medication in its originally labeled, light-resistant container, away from heat and moisture. Heat and moisture may precipitate breakdown of your medication, and the medication may lose its therapeutic effects.
- Keep your medication out of reach of children. TCAs are extremely dangerous in acute overdose in young children.

If you have any questions about your medication, consult your physician or pharmacist.

Notes

_____

_____

_____

_____

_____

_____

_____

From Chew RH, Hales RE, Yudofsky SC: *What Your Patients Need to Know About Psychiatric Medications*, Second Edition. Washington, DC, American Psychiatric Publishing, 2009

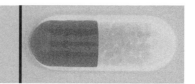

Norpramin (desipramine)

Generic name: Desipramine
Available strengths: 10 mg, 25 mg, 50 mg, 75 mg,
   100 mg, 150 mg tablets
Available in generic: Yes
Drug class: Tricyclic antidepressant

General Information

Norpramin (desipramine) exerts its antidepressant action principally by inhibiting the reuptake of **norepinephrine** and, to a lesser extent, **serotonin,** two important neurotransmitters in the central nervous system, and thereby boosting neurotransmission. Norpramin also has other pharmacological effects, which are associated with its side effects. Depression and other mental disorders may be due to abnormally low levels of certain neurotransmitters in the brain. This abnormality may in turn produce changes in affected areas of the brain, resulting in psychiatric symptoms such as depression or anxiety. Norpramin exerts its antidepressant action presumably by boosting the levels of serotonin and norepinephrine. There is usually a time lag of 3–4 weeks for antidepressants to achieve their optimal effect, which may be the time needed for the brain to restore normal functioning before reducing the symptoms of the illness.

Norpramin was approved by the U.S. Food and Drug Administration (FDA) for the treatment of depression. The use of a medication for its approved indications is called its *labeled use.* In clinical practice, however, physicians often prescribe medications for *unlabeled* ("off-label") uses when published clinical studies, case reports, or their own clinical experiences support the efficacy and safety of those treatments. Unlabeled uses of Norpramin include treatment of chronic pain syndromes (e.g., migraine, diabetic neuropathy, cancer pain), eating disorders (bulimia nervosa), panic disorder, premenstrual dysphoric disorder, posttraumatic stress disorder, and insomnia, and facilitation of cocaine withdrawal. Physicians may also use Norpramin in combination with another antidepressant, such as a **selective serotonin reuptake inhibitor** (SSRI), to augment the antidepressant effect. This augmentation strategy is often successful in treating refractory depression when response to a single antidepressant is inadequate.

Dosing Information

The recommended starting dose is 75 mg, taken once a day, preferably at bedtime. The dosage is increased by 25–50 mg weekly, depending on tolerability, to 100–200 mg/day, which may be taken in a single bedtime dose or in divided doses. If depressive symptoms persist after 8 weeks, the physician may further increase the dosage up to a maximum of 300 mg/day or switch the patient's medication to another antidepressant. Seniors and adolescents generally require lower dosages of 25–100 mg/day, and dosages greater than 150 mg/day are not recommended for those patients.

Common Side Effects

Because the tricyclic antidepressants (TCAs) inhibit **cholinergic neurons** in the nervous system, they frequently produce a cluster of symptoms called **anticholinergic** side effects, which include dry mouth and skin, blurred vision, constipation, and difficulty urinating. Usually, individuals become tolerant to these side effects, but excessive anticholinergic effects may lead to confusion and a psychiatric disorder called delirium if not monitored closely. Sometimes the physician may prescribe another medication to counteract the anticholinergic action of the antidepressant. For example, a physician may prescribe a 1% pilocarpine eye drop to treat blurred vision and bethanechol (e.g., Urecholine), a cholinergic agent, to treat urinary difficulties. For constipation, an over-the-counter stool softener such as Colace (docusate) is usually helpful.

Individuals may experience dizziness from TCAs. Dizziness may be caused by the drugs' effect in momentarily dropping blood pressure; they block the body's compensatory response to maintain a stable blood pressure when a person moves from lying down to a sitting position or from sitting to standing. This reaction is known in medical terms as **orthostatic hypotension.** Seniors and those taking other medications to lower blood pressure may be more susceptible to orthostatic hypotension from these antidepressants.

Weight gain is another common problem. Most individuals gain several pounds while taking TCAs, including Norpramin. If the individual's weight does not stabilize, the physician may switch the patient's medication to one of the newer, weight-neutral antidepressants, such as the SSRIs.

Norpramin may also produce sexual difficulties, including impotence and ejaculatory difficulty in men and decreased sexual drive in both men and women. If this is a problem, the physician may switch the patient's medication to another antidepressant, such as bupropion (Wellbutrin SR or Wellbutrin XL), that does not interfere with sexual functioning.

Adverse Reactions and Precautions

Norpramin may cause significant drowsiness and blurred vision in some people. Patients should not drive, operate machinery, or perform other potentially hazardous tasks until they are certain that their vision, alertness, or coordination is not affected by the medication. Patients with a known allergy to Norpramin or who have experienced a severe reaction after taking it should not take Norpramin.

Norpramin may affect cardiac conduction by slowing the electrical impulses that travel across cardiac tissues, leading to a disturbance in heart rhythms called an arrhythmia. This side effect is common in seniors and in people with a history of arrhythmias or cardiovascular disease. Therefore, patients over 65 years of age and those with a history of heart disease should obtain a pretreatment electrocardiogram and periodic checks (at least annually).

As previously stated, seniors and individuals taking medications to lower blood pressure may be particularly susceptible to Norpramin-induced orthostatic hypotension. In such susceptible individuals, the sudden drop in blood pressure from rising too rapidly may cause fainting. To prevent this from occurring, the individual should rise slowly, allowing blood pressure to adjust gradually.

Use in Pregnancy and Breastfeeding: Pregnancy Category C

Norpramin has not been tested in women to determine its safety in pregnancy. TCAs are *not* recommended during pregnancy, especially during the first 3 months. The anticholinergic side effects induced by TCAs may also affect the baby (these effects are known as **fetal anticholinergic syndrome**). Thus, use during pregnancy must be clearly weighed against the potential risk of the medication to the fetus. Women who are pregnant or may become pregnant should discuss this with their physician. Some women may experience a recurrence of their depression when they stop their antidepressant. In these circumstances it may be necessary to restart the medication or seek an alternative medication or treatment.

Nursing mothers should not take Norpramin, because small amounts will pass into breast milk and be ingested by the baby. If stopping the drug is not an alternative, breastfeeding should not be started or should be discontinued.

Possible Drug Interactions

The combined use of Norpramin with certain other medications may result in adverse drug interactions, because one medication may alter the blood levels of the other. The significant drug interactions with Norpramin are summarized in the table below.

Selective serotonin reuptake inhibitors (SSRIs)	The combination of Norpramin and an SSRI may significantly increase the level of Norpramin, resulting in adverse or toxic reactions.
Tegretol (carbamazepine)	This combination may result in decreased levels of Norpramin and may lower its positive pharmacological effects; the combination may also increase Tegretol levels, resulting in more side effects and increased toxicity.
Coumadin (warfarin)	Norpramin may increase Coumadin levels and its anticoagulant effect, resulting in bleeding.
Catapres (clonidine)	This combination may result in dangerous elevation of blood pressure and should be avoided.
Quinidine	The combination of Norpramin and quinidine, an antiarrhythmia medication, may increase the risk of arrhythmias and should be avoided.
Depakote, Depakote ER, or Depakene	The combination of Depakote, Depakote ER, or Depakene and Norpramin may elevate Norpramin levels, which may increase side effects.
Anticholinergic agents (e.g., Cogentin, Benadryl)	Anticholinergic side effects may increase when Norpramin is combined with an anticholinergic agent or another medication with anticholinergic side effects.
Antabuse (disulfiram)	The combination of Antabuse and TCAs has been reported to cause a rare but potentially serious reaction called *organic brain syndrome*, which affects mental function.

Antidepressants known as **monoamine oxidase inhibitors** (MAOIs) should not be taken together with Norpramin, because the combination may potentially produce a toxic reaction that includes elevated temperature, high blood pressure, and extreme excitation and agitation. Patients should consult their physician or pharmacist before taking any new medications, including over-the-counter medications and herbal supplements, with Norpramin.

Patients taking Norpramin should avoid alcohol or should consume it in moderation because the combination may worsen depression.

Overdose

Norpramin, like other TCAs, is extremely lethal in acute overdose, especially in children. Overdoses may result in death, especially when the antidepressant is combined with other medications or alcohol. Disturbance of cardiac rhythm is usually the leading cause of death.

Any suspected overdose should be treated as an emergency. The person should be taken to the emergency room for observation and treatment. The prescription bottle of medication (and any other medication suspected in the overdose) should be brought as well, because the information on the prescription label can be helpful to the treating physician in determining the number of pills ingested.

Special Considerations

Most cases of major depression can be treated successfully, usually with medication, psychotherapy, or both. The combination of psychotherapy and antidepressants is very effective in treating moderate to severe depression. The medications improve mood, sleep, energy, and appetite, while therapy strengthens coping skills, deals with possible underlying issues, and improves thought patterns and behavior.

In general, antidepressants alone help about 60%–70% of those taking them. Although a few individuals may experience some improvement from antidepressants by the end of the first week, most people do not see significant benefits from their antidepressants until after 3–4 weeks, and it can sometimes take as long as 8 weeks for the medication to produce its full effects. Thus it is critical that patients continue to take their antidepressant long enough for the medication to be beneficial and that patients not get discouraged and stop their medication prematurely if they do not feel better immediately.

In short-term studies, antidepressants were found to increase the risk of suicidal thinking and behavior in children and adolescents with major depression and other psychiatric disorders. The FDA requires the prescriber to warn of this risk in children and adolescents when starting antidepressant therapy. According to the FDA findings, the risk of suicidal thoughts and behaviors associated with antidepressants is age-related. This phenomenon tends to occur in the younger population and is most likely to occur early in the course of treatment. In adults over 24 years of age, there did not appear to be an increased risk of suicidality with antidepressants compared with placebo. In patients over age 65, the findings showed that antidepressants had a "protective effect" against suicidal thoughts and behavior. Other studies have found that when more people in a community are taking antidepressants, the suicide rate is lower.

The risk of suicide is inherent in depression and may persist until the individual responds to treatment. After starting or changing antidepressant therapy, the person, especially a child or adolescent, should be closely observed for worsening signs of depression, and the family or caregiver should communicate any concerns to the physician.

- **Warning:** Always let your physician or a family member know if you have suicidal thoughts. Notify your psychiatrist or your family physician whenever your depressive symptoms worsen or whenever you feel unable to control suicidal urges or thoughts.
- Do not discontinue Norpramin without consulting your physician. Norpramin should not be stopped abruptly, but gradually tapered down before discontinuation. Abrupt discontinuation of Norpramin may cause nausea, headache, and malaise.
- If you miss a dose, take it as soon as possible. If it is close to the next scheduled dose, skip the missed dose and continue on your regular dosing schedule. Do not take double doses.

- Norpramin may cause significant drowsiness. Until you are certain that your alertness and coordination are not affected by your medication, you should avoid driving and operating machinery.
- If you experience blurred vision, you should avoid driving, operating machinery, or performing potentially hazardous tasks. Consult your physician if you experience blurred vision.
- Do not take Norpramin if you have a known allergy to Norpramin or have experienced a severe reaction to it.
- Store the medication in its originally labeled, light-resistant container, away from heat and moisture. Heat and moisture may precipitate breakdown of your medication, and the medication may lose its therapeutic effects.
- Keep your medication out of reach of children. TCAs are extremely dangerous in acute overdose in young children.

If you have any questions about your medication, consult your physician or pharmacist.

Notes

From Chew RH, Hales RE, Yudofsky SC: *What Your Patients Need to Know About Psychiatric Medications*, Second Edition. Washington, DC, American Psychiatric Publishing, 2009

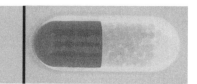

Pamelor (nortriptyline)

Generic name: Nortriptyline
Available strengths: 10 mg, 25 mg, 50 mg,
   75 mg capsules; 10 mg/5 mL oral solution
Available in generic: Yes
Drug class: Tricyclic antidepressant

General Information

Pamelor (nortriptyline) exerts its antidepressant action principally by inhibiting the reuptake of **norepinephrine** and, to a lesser extent, **serotonin,** two important neurotransmitters in the central nervous system, and thereby boosting neurotransmission. Pamelor also has other pharmacological effects, which are associated with its side effects. Depression and other mental disorders may be due to abnormally low levels of certain neurotransmitters in the brain. This abnormality may in turn produce changes in affected areas of the brain, resulting in psychiatric symptoms such as depression or anxiety. Pamelor exerts its antidepressant action presumably by boosting the levels of serotonin and norepinephrine. There is usually a time lag of 3–4 weeks for antidepressants to achieve their optimal effect, which may be the time needed for the brain to restore normal functioning before reducing the symptoms of the illness.

Pamelor was approved by the U.S. Food and Drug Administration (FDA) for the treatment of depression. The use of a medication for its approved indications is called its *labeled use*. In clinical practice, however, physicians often prescribe medications for *unlabeled* ("off-label") uses when published clinical studies, case reports, or their own clinical experiences support the efficacy and safety of those treatments. Unlabeled uses of Pamelor include treatment of panic disorder, premenstrual dysphoric disorder, posttraumatic stress disorder, and insomnia. Physicians may also use Pamelor in combination with another antidepressant, such as a **selective serotonin reuptake inhibitor** (SSRI), to augment the antidepressant effect. This augmentation strategy is often successful in treating refractory depression when response to a single antidepressant is inadequate.

Dosing Information

The usual starting dosage is 50 mg/day, which may be taken in divided doses or as a single bedtime dose. The dosage may be increased by 25–50 mg every week, but the maximum dosage should not exceed 150 mg/day. Seniors may require lower dosages of 25–50 mg/day, and dosages greater than 100 mg/day are not recommended. Nortriptyline (available under the brand name Aventyl) is the only tricyclic antidepressant (TCA) known to have a "therapeutic window" in which the optimal dosage is associated with achieving a certain blood level of the medication in the patient. The treating physician may periodically order blood tests to determine whether the patient's blood levels of the medication are within the optimal range to achieve the normal beneficial effect.

Common Side Effects

Compared with other TCAs (e.g., amitriptyline), Pamelor is generally better tolerated. The dosage and the individual's tolerability to the side effects are also factors. Pamelor may induce sedation. This side effect may be minimized by taking the medication close to bedtime.

Because the TCAs inhibit **cholinergic neurons** in the nervous system, they frequently produce a cluster of symptoms called **anticholinergic** side effects, which include dry mouth and skin, blurred vision, constipation, and difficulty urinating. Usually, individuals become tolerant to these side effects, but excessive anticholinergic effects may lead to confusion and a psychiatric disorder called delirium if not monitored closely. Sometimes the physician may prescribe another medication to counteract the anticholinergic action of the antidepressant. For example, a physician may prescribe a 1% pilocarpine eyedrop to treat blurred vision and bethanechol (e.g., Urecholine), a cholinergic agent, to treat urinary difficulties. For constipation, an over-the-counter stool softener such as Colace (docusate) is usually helpful.

Individuals may experience dizziness from TCAs. Dizziness may be caused by the drugs' effect in momentarily dropping blood pressure; they block the body's compensatory response to maintain a stable blood pressure when a person moves from lying down to a sitting position or from sitting to standing. This reaction is known in medical terms as **orthostatic hypotension.** Seniors and those taking other medications to lower blood pressure may be more susceptible to orthostatic hypotension from these antidepressants.

Weight gain is another common problem. Most individuals gain several pounds while taking TCAs, including Pamelor. If the individual's weight does not stabilize, the physician may switch the patient's medication to one of the newer, weight-neutral antidepressants, such as the SSRIs.

Pamelor may also produce sexual difficulties, including impotence and ejaculatory difficulty in men and decreased sexual drive in both men and women. If this is a problem, the physician may switch the patient's medication to another antidepressant, such as bupropion (Wellbutrin SR or Wellbutrin XL), that does not interfere with sexual functioning.

Adverse Reactions and Precautions

Pamelor may cause significant drowsiness and blurred vision in some people. Patients should not drive, operate machinery, or perform other potentially hazardous tasks until they are certain that their vision, alertness, or coordination is not affected by the medication. Patients with a known allergy to Pamelor or who have experienced a severe reaction after taking it should not take Pamelor.

Pamelor may affect cardiac conduction by slowing the electrical impulses that travel across cardiac tissues, leading to a disturbance in heart rhythms called an arrhythmia. This side effect is common in seniors and in people with a history of arrhythmias or cardiovascular disease. Therefore, patients over 65 years of age and those with a history of heart disease should obtain a pretreatment electrocardiogram and periodic checks (at least annually). Patients with a recent history of heart attack or a history of arrhythmias should *not* take Pamelor (or Aventyl) because of the increased risk for dangerous irregular heartbeats.

As previously stated, seniors and individuals taking medications to lower blood pressure may be particularly susceptible to Pamelor-induced **orthostatic hypotension.** In such susceptible individuals, the sudden drop in blood pressure from rising too rapidly may cause fainting. To prevent this from occurring, the individual should rise slowly, allowing blood pressure to adjust gradually.

Use in Pregnancy and Breastfeeding: Pregnancy Category D

TCAs are not recommended during pregnancy, especially during the first 3 months. The anticholinergic side effects induced by TCAs may also affect the baby (these effects are known as **fetal anticholinergic syndrome**). Congenital malformations associated with nortriptyline have been reported, but the use of Pamelor in pregnancy has not been clinically studied. Thus, use during pregnancy must be clearly weighed against the potential risk to the developing fetus. Women who are pregnant or may become pregnant should discuss this with their physician. Some women may experience a recurrence of their depression when they stop their antidepressant. In these circumstances it may be necessary to restart the medication or seek an alternative medication or treatment.

Nursing mothers should not take Pamelor, because small amounts will pass into breast milk and be ingested by the baby. If stopping the antidepressant is not an alternative, breastfeeding should not be started or should be discontinued.

Possible Drug Interactions

The combined use of Pamelor with certain other medications may result in adverse drug interactions, because one medication may alter the blood levels of the other. The significant drug interactions with Pamelor are summarized in the table below.

Selective serotonin reuptake inhibitors (SSRIs)	The combination of Pamelor and an SSRI may significantly increase the level of Pamelor, resulting in adverse or toxic reactions.
Tegretol (carbamazepine)	This combination may result in decreased levels of Pamelor and may lower its positive pharmacological effects; the combination may also increase Tegretol levels, resulting in more side effects and increased toxicity.
Coumadin (warfarin)	Pamelor may increase Coumadin levels and its anticoagulant effect, resulting in bleeding.
Catapres (clonidine)	This combination may result in dangerous elevation of blood pressure and should be avoided.
Quinidine	The combination of Pamelor and quinidine, an anti-arrhythmia medication, may increase the risk of arrhythmias and should be avoided.
Depakote, Depakote ER, or Depakene	The combination of Depakote, Depakote ER, or Depakene and Pamelor may elevate Pamelor levels, which may increase the likelihood of side effects.
Anticholinergic agents (e.g., Cogentin, Benadryl)	Anticholinergic side effects may increase when Pamelor is combined with an anticholinergic agent or another medication with anticholinergic side effects.
Antabuse (disulfiram)	The combination of Antabuse and TCAs has been reported to cause a rare but potentially serious reaction called *organic brain syndrome*, which affects mental function.

Antidepressants known as **monoamine oxidase inhibitors** (MAOIs) should not be taken together with Pamelor, because the combination may potentially produce a toxic reaction that includes elevated temperature, high blood pressure, and extreme excitation and agitation. Patients should consult their physician or pharmacist before taking any new medications, including over-the-counter medications and herbal supplements, with Pamelor.

Patients taking Pamelor should avoid alcohol or should consume it in moderation because the combination may worsen depression.

Overdose

Pamelor, like other TCAs, is extremely lethal in acute overdose, especially in children. Overdoses may result in death, especially when the antidepressant is combined with other medications or alcohol. Disturbance of cardiac rhythm is usually the leading cause of death.

Any suspected overdose should be treated as an emergency. The person should be taken to the emergency room for observation and treatment. The prescription bottle of medication (and any other medication suspected in the overdose) should be brought as well, because the information on the prescription label can be helpful to the treating physician in determining the number of pills ingested.

Special Considerations

Most cases of major depression can be treated successfully, usually with medication, psychotherapy, or both. The combination of psychotherapy and antidepressants is very effective in treating moderate to severe depression. The medications improve mood, sleep, energy, and appetite, while therapy strengthens coping skills, deals with possible underlying issues, and improves thought patterns and behavior.

In general, antidepressants alone help about 60%–70% of those taking them. Although a few individuals may experience some improvement from antidepressants by the end of the first week, most people do not see significant benefits from their antidepressants until after 3–4 weeks, and it can sometimes take as long as 8 weeks for the medication to produce its full effects. Thus it is critical that patients continue to take their antidepressant long enough for the medication to be beneficial and that patients not get discouraged and stop their medication prematurely if they do not feel better immediately.

In short-term studies, antidepressants were found to increase the risk of suicidal thinking and behavior in children and adolescents with major depression and other psychiatric disorders. The FDA requires the prescriber to warn of this risk in children and adolescents when starting antidepressant therapy. According to the FDA findings, the risk of suicidal thoughts and behaviors associated with antidepressants is age-related. This phenomenon tends to occur in the younger population and is most likely to occur early in the course of treatment. In adults over 24 years of age, there did not appear to be an increased risk of suicidality with antidepressants compared with placebo. In patients over age 65, the findings showed that antidepressants had a "protective effect" against suicidal thoughts and behavior. Other studies have found that when more people in a community are taking antidepressants, the suicide rate is lower.

The risk of suicide is inherent in depression and may persist until the individual responds to treatment. After starting or changing antidepressant therapy, the person, especially a child or adolescent, should be closely observed for worsening signs of depression, and the family or caregiver should communicate any concerns to the physician.

- **Warning:** Always let your physician or a family member know if you have suicidal thoughts. Notify your psychiatrist or your family physician whenever your depressive symptoms worsen or whenever you feel unable to control suicidal urges or thoughts.

- Do not discontinue Pamelor without consulting your physician. Pamelor should not be stopped abruptly, but gradually tapered down before discontinuation. Abrupt discontinuation of Pamelor may cause nausea, headache, and malaise.
- If you miss a dose, take it as soon as possible. If it is close to the next scheduled dose, skip the missed dose and continue on your regular dosing schedule. Do not take double doses.
- Pamelor may cause significant drowsiness. Until you are certain that your alertness and coordination are not affected by your medication, you should avoid driving and operating machinery.
- If you experience blurred vision, you should avoid driving, operating machinery, or performing potentially hazardous tasks. Consult your physician if you experience blurred vision.
- Do not take Pamelor if you have a known allergy to Pamelor or have experienced a severe reaction to it.
- Store the medication in its originally labeled, light-resistant container, away from heat and moisture. Heat and moisture may precipitate breakdown of your medication, and the medication may lose its therapeutic effects.
- Keep your medication out of reach of children. TCAs are extremely dangerous in acute overdose in young children.

If you have any questions about your medication, consult your physician or pharmacist.

Notes

_____

_____

_____

_____

_____

_____

_____

From Chew RH, Hales RE, Yudofsky SC: *What Your Patients Need to Know About Psychiatric Medications*, Second Edition. Washington, DC, American Psychiatric Publishing, 2009

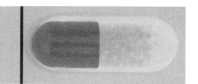

Sinequan (doxepin)

Generic name: Doxepin
Available strengths: 10 mg, 25 mg, 50 mg, 75 mg, 100 mg,
    150 mg capsules; 10 mg/mL oral concentrate
Available in generic: Yes
Drug class: Tricyclic antidepressant

General Information

Sinequan (doxepin) exerts its antidepressant action principally by inhibiting the reuptake of **serotonin** and **norepinephrine,** two important neurotransmitters in the central nervous system, and thereby boosting neurotransmission. Sinequan also has other pharmacological effects, which are associated with its side effects. Depression and other mental disorders may be due to abnormally low levels of certain neurotransmitters in the brain. This abnormality may in turn produce changes in affected areas of the brain, resulting in psychiatric symptoms such as depression or anxiety. Sinequan exerts its antidepressant action presumably by boosting the levels of serotonin and norepinephrine. There is usually a time lag of 3–4 weeks for antidepressants to achieve their optimal effect, which may be the time needed for the brain to restore normal functioning before reducing the symptoms of the illness.

Sinequan was approved by the U.S. Food and Drug Administration (FDA) for the treatment of depression and anxiety. The use of a medication for its approved indications is called its *labeled use.* In clinical practice, however, physicians often prescribe medications for *unlabeled* ("off-label") uses when published clinical studies, case reports, or their own clinical experiences support the efficacy and safety of those treatments. Unlabeled uses of Sinequan include treatment of chronic pain syndromes (e.g., migraine headaches, diabetic neuropathy, cancer pain), eating disorders (bulimia nervosa), panic disorder, premenstrual dysphoric disorder, posttraumatic stress disorder, and insomnia. Physicians may also use Sinequan in combination with another antidepressant, such as a **selective serotonin reuptake inhibitor** (SSRI), to augment the antidepressant effect. This augmentation strategy is often successful in treating refractory depression when response to a single antidepressant is inadequate.

Dosing Information

The recommended starting dosage is 75 mg/day, preferably taken at bedtime. The dosage is increased by 25–50 mg weekly, as needed, to 150–200 mg/day, which may be taken in a single bedtime dose or in divided doses.

If depressive symptoms persist after 8 weeks, the physician may further increase the dosage up to a maximum of 300 mg/day or switch the patient's medication to another antidepressant. Seniors and adolescents generally require lower dosages.

Common Side Effects

Because the tricyclic antidepressants (TCAs) inhibit **cholinergic neurons** in the nervous system, they frequently produce a cluster of symptoms called **anticholinergic** side effects, which include dry mouth and skin, blurred vision, constipation, and difficulty urinating. Usually, individuals become tolerant to these side effects, but excessive anticholinergic effects may lead to confusion and a psychiatric disorder called delirium if not monitored closely. Sometimes the physician may prescribe another medication to counteract the anticholinergic action of the antidepressant. For example, a physician may prescribe a 1% pilocarpine eyedrop to treat blurred vision and bethanechol (e.g., Urecholine), a cholinergic agent, to treat urinary difficulties. For constipation, an over-the-counter stool softener such as Colace (docusate) is usually helpful.

Individuals may experience dizziness from TCAs. Dizziness may be caused by the drugs' effect in momentarily dropping blood pressure; they block the body's compensatory response to maintain a stable blood pressure when a person moves from lying down to a sitting position or from sitting to standing. This reaction is known in medical terms as **orthostatic hypotension.** Seniors and those taking other medications to lower blood pressure may be more susceptible to orthostatic hypotension from these antidepressants.

Weight gain is another common problem. Most individuals gain several pounds while taking TCAs, including Sinequan. If the individual's weight does not stabilize, the physician may switch the patient's medication to one of the newer, weight-neutral antidepressants, such as the SSRIs.

Sinequan may also produce sexual difficulties, including impotence and ejaculatory difficulty in men and decreased sexual drive in both men and women. If this is a problem, the physician may switch the patient's medication to another antidepressant, such as bupropion (Wellbutrin SR or Wellbutrin XL), that does not interfere with sexual functioning.

Adverse Reactions and Precautions

Sinequan may cause significant drowsiness and blurred vision in some people. Patients should not drive, operate machinery, or perform other potentially hazardous tasks until they are certain that their vision, alertness, or coordination is not affected by the medication. Patients with a known allergy to Sinequan or who have experienced a severe reaction after taking it should not take Sinequan.

Sinequan may affect cardiac conduction by slowing the electrical impulses that travel across cardiac tissues, leading to a disturbance in heart rhythms called an arrhythmia. This side effect is common in seniors and in people with a history of arrhythmias or cardiovascular disease. Therefore, patients over 65 years of age and those with a history of heart disease should obtain a pretreatment electrocardiogram and periodic checks (at least annually).

As previously stated, seniors and individuals taking medications to lower blood pressure may be susceptible to Sinequan-induced orthostatic hypotension. In such susceptible individuals, the sudden drop in blood pressure from rising too rapidly may cause fainting. To prevent this from occurring, the individual should rise slowly, allowing blood pressure to adjust gradually.

Use in Pregnancy and Breastfeeding: Pregnancy Category C

Sinequan has not been tested in women to determine its safety in pregnancy. TCAs are *not* recommended during pregnancy, especially during the first 3 months. The anticholinergic side effects induced by these drugs may also affect the baby (these effects are known as **fetal anticholinergic syndrome**). Thus, use during pregnancy must be clearly weighed against the potential risk of the medication to the developing fetus. Women who are pregnant or may become pregnant should discuss this with their physician. Some women may experience a recurrence of their depression when they stop their antidepressant. In these circumstances it may be necessary to restart the medication or seek an alternative medication or treatment.

Nursing mothers should not take Sinequan, because small amounts will pass into breast milk and be ingested by the baby. If stopping the antidepressant is not an alternative, breastfeeding should not be started or should be discontinued.

Possible Drug Interactions

The combined use of Sinequan with certain other medications may result in adverse drug interactions, because one medication may alter the blood levels of the other. The significant drug interactions with Sinequan are summarized in the table below.

Selective serotonin reuptake inhibitors (SSRIs)	The combination of Sinequan and an SSRI may significantly increase the level of Sinequan, resulting in adverse or toxic reactions.
Tegretol (carbamazepine)	This combination may result in decreased levels of Sinequan and may lower its positive pharmacological effects; the combination may also increase Tegretol levels, resulting in more side effects and increased toxicity.
Coumadin (warfarin)	Sinequan may increase Coumadin levels and its anticoagulant effects, resulting in bleeding.
Catapres (clonidine)	This combination may result in dangerous elevation of blood pressure and should be avoided.
Quinidine	The combination of Sinequan and quinidine, an antiarrhythmia medication, may increase the risk of arrhythmias and should be avoided.
Depakote, Depakote ER, or Depakene	The combination of Depakote, Depakote ER, or Depakene and Sinequan may elevate Sinequan levels, which may increase the likelihood of side effects.
Anticholinergic agents (e.g., Cogentin, Benadryl)	Anticholinergic side effects may increase when Sinequan is combined with an anticholinergic agent or another medication with anticholinergic side effects.
Antabuse (disulfiram)	The combination of Antabuse and TCAs has been reported to cause a rare but potentially serious reaction called *organic brain syndrome*, which affects mental function.

Antidepressants known as **monoamine oxidase inhibitors** (MAOIs) should not be taken together with Sinequan, because the combination may potentially produce a toxic reaction that includes elevated temperature, high blood pressure, and extreme excitation and agitation. Patients should consult their physician or pharmacist before taking any new medications, including over-the-counter medications and herbal supplements, with Sinequan.

Patients taking Sinequan should avoid alcohol or should consume it in moderation because the combination may worsen depression.

Overdose

Sinequan, like other TCAs, is extremely lethal in acute overdose, especially in children. Overdoses may result in death, especially when the antidepressant is combined with other medications or alcohol. Disturbance of cardiac rhythm is usually the leading cause of death.

Any suspected overdose should be treated as an emergency. The person should be taken to the emergency room for observation and treatment. The prescription bottle of medication (and any other medication suspected in the overdose) should be brought as well, because the information on the prescription label can be helpful to the treating physician in determining the number of pills ingested.

Special Considerations

Most cases of major depression can be treated successfully, usually with medication, psychotherapy, or both. The combination of psychotherapy and antidepressants is very effective in treating moderate to severe depression. The medications improve mood, sleep, energy, and appetite, while therapy strengthens coping skills, deals with possible underlying issues, and improves thought patterns and behavior.

In general, antidepressants alone help about 60%–70% of those taking them. Although a few individuals may experience some improvement from antidepressants by the end of the first week, most people do not see significant benefits from their antidepressants until after 3–4 weeks, and it can sometimes take as long as 8 weeks for the medication to produce its full effects. Thus it is critical that patients continue to take their antidepressant long enough for the medication to be beneficial and that patients not get discouraged and stop their medication prematurely if they do not feel better immediately.

In short-term studies, antidepressants were found to increase the risk of suicidal thinking and behavior in children and adolescents with major depression and other psychiatric disorders. The FDA requires the prescriber to warn of this risk in children and adolescents when starting antidepressant therapy. According to the FDA findings, the risk of suicidal thoughts and behaviors associated with antidepressants is age-related. This phenomenon tends to occur in the younger population and is most likely to occur early in the course of treatment. In adults over 24 years of age, there did not appear to be an increased risk of suicidality with antidepressants compared with placebo. In patients over age 65, the findings showed that antidepressants had a "protective effect" against suicidal thoughts and behavior. Other studies have found that when more people in a community are taking antidepressants, the suicide rate is lower.

The risk of suicide is inherent in depression and may persist until the individual responds to treatment. After starting or changing antidepressant therapy, the person, especially a child or adolescent, should be closely observed for worsening signs of depression, and the family or caregiver should communicate any concerns to the physician.

- **Warning:** Always let your physician or a family member know if you have suicidal thoughts. Notify your psychiatrist or your family physician whenever your depressive symptoms worsen or whenever you feel unable to control suicidal urges or thoughts.
- Do not discontinue Sinequan without consulting your physician. Sinequan should not be stopped abruptly, but gradually tapered down before discontinuation. Abrupt discontinuation of Sinequan may cause nausea, headache, and malaise.
- If you miss a dose, take it as soon as possible. If it is close to the next scheduled dose, skip the missed dose and continue on your regular dosing schedule. Do not take double doses.

- Sinequan may cause significant drowsiness. Until you are certain that your alertness and coordination are not affected by your medication, you should avoid driving and operating machinery.
- If you experience blurred vision, you should avoid driving, operating machinery, or performing potentially hazardous tasks. Consult your physician if you experience blurred vision.
- Do not take Sinequan if you have a known allergy to Sinequan or have experienced a severe reaction to it.
- Store the medication in its originally labeled, light-resistant container, away from heat and moisture. Heat and moisture may precipitate breakdown of your medication, and the medication may lose its therapeutic effects.
- Keep your medication out of reach of children. TCAs are extremely dangerous in acute overdose in young children.

If you have any questions about your medication, consult your physician or pharmacist.

Notes

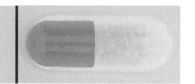

Tofranil and Tofranil-PM (imipramine)

Generic name: Imipramine
Available strengths: 10 mg, 25 mg, 50 mg tablets;
    75 mg, 100 mg, 125 mg, 150 mg capsules (Tofranil-PM)
Available in generic: Yes
Drug class: Tricyclic antidepressant

General Information

Tofranil (imipramine) exerts its antidepressant action principally by inhibiting the reuptake of **serotonin** and, to a lesser extent, **norepinephrine,** two important neurotransmitters in the central nervous system, and thereby boosting neurotransmission. Tofranil also has other pharmacological effects, which are associated with its side effects. Depression and other mental disorders may be due to abnormally low levels of certain neurotransmitters in the brain. This abnormality may in turn produce changes in affected areas of the brain, resulting in psychiatric symptoms such as depression or anxiety. Tofranil exerts its antidepressant action presumably by boosting the levels of serotonin and norepinephrine. There is usually a time lag of 3–4 weeks for antidepressants to achieve their optimal effect, which may be the time needed for the brain to restore normal functioning before reducing the symptoms of the illness.

Tofranil was approved by the U.S. Food and Drug Administration (FDA) for the treatment of depression and for the treatment of bedwetting (enuresis) in children over 6 years of age. The use of a medication for its approved indications is called its *labeled use*. In clinical practice, however, physicians often prescribe medications for *unlabeled* ("off-label") uses when published clinical studies, case reports, or their own clinical experiences support the efficacy and safety of those treatments. Unlabeled uses of Tofranil include treatment of chronic pain syndromes (e.g., migraine headaches, diabetic neuropathy, cancer pain), eating disorders (bulimia nervosa), panic disorder, premenstrual dysphoric disorder, posttraumatic stress disorder, and insomnia, and facilitation of cocaine withdrawal. Physicians may also use Tofranil in combination with another antidepressant, such as a **selective serotonin reuptake inhibitor** (SSRI), to augment the antidepressant effect. This augmentation strategy is often successful in treating refractory depression when response to a single antidepressant is inadequate.

Dosing Information

The recommended starting dosage is 75 mg/day, preferably taken at bedtime. The dosage is increased, as needed, to 150 mg/day in week 2 and may be taken in a single bedtime dose or in divided doses. If depressive symptoms persist, the physician may further increase the dosage up to a maximum of 300 mg/day or switch the patient's medication to another antidepressant. Seniors and adolescents generally require lower dosages of 25–100 mg/day, and dosages greater than 100 mg/day are not recommended for these patients.

Tofranil-PM sustained-release capsules offer the convenience of once-a-day dosing, preferably in the evening or at bedtime. A single dose at bedtime is convenient and will minimize daytime sedation and bothersome anticholinergic side effects. With higher dosages, a single dose of regular Tofranil produces high peak blood levels that may result in more side effects for most people. The sustained-release preparation of Tofranil-PM, however, may improve the tolerability of single daily dosing.

Common Side Effects

Because the tricyclic antidepressants (TCAs) inhibit **cholinergic neurons** in the nervous system, they frequently produce a cluster of symptoms called **anticholinergic** side effects, which include dry mouth and skin, blurred vision, constipation, and difficulty urinating. Usually, individuals become tolerant to these side effects, but excessive anticholinergic effects may lead to confusion and a psychiatric disorder called delirium if not monitored closely. Sometimes the physician may prescribe another medication to counteract the anticholinergic action of the antidepressant. For example, a physician may prescribe a 1% pilocarpine eyedrop to treat blurred vision and bethanechol (e.g., Urecholine), a cholinergic agent, to treat urinary difficulties. For constipation, an over-the-counter stool softener such as Colace (docusate) is usually helpful.

Individuals may experience dizziness from TCAs. Dizziness may be caused by the drugs' effect in momentarily dropping blood pressure; they block the body's compensatory response to maintain a stable blood pressure when a person moves from lying down to a sitting position or from sitting to standing. This reaction is known in medical terms as **orthostatic hypotension.** Seniors and those taking other medications to lower blood pressure may be more susceptible to orthostatic hypotension from these antidepressants.

Weight gain is another common problem. Most individuals gain several pounds while taking TCAs, including Tofranil. If the individual's weight does not stabilize, the physician may switch the patient's medication to one of the newer, weight-neutral antidepressants, such as the SSRIs.

Tofranil may also produce sexual difficulties, including impotence and ejaculatory difficulty in men and decreased sexual drive in both men and women. If this is a problem, the physician may switch the patient's medication to another antidepressant, such as bupropion (Wellbutrin SR or Wellbutrin XL), that does not interfere with sexual functioning.

Adverse Reactions and Precautions

Tofranil may cause significant drowsiness and blurred vision in some people. Patients should not drive, operate machinery, or perform other potentially hazardous tasks until they are certain that their vision, alertness, or coordination is not affected by the medication. Patients with a known allergy to Tofranil or who have experienced a severe reaction after taking it should not take Tofranil.

Tofranil may affect cardiac conduction by slowing the electrical impulses that travel across cardiac tissues, leading to a disturbance in heart rhythms called an arrhythmia. This side effect is common in seniors and in people with a history of arrhythmias or cardiovascular disease. Therefore, patients over 65 years of age and those with a history of heart disease should obtain a pretreatment electrocardiogram and periodic checks (at least annually). Moreover, because of the increased risk of cardiovascular complications and side effects, seniors may not tolerate single daily doses.

As previously stated, seniors and individuals taking medications to lower blood pressure may be susceptible to Tofranil-induced orthostatic hypotension. In such susceptible individuals, the sudden drop in blood pressure from rising too rapidly may cause fainting. To prevent this from occurring, the individual should rise slowly, allowing blood pressure to adjust gradually.

Use in Pregnancy and Breastfeeding: Pregnancy Category D

There have been reports of congenital malformations associated with Tofranil, and thus it is placed in a higher-risk category. The exposure of Tofranil during pregnancy in these women, however, was not confirmed as having a definite association with the defect. TCAs are *not* recommended during pregnancy, especially during the first 3 months. The anticholinergic side effects induced by TCAs may also affect the baby (these effects are known as **fetal anticholinergic syndrome**). Thus, use during pregnancy must be clearly weighed against the potential risk to the developing fetus. Women who are pregnant or may become pregnant should discuss this with their physician. Some women may experience a recurrence of their depression when they stop their antidepressant. In these circumstances it may be necessary to restart the medication or seek an alternative medication or treatment.

Nursing mothers should not take Tofranil, because small amounts will pass into breast milk and be ingested by the baby. If stopping the antidepressant is not an alternative, breastfeeding should not be started or should be discontinued.

Possible Drug Interactions

Combined use of Tofranil with certain medications may result in adverse drug interactions, because one medication may alter the blood levels of the other. The significant drug interactions with Tofranil are summarized below.

Selective serotonin reuptake inhibitors (SSRIs)	The combination of Tofranil and an SSRI may significantly increase the level of Tofranil, resulting in adverse or toxic reactions.
Tegretol (carbamazepine)	The combination of Tofranil and Tegretol may result in decreased levels of Tofranil and may lower its positive pharmacological effects; the combination may also increase Tegretol levels, resulting in more side effects and increased toxicity.
Coumadin (warfarin)	Tofranil may increase Coumadin levels and its anticoagulant effects, resulting in bleeding.
Catapres (clonidine)	The combination of Tofranil and Catapres may result in dangerous elevation of blood pressure and should be avoided.
Quinidine	The combination of Tofranil and quinidine, an antiarrhythmia medication, may increase the risk of arrhythmias and should be avoided.
Depakote, Depakote ER, or Depakene	The combination of Tofranil and Depakote, Depakote ER, or Depakene may elevate Tofranil levels, which may increase the likelihood of side effects.
Anticholinergic agents (e.g., Cogentin, Benadryl)	Anticholinergic side effects may increase when Tofranil is combined with an anticholinergic agent or another medication with anticholinergic side effects.
Antabuse (disulfiram)	The combination of Antabuse and TCAs has been reported to cause a rare but potentially serious reaction called *organic brain syndrome*, which affects mental function.

Antidepressants known as **monoamine oxidase inhibitors** (MAOIs) should not be taken together with Tofranil, because the combination may potentially produce a toxic reaction that includes elevated temperature, high blood pressure, and extreme excitation and agitation. Patients should consult their physician or pharmacist before taking any new medications, including over-the-counter medications and herbal supplements, with Tofranil.

Patients taking Tofranil should avoid alcohol or should consume it in moderation because the combination may worsen depression.

Overdose

Tofranil, like other tricyclic antidepressants (TCAs), is extremely lethal in acute overdose, especially in children. Overdoses may result in death, especially when the antidepressant is combined with other medications or alcohol. Disturbance of cardiac rhythm is usually the leading cause of death.

Any suspected overdose should be treated as an emergency. The person should be taken to the emergency room for observation and treatment. The prescription bottle of medication (and any other medication suspected in the overdose) should be brought as well, because the information on the prescription label can be helpful to the treating physician in determining the number of pills ingested.

Special Considerations

Most cases of major depression can be treated successfully, usually with medication, psychotherapy, or both. The combination of psychotherapy and antidepressants is very effective in treating moderate to severe depression. The medications improve mood, sleep, energy, and appetite, while therapy strengthens coping skills, deals with possible underlying issues, and improves thought patterns and behavior.

In general, antidepressants alone help about 60%–70% of those taking them. Although a few individuals may experience some improvement from antidepressants by the end of the first week, most people do not see significant benefits from their antidepressants until after 3–4 weeks, and it can sometimes take as long as 8 weeks for the medication to produce its full effects. Thus it is critical that patients continue to take their antidepressant long enough for the medication to be beneficial and that patients not get discouraged and stop their medication prematurely if they do not feel better immediately.

In short-term studies, antidepressants were found to increase the risk of suicidal thinking and behavior in children and adolescents with major depression and other psychiatric disorders. The FDA requires the prescriber to warn of this risk in children and adolescents when starting antidepressant therapy. According to the FDA findings, the risk of suicidal thoughts and behaviors associated with antidepressants is age-related. This phenomenon tends to occur in the younger population and is most likely to occur early in the course of treatment. In adults over 24 years of age, there did not appear to be an increased risk of suicidality with antidepressants compared with placebo. In patients over age 65, the findings showed that antidepressants had a "protective effect" against suicidal thoughts and behavior. Other studies have found that when more people in a community are taking antidepressants, the suicide rate is lower.

The risk of suicide is inherent in depression and may persist until the individual responds to treatment. After starting or changing antidepressant therapy, the person, especially a child or adolescent, should be closely observed for worsening signs of depression, and the family or caregiver should communicate any concerns to the physician.

- **Warning:** Always let your physician or a family member know if you have suicidal thoughts. Notify your psychiatrist or your family physician whenever your depressive symptoms worsen or whenever you feel unable to control suicidal urges or thoughts.

- Do not discontinue Tofranil without consulting with your physician. Tofranil should not be stopped abruptly, but gradually tapered down before discontinuation. Abrupt discontinuation of Tofranil may cause nausea, headache, and malaise.
- If you miss a dose, take it as soon as possible. If it is close to the next scheduled dose, skip the missed dose and continue on your regular dosing schedule. Do not take double doses.
- Tofranil may cause significant drowsiness. Until you are certain that your alertness and coordination are not affected by your medication, you should avoid driving and operating machinery.
- If you experience blurred vision, you should avoid driving, operating machinery, or performing potentially hazardous tasks. Consult your physician if you experience blurred vision.
- Do not take Tofranil if you have a known allergy to Tofranil or have experienced a severe reaction to it.
- Store the medication in its originally labeled, light-resistant container, away from heat and moisture. Heat and moisture may precipitate breakdown of your medication, and the medication may lose its therapeutic effects.
- Keep your medication out of reach of children. TCAs are extremely dangerous in acute overdose in young children.

If you have any questions about your medication, consult your physician or pharmacist.

Notes

From Chew RH, Hales RE, Yudofsky SC: *What Your Patients Need to Know About Psychiatric Medications*, Second Edition. Washington, DC, American Psychiatric Publishing, 2009

Monoamine Oxidase Inhibitors

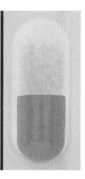

Eldepryl (selegiline)
Emsam (selegiline skin patch)
Marplan (isocarboxazid)
Nardil (phenelzine)
Parnate (tranylcypromine)

The **monoamine oxidase inhibitors** (MAOIs) represent a group of older antidepressants that have limited, but selective, use for treatment of depression. These agents have been replaced by newer and safer agents such as **selective serotonin reuptake inhibitors** (SSRIs) as well as other non-SSRIs such as Wellbutrin (bupropion), Effexor (venlafaxine), and Remeron (mirtazapine) for treating depression. The MAOIs include Marplan (isocarboxazid), Nardil (phenelzine), Parnate (tranylcypromine), and Eldepryl (selegiline), which was developed for treatment of Parkinson's disease rather than depression.

Neurotransmission is the process by which brain cells (neurons) communicate with each other. It starts with an electrical impulse that travels down the nerve cell, causing release of a *neurotransmitter*, such as serotonin, norepinephrine, or dopamine, from the neuron into the space between that neuron and the next neuron, thus allowing the electrical stimulus to continue into the neighboring neuron. The actions of neurotransmitters are terminated primarily by 1) reuptake of neurotransmitters back into neurons and 2) breakdown of neurotransmitters by enzymes prior to reuptake back into the neuron. A type of enzyme that breaks down neurotransmitters is **monoamine oxidase** (MAO), a complex enzyme system widely distributed throughout the body and found in the brain. MAOIs work differently from SSRIs and other antidepressants. They block MAO from breaking down neurotransmitters, resulting in an increase in the neurotransmitter concentration in the space between neurons. The older MAOIs Nardil, Parnate, and Marplan inhibit MAO enzymes nonselectively and irreversibly, whereas Eldepryl is relatively more selective for a specific type of MAO enzyme, and its inhibition is terminated more rapidly once the patient stops taking the medication.

Depression and other mental disorders may be caused by abnormally low levels of certain neurotransmitters in the brain. This abnormality may in turn produce changes in affected areas of the brain, resulting in psychiatric symptoms such as depression or anxiety. When neurotransmission is altered by the antidepressant, the affected brain areas may be restored to normal functioning, decreasing or eliminating the symptoms of the illness.

With many safe and effective antidepressants currently available, the use of MAOIs has been limited to treating refractory and severe forms of depression. Physicians usually prescribe MAOIs when trials with other antidepressants fail. MAOIs may also be used outside their indication for depression. The use of a medication for its approved indications is called its *labeled use*. In clinical practice, however, physicians often prescribe medications for *unlabeled* ("off-label") uses when published clinical studies, case reports, or their own clinical experiences support the efficacy and safety of those treatments. MAOIs, for example, may be prescribed to treat panic disorder, generalized anxiety disorder, specific phobias, posttraumatic stress disorder, and migraine headaches resistant to other therapies. Eldepryl oral tablets are not approved for treatment of depression but are approved by the U.S. Food and Drug Administration (FDA) for treatment of Parkinson's disease, a progressive neurological disease affecting movement and mobility. A selegiline skin patch (Emsam) was recently developed and subsequently was approved for treating depression.

Dosing Information

Nardil and Parnate are the most commonly prescribed MAOIs. The recommended starting dosage for Nardil is 15 mg two or three times a day, with the dosage increasing by 15 mg weekly as needed to a therapeutic range of 45–60 mg/day. The recommended starting dosage of Parnate is 10 mg two or three times a day, with the dosage increasing by 10 mg weekly as needed to a therapeutic range of 40–60 mg/day. Marplan is usually started at a dosage of 20 mg/day, taken in two doses of 10 mg each, and the dosage is increased by 10 mg every 2–4 days to achieve a therapeutic range of 30–60 mg/day.

Common Side Effects

The MAOIs are associated with numerous side effects that often limit their usefulness and tolerability. Potential side effects may be reduced by increasing the dosage slowly or by reducing the dosage. Common side effects associated with MAOIs are daytime sedation, dizziness, dry mouth, altered taste, nervousness, muscle aches, insomnia, weight gain, sexual dysfunction, and urinary difficulty. Sexual side effects induced by MAOIs include anorgasmia (inability to achieve orgasm) and impotency, which are apparently more frequent with Nardil than Parnate. Some patients may be bothered by paresthesia (pricking or tingling sensation). This may be from the MAOI's interference with pyridoxine (vitamin B_6) metabolism. Taking a daily dose of 100 mg of vitamin B_6 may reduce or eliminate these symptoms.

Adverse Reactions and Precautions

The combination of other medications that boost serotonin, such as SSRIs and tricyclic antidepressants, with MAOIs may precipitate a potentially hazardous condition called **serotonin syndrome,** a reaction caused by excessive serotonin stimulation in the brain. The early signs of serotonin syndrome are restlessness, confusion, tremors, flushing, excessive sweating, and involuntary muscle jerks. If the medications are not stopped, the individual may develop more life-threatening complications resulting in severe muscle contractions, high fever, respiratory problems, clotting problems, destruction of red blood cells (that may lead to acute renal failure), coma, and death. Patients taking MAOIs should be alerted to the possible signs of serotonin syndrome, which require immediate medical attention and discontinuation of the serotonin-boosting medications. They should be cautious of any other medications they may take with MAOIs, including over-the-counter medications and herbal supplements.

Dizziness may be caused by MAOIs' effect in momentarily dropping blood pressure. MAOIs block the body's compensatory response to maintain a stable blood pressure when a person moves from lying down to a sitting position or from sitting to standing. This reaction is known in medical terms as **orthostatic hypotension.** Seniors and those taking other medications to lower blood pressure may be particularly susceptible to orthostatic hypotension from MAOIs. Patients should be cautious when rising to their feet suddenly. When lying down, they should get up gradually to a sitting position before standing. If feeling lightheaded or dizzy, they should sit and wait for a minute or two before standing up, to allow the blood pressure to adjust.

Other important precautions for patients taking MAOIs are to avoid foods high in **tyramine** and to restrict certain medications (especially cold and allergy preparations containing decongestants) that may produce dangerously elevated blood pressure and perhaps cause a stroke. Tyramine is a naturally occurring substance derived from the aging process of foods and alcohol. In the intestines, tyramine is metabolized by MAO enzymes before any significant amount is absorbed and distributed in the body. In the presence of MAOIs, tyramine is not broken down and large amounts may get absorbed. High levels of tyramine can suddenly and dangerously elevate blood pressure. Certain medications (and illicit drugs) may interact with MAOIs and elevate blood pressure. When blood pressure becomes dangerously elevated and goes untreated, a *hypertensive crisis* ensues. Food and medication restrictions for patients taking MAOIs are listed in the table below.

Foods that must be avoided	Foods that may be consumed in small amounts, but large amounts may be unsafe	Medications that must be avoided
Aged cheese (cottage and cream cheese are allowed)	Yogurt Chocolate	Cold and allergy medications containing decongestants
Liver (from any animal source), liverwurst	Caffeinated beverages Ripe fruits (e.g., bananas, avocado)	Nasal decongestants and sinus medications
Aged foods, smoked meats (e.g., salami, sausage, salami, pepperoni, and corned beef), smoked fish		Inhalants for bronchial dilatation (e.g., Atrovent)
		Epinephrine (e.g., bee-sting kits)
Beer and red wine		Demerol (meperidine)
Fava or broad bean pods		Stimulants (e.g., appetite suppressants, Ritalin, amphetamine, cocaine)
Meat extracts or yeast extracts (baked goods containing yeasts are safe)		
Soy sauce, tofu, fermented bean curd (found in soybean paste and miso soup)		Levodopa and dopamine medications used to treat Parkinson's disease

Use in Pregnancy and Breastfeeding: Pregnancy Category C

The safety of MAOIs during pregnancy has not been established. However, because of the risk of hypertensive crisis, MAOIs are not recommended during pregnancy. Moreover, when a pregnant woman is taking an MAOI, the potential of drug interactions may preclude use of certain medications or may complicate use of anesthesia during an emergency. Women who are taking an MAOI should always consult their physician if contemplating pregnancy or if they become pregnant. Some women may experience a recurrence of depression when they stop their antidepressant. In these circumstances, the physician will discuss the treatment options with the patient, including continuing to take the MAOI under close surveillance, if necessary.

Women taking MAOIs should not breastfeed, because small amounts will pass into breast milk and be ingested by the baby. If stopping the MAOI is not an alternative, breastfeeding should not be started or should be discontinued.

Possible Drug Interactions

There are numerous possible drug interactions with MAOIs. The interactions of greatest concern are with those drugs that may precipitate a hypertensive crisis or serotonin syndrome when combined with MAOIs; these are listed in the table on the next page.

Demerol (meperidine)	The combination of MAOIs and Demerol may result in agitation, seizures, and fever, which may lead to coma and death. This reaction is possible weeks after the MAOI is stopped.
Anesthetics	MAOIs should be discontinued at least 10 days before elective surgery requiring general anesthesia. Local anesthesia with epinephrine or cocaine should also be avoided.
Antidepressants	MAOIs in combination with another antidepressant, or shortly after beginning any of these agents, may result in a serious serotonin syndrome reaction or hypertensive crisis.
Tegretol (carbamazepine) and Trileptal (oxcarbazepine)	Hypertensive crisis, seizures, and circulatory collapse may ensue with this combination.
Wellbutrin or Zyban (bupropion)	Bupropion in Wellbutrin antidepressants or Zyban (for smoking cessation) should not be combined with an MAOI. The combination may trigger a dangerous reaction.
Dextromethorphan (e.g., Robitussin)	The ingredient dextromethorphan in many cough preparations should not be combined with MAOIs. The combination may be dangerous.
Decongestants	Decongestants such as phenylpropanolamine and pseudoephedrine, commonly found in cold and allergy over-the-counter medications, should not be combined with MAOIs. The combination may precipitate a hypertensive crisis.
Bronchodilators (e.g., Ventolin, Primatene)	The combination of MAOIs and bronchodilators used for breathing should be avoided. The combination may trigger a hypertensive crisis.
Antiparkinson medications (e.g., levodopa, Sinemet)	The combination of these medications may precipitate a hypertensive crisis.
BuSpar (buspirone)	MAOIs should not be combined with BuSpar. There have been reports of elevated blood pressure when BuSpar was added to medication regimens including an MAOI.

Other medications and herbal products that can interact with MAOIs include Flexeril (cyclobenzaprine), diet pills and herbal weight-loss products, St. John's wort, and stimulants, among others.

Overdose

Early signs and symptoms of MAOI overdose include drowsiness, irritability, low blood pressure, restlessness, and breathing difficulties. The person may develop rapid breathing and rapid heart rate, movement disorders, severe headaches, and hypertensive crisis. Convulsions and coma may follow, and death may occur. The severity of symptoms depends on the amount of MAOI ingested and whether other medications are involved.

Any suspected overdose should be treated as an emergency. The person should be taken to the emergency room for observation and treatment. The prescription bottle of medication (and any other medication suspected in the overdose) should be brought as well, because the information on the prescription label can be helpful to the treating physician in determining the number of pills ingested.

Special Considerations

Most cases of major depression can be treated successfully, usually with medication, psychotherapy, or both. The combination of psychotherapy and antidepressants is very effective in treating moderate to severe depression. The medications improve mood, sleep, energy, and appetite, while therapy strengthens coping skills, deals with possible underlying issues, and improves thought patterns and behavior.

In general, antidepressants alone help about 60%–70% of those taking them. Although a few individuals may experience some improvement from antidepressants by the end of the first week, most people do not see significant benefits from their antidepressants until after 3–4 weeks, and it can sometimes take as long as 8 weeks for the medication to produce its full effects. Thus it is critical that patients continue to take their antidepressant long enough for the medication to be beneficial and that patients not get discouraged and stop their medication prematurely if they do not feel better immediately.

In short-term studies, antidepressants were found to increase the risk of suicidal thinking and behavior in children and adolescents with major depression and other psychiatric disorders. The FDA requires the prescriber to warn of this risk in children and adolescents when starting antidepressant therapy. According to the FDA findings, the risk of suicidal thoughts and behaviors associated with antidepressants is age-related. This phenomenon tends to occur in the younger population and is most likely to occur early in the course of treatment. In adults over 24 years of age, there did not appear to be an increased risk of suicidality with antidepressants compared with placebo. In patients over age 65, the findings showed that antidepressants had a "protective effect" against suicidal thoughts and behavior. Other studies have found that when more people in a community are taking antidepressants, the suicide rate is lower.

The risk of suicide is inherent in depression and may persist until the individual responds to treatment. After starting or changing antidepressant therapy, the person, especially a child or adolescent, should be closely observed for worsening signs of depression, and the family or caregiver should communicate any concerns to the physician.

- **Warning:** Always let your physician or a family member know if you have suicidal thoughts. Notify your psychiatrist or your family physician whenever your depressive symptoms worsen or whenever you feel unable to control suicidal urges or thoughts.
- Do not discontinue your MAOI abruptly. The medication should be tapered gradually before completely stopping it.
- If you miss a dose, take it as soon as possible, within 2–3 hours of the scheduled dose. If it is close to the next scheduled dose, skip the missed dose and continue on your regular dosing schedule. Do not take double doses.
- Your MAOI may be taken with or without food.
- It is recommended that you carry an identification card or wear a MedicAlert bracelet to alert health care professionals that you are taking an MAOI. Inform other physicians and your dentist that you are taking an MAOI.
- Avoid foods that are high in tyramine. If you are unsure of the food, avoid it until you check with your physician or pharmacist. Furthermore, even after stopping your MAOI, it takes about 2 weeks before it is safe to resume a regular diet or take certain medications; therefore, it is very important to maintain your dietary and medication restrictions for 2 weeks after discontinuation of your MAOI.
- Store the medication in its originally labeled, light-resistant container, away from heat and moisture. Heat and moisture may precipitate breakdown of your medication, and the medication may lose its therapeutic effects.
- Keep your medication out of reach of children.

If you have any questions about your medication, consult your physician or pharmacist.

Notes

_____

_____

_____

_____

_____

_____

_____

_____

_____

_____

_____

From Chew RH, Hales RE, Yudofsky SC: *What Your Patients Need to Know About Psychiatric Medications*, Second Edition. Washington, DC, American Psychiatric Publishing, 2009

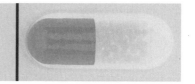

Emsam (selegiline skin patch)

Generic name: Selegiline transdermal patches
Available strengths: 6 mg/24 hr, 9 mg/24 hr,
    12 mg/24 hr
Available in generic: No
Drug class: Antidepressant/monoamine oxidase inhibitor

General Information

Emsam (selegiline) is a **monoamine oxidase inhibitor (MAOI)** antidepressant. It incorporates the antidepressant selegiline in a transdermal delivery system that allows the medication to be absorbed through the skin and into the bloodstream, where it is delivered to the brain for its therapeutic action. The transdermal patch was developed to reduce the serious side effects associated with MAOIs, which limited the usefulness of these medications for the treatment of depression.

The oral MAOIs (Marplan, Nardil, and Parnate) require dietary restriction of foods and drinks that contain high levels of a substance called **tyramine,** which is commonly found in aged cheese, red wine, fava beans, and other products. Monoamine oxidase enzymes in the intestines normally break down tyramine in ingested foods and prevent any appreciable amount from being absorbed into the bloodstream. However, when a patient takes an MAOI and consumes a food or beverage high in tyramine, the normal process of breaking down tyramine by the enzyme is blocked, and tyramine is absorbed into the bloodstream, where it can cause vasoconstriction of blood vessels and severely elevate blood pressure. This adverse reaction is known as a **hypertensive crisis,** which can lead to a stroke and death.

Emsam delivers the MAOI through the skin directly into the bloodstream, bypassing the gut. With less of the MAOI getting into the intestines and interfering with the breakdown of tyramine, there is less danger of a hypertensive crisis. However, the advantage of Emsam over the oral MAOI is only relative: with the lower-dose Emsam patch (6 mg/24 hours), patients do not have to adhere to dietary restrictions; with the 9 mg and 12 mg patches, patients are advised to avoid tyramine-rich foods and beverages, because at these higher strengths, significant amounts of selegiline can get to the gut and interfere with tyramine breakdown.

Dosing Information

The recommended starting and target dosage for Emsam is a 6 mg patch applied every 24 hours. The patch should be applied to the upper torso, the upper thigh, or the outer surface of the upper arm. The full antidepressant effect may not be apparent for up to 2 weeks. If clinical response is inadequate after 2 weeks or an appropriate trial of different duration, your physician may increase Emsam to 9 mg/24 hours. The maximum dose is 12 mg/24 hours.

Patients receiving the 9 mg or 12 mg dose must follow the dietary restrictions mentioned in the previous section (for more information, refer to the handout on monoamine oxidase inhibitors). The patient must start the dietary restrictions on the first day of using the 9 mg or 12 mg patch and continue them for 2 weeks following discontinuation of the higher strengths or after a dose reduction to the 6 mg patch.

Common Side Effects

Common side effects associated with MAOIs are daytime sedation, dizziness, dry mouth, altered taste, nervousness, muscle aches, insomnia, weight gain, sexual dysfunction, and urinary difficulty. Sexual side effects induced by MAOIs include anorgasmia (inability to achieve orgasm) and impotency, which are apparently more frequent with oral MAOIs than with Emsam. Some patients may be bothered by paresthesia (pricking or tingling sensation). With continued therapy, these side effects subside and become less bothersome. With the topical patch, some patients report skin reactions at the site of application that consist of redness and localized rash. In most cases, the local reaction resolves and requires no treatment. If needed, topical hydrocortisone cream 1% may be used.

Adverse Reactions and Precautions

The combination of other medications that boost serotonin, such as selective serotonin reuptake inhibitor (SSRI) antidepressants and tricyclic antidepressants, with Emsam may precipitate a potentially hazardous condition called **serotonin syndrome,** a reaction caused by excessive serotonin stimulation in the brain. The early signs of serotonin syndrome are restlessness, confusion, tremors, flushing, excessive sweating, and involuntary muscle jerks. If the medications are not stopped, the individual may develop more life-threatening complications resulting in severe muscle contractions, high fever, respiratory problems, clotting problems, destruction of red blood cells (that may lead to acute renal failure), coma, and death. Patients taking Emsam should be alerted to the possible signs of serotonin syndrome, which require immediate medical attention and discontinuation of the serotonin-boosting medications.

Emsam must not be combined with products that contain phenylephrine, pseudoephedrine, phenylpropanolamine, and ephedrine, such as cold and cough remedies and weight-reducing preparations. Most of these stimulants have been discontinued in the United States but can still be found in products when traveling abroad. Emsam should not be combined with some pain medications, including Demerol (meperidine), methadone, Darvon (propoxyphene), or Ultram (tramadol). Always consult your physician or pharmacist before taking another medication or herbal supplement with Emsam.

Emsam's effect of momentarily dropping blood pressure may cause dizziness. MAOIs block the body's compensatory response to maintain a stable blood pressure when a person moves from lying down to a sitting position or from sitting to standing. This reaction is known as **orthostatic hypotension.** Seniors and those taking other medications to lower blood pressure may be particularly susceptible to orthostatic hypotension from MAOIs. Patients should be cautious when rising to their feet suddenly. When lying down, they should get up gradually to a sitting position before standing. If feeling lightheaded or dizzy, they should sit and wait for a minute or two before standing up, to allow the blood pressure to adjust.

Patients using 9 mg/24 hours and 12 mg/24 hours dosages must avoid the following foods and beverages:

- Aged cheese (cottage and cream cheese are allowed)
- Liver (from any animal source), liverwurst
- Aged foods, smoked meats (e.g., salami, sausage, pepperoni, and corned beef), smoked fish

- Beer and red wine
- Fava or broad bean pods
- Meat or yeast extracts (baked goods containing yeasts are safe)
- Soy sauce, tofu, fermented bean curd (found in soybean paste and miso soup)

   The following foods may be consumed in small amounts, but large amounts may be unsafe:

- Yogurt
- Chocolate
- Caffeinated beverages
- Ripe fruits (e.g., bananas, avocado)

Use in Pregnancy and Breastfeeding: Pregnancy Category C

The safety of taking Emsam during pregnancy has not been established. However, because of the risk of a hypertensive crisis, Emsam is *not* recommended during pregnancy. Moreover, when a pregnant woman is taking Emsam, the potential of drug interactions may preclude use of certain medications or may complicate use of anesthesia during an emergency. Women who are taking Emsam should always consult their physician if contemplating pregnancy or if they become pregnant. Some women may experience a recurrence of depression when they stop their antidepressant. In these circumstances, the physician will discuss the treatment options with the patient, including continuing to take Emsam under close surveillance, if necessary.

   It is not known if selegiline is excreted in human breast milk. Therefore, it is not recommended that nursing mothers take Emsam. If stopping the drug is not an alternative, breastfeeding should not be started or should be discontinued.

Possible Drug Interactions

There are numerous possible drug interactions with MAOIs. The interactions of greatest concern are with those drugs that may precipitate a hypertensive crisis or serotonin syndrome when combined with MAOIs. Do not take the following medications while using Emsam (for all three strengths) and for 2 weeks after stopping Emsam:

- Other medications used for treating depression, including other MAOIs (Marplan, Nardil, or Parnate), SSRIs, and serotonin-norepinephrine reuptake inhibitors
- Tricyclic antidepressants (e.g., Elavil), which may also be prescribed for pain
- Demerol (meperidine) and other pain medications such as Ultram (tramadol), Darvon and Darvocet (propoxyphene), or methadone
- Tegretol (carbamazepine) and Trileptal (oxcarbazepine) for seizures and mania
- Flexeril (cyclobenzaprine) for muscle spasm
- Cough preparations containing dextromethorphan
- Decongestant preparations containing pseudoephedrine (Sudafed), phenylephrine, phenylpropanolamine, and ephedrine
- Diet pills and herbal weight-loss products
- St. John's wort
- Stimulants, including amphetamines and methylphenidate
- BuSpar (buspirone) for anxiety

   Always consult your physician or pharmacist before taking an over-the-counter medication or herbal supplement while using Emsam.

Overdose

It would be unusual to have an acute overdose with Emsam patches. However, patients should be able to recognize signs and symptoms of an MAOI overdose, which include drowsiness, irritability, low blood pressure, restlessness, and breathing difficulties. The person may develop rapid breathing and rapid heart rate, movement disorders, severe headaches, and hypertensive crisis. Convulsions and coma may follow, and death may occur. The severity of symptoms depends on the amount of MAOI ingested and whether other medications are involved.

Any suspected overdose should be treated as an emergency. The person should be taken to the emergency room for observation and treatment. The prescription bottle of medication (and any other medication suspected in the overdose) should be brought as well, because the information on the prescription label can be helpful to the treating physician in determining the number of pills ingested.

Special Considerations

Most cases of major depression can be treated successfully, usually with medication, psychotherapy, or both. The combination of psychotherapy and antidepressants is very effective in treating moderate to severe depression. The medications improve mood, sleep, energy, and appetite, while therapy strengthens coping skills, deals with possible underlying issues, and improves thought patterns and behavior.

In general, antidepressants alone help about 60%–70% of those taking them. Although a few individuals may experience some improvement from antidepressants by the end of the first week, most people do not see significant benefits from their antidepressants until after 3–4 weeks, and it can sometimes take as long as 8 weeks for the medication to produce its full effects. Thus, it is critical that patients continue to take their antidepressant long enough for the medication to be beneficial and that patients not get discouraged and stop their medication prematurely if they do not feel better immediately.

In short-term studies, antidepressants were found to increase the risk of suicidal thinking and behavior in children and adolescents with major depression and other psychiatric disorders. The U.S. Food and Drug Administration (FDA) requires the prescriber to warn of this risk in children and adolescents when starting antidepressant therapy. According to the FDA findings, the risk of suicidal thoughts and behaviors associated with antidepressants is age-related. This phenomenon tends to occur in the younger population and is most likely to occur early in the course of treatment. In adults over 24 years of age, there did not appear to be an increased risk of suicidality with antidepressants compared with placebo. In patients over age 65, the findings showed that antidepressants had a "protective effect" against suicidal thoughts and behavior. Other studies have found that when more people in a community are taking antidepressants, the suicide rate is lower.

The risk of suicide is inherent in depression and may persist until the individual responds to treatment. After starting or changing antidepressant therapy, the person, especially a child or adolescent, should be closely observed for worsening signs of depression, and the family or caregiver should communicate any concerns to the physician.

- **Warning:** Always let your physician or a family member know if you have suicidal thoughts. Notify your psychiatrist or your family physician whenever your depressive symptoms worsen or whenever you feel unable to control suicidal urges or thoughts.
- Apply Emsam to clean, dry skin on the upper torso (below the neck and above the waist), the upper thigh, or the outer surface of the upper arm. Do not apply to areas of the skin that are hairy, oily, irritated, broken, calloused, or scarred.
- Apply a new patch every 24 hours on a new application site. Wash your hands after application, and do not rub your eyes until after you wash your hands.
- Apply the patch at about the same time each day.

- If you forget to apply a patch at the scheduled time, apply it as soon as possible. However, if it is close to the next scheduled dose, skip the missed dose and continue on your regular dosing schedule. Do not wear more than one patch at a time.
- Do not discontinue Emsam without consulting your physician.
- Inform other physicians and your dentist that you are taking an MAOI.
- When taking the 9 mg or 12 mg patches, avoid foods that are high in tyramine. If you are unsure of the food, avoid it until you check with your physician or pharmacist. Furthermore, even after stopping Emsam, it takes about 2 weeks before it is safe to resume a regular diet or take certain medications. Therefore, it is very important to maintain your dietary and medication restrictions for 2 weeks after discontinuation of Emsam.
- Store the medication in its originally labeled, light-resistant container, away from heat and moisture. Heat and moisture may precipitate breakdown of your medication, and the medication may lose its therapeutic effects.
- Keep your medication out of reach of children.

If you have any questions about your medication, consult your physician or pharmacist.

Notes

Mood Stabilizers

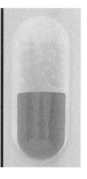

Anticonvulsants

Depakene/Stavzor (valproic acid) and
Depakote/Depakote ER (divalproex sodium)
Equetro, Tegretol, and Tegretol-XR (carbamazepine)
Lamictal (lamotrigine)
Lyrica (pregabalin)
Neurontin (gabapentin)
Topamax (topiramate)
Trileptal (oxcarbazepine)

Lithium Carbonate and Lithium Citrate

Lithium carbonate
Lithium Citrate
Lithobid

Second-Generation Antipsychotics

Abilify (aripiprazole)
Clozaril (clozapine)
Geodon (ziprasidone)
Invega (paliperidone)
Risperdal, Risperdal M-Tab, and Risperdal Consta (risperidone)
Seroquel (quetiapine)
Zyprexa and Zyprexa Zydis (olanzapine)

Simply defined, mood stabilizers are medicines used in treating mood disorders such as bipolar disorder and depression. Bipolar disorder is characterized by mood swings in which the individual cycles between mania and depression. The symptoms fluctuate from euphoria and limitless energy in the manic phase to the depths of depression with little energy, guilt, sadness, decreased concentration, lack of appetite, and sleep disturbance. Because of the wide range of symptoms, from mania to depression, bipolar disorder is often called **manic depression.**

Mood stabilizers are used to treat acute mania, hypomania (a mild form of mania), mixed episodes (when mania and depression coexist in an episode), and depression. Following the acute episode, mood stabilizers are used in maintenance therapy to prevent the cyclical relapse of abnormal mood elevations and depressions. The goals of maintenance treatment with a mood stabilizer are to 1) reduce residual symptoms, 2) prevent manic or depressive relapse, 3) reduce the frequency of cycling into the next manic or depressive episode, 4) improve functioning, and 5) reduce the risk of suicide.

Lithium

Lithium was one of the first mood stabilizers used in the treatment of bipolar disorder. Lithium is a simple ion, not unlike sodium found in table salt (sodium chloride). Lithium comes in two forms—lithium carbonate and lithium citrate. Lithium carbonate is available in immediate- and controlled-release capsules and tablets. Lithium also comes in a liquid preparation in the form of lithium citrate. Over several decades of clinical experience, lithium has been shown to be effective not only in treating mania but also in preventing relapse of mania and depression in bipolar disorder. Lithium was the most important mood stabilizer for many years, but another mood stabilizer—Depakote (divalproex sodium)—has since surpassed lithium for the treatment of bipolar disorder. The reason is that lithium has many troublesome side effects, including nausea, diarrhea, weight gain, and mental sluggishness, and there is a risk of lithium toxicity when the amount of lithium, as measured by serum levels, exceeds its narrow therapeutic range. Monitoring of lithium blood levels is very important to prevent lithium toxicity (for more information, refer to the handout on lithium).

Anticonvulsants as Mood Stabilizers

The introduction of anticonvulsants to the treatment of mood disorders emerged as one of the most significant advances in modern psychiatry. Tegretol (carbamazepine) has been used for more than two decades to treat bipolar disorder without an approved indication for this purpose from the U.S. Food and Drug Administration (FDA). Equetro (carbamazepine) is FDA-approved for the treatment of acute manic and mixed episodes associated with bipolar disorder. Depakote and Depakote ER (divalproex), Stavzor (valproic acid), and Lamictal (lamotrigine) are approved by the FDA for the treatment of seizures and of acute manic episodes associated with bipolar disorder. The other anticonvulsants are indicated primarily for treatment of epilepsy. The use of a medication for its approved indications is called its *labeled use*. In clinical practice, however, physicians often prescribe medications for *unlabeled* ("off-label") uses when published clinical studies, case reports, or their own clinical experiences support the efficacy and safety of those treatments. Based on a number of clinical studies, some medications with anti-epileptic properties are also effective for treating bipolar disorder, despite the lack of an FDA-approved indication for this purpose.

Some may wonder why an anticonvulsant that is effective for controlling seizures also works for bipolar disorder. How is this paradox explained? The application of anticonvulsants in psychiatry was due in part to serendipity. With certain types of epilepsy, individuals sometimes manifest psychiatric symptoms, including hallucinations, agitation, and changes in mood. When such patients were treated with phenytoin (Dilantin), an anticonvulsant, their seizures, as well as their psychiatric symptoms, were stabilized. These observations spurred clinical investigations of other anticonvulsants, including carbamazepine and valproic acid (and valproate), to determine if they also offered benefits in treating mood disorders. A number of clinical studies have shown that Depakote, Lamictal, and carbamazepine are effective for bipolar disorder.

It is not clear why some anticonvulsants are effective for seizures and bipolar disorder. The anticonvulsants, which have very complex effects on the central nervous system, may be effective by controlling "kindling" in the areas of the brain from which the psychiatric disorder emanates. Kindling is a phenomenon that occurs when repeated subthreshold stimulation is applied to certain regions of the brain and sensitizes them, setting off a cascade of events leading to seizures or manic behavior. By decreasing electrical conduction or neurotransmitter activity in unstable brain cells, anticonvulsants are effective in controlling seizures and bipolar illness.

Second-Generation Antipsychotics as Mood Stabilizers

Antipsychotics are frequently prescribed in combination with a mood stabilizer, such as lithium or Depakote, to treat acute mania. An antipsychotic is helpful for rapidly reducing mania, especially during the interval of time until the mood stabilizer, which has a slower onset of action, takes effect. Generally, the psychiatrist would discontinue the antipsychotic after mania abates, maintaining mood stabilization with the mood stabilizer alone. This was the conventional practice when only the older, first-generation antipsychotics—for example, chlorpromazine, fluphenazine, Haldol (haloperidol), and thioridazine—were available. The long-term use of conventional antipsychotics was not advisable then because the older agents were associated with significant risks of **tardive dyskinesia** (disabling, late-onset movement disorders) and **extrapyramidal symptoms,** which are side effects that affect coordination and movement. Moreover, the conventional agents can exacerbate depressive symptoms in some patients.

The strategy of only using antipsychotics for short-term to treat bipolar disorders changed when the newer, second-generation antipsychotics became available. These antipsychotics have significantly reduced the risk of tardive dyskinesia and extrapyramidal symptoms and have fewer of the bothersome side effects commonly seen with the conventional agents. Furthermore, they appear to have a wider spectrum of therapeutic activity than the conventional agents. They can do more than just reduce mania; they appear to have mood-stabilizing properties and can prevent relapse when used in maintenance therapy. Zyprexa (olanzapine), Seroquel (quetiapine), and Abilify (aripiprazole) are the second-generation antipsychotics approved by the FDA for both acute mania and maintenance therapy for relapse prevention in bipolar illness. The others are also effective antimanic agents, but it is not clear whether they also possess mood-stabilizing properties for long-term maintenance therapy. Furthermore, the FDA recently approved use of Risperdal (risperidone) and Abilify for treatment of bipolar illness in children and adolescents 10–17 years of age; however, Risperdal is approved for use only in acute episodes, whereas Abilify is indicated for acute and maintenance treatment of bipolar disorder. (Handouts for these antipsychotics can be found in "Second-Generation Antipsychotics.")

For more information about a particular mood stabilizer, refer to the handout for that medication.

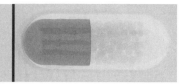

Depakene/Stavzor (valproic acid) Depakote/Depakote ER (divalproex sodium)

Generic name: Valproic acid (Depakene, Stavzor),
divalproex sodium (Depakote, Depakote ER)
Available strengths: **Valproic acid:** 250 mg capsule (Depakene);
125 mg, 250 mg, 500 mg delayed-release capsules (Stavzor);
250 mg/5 mL liquid (Depakene Liquid);
Divalproex sodium: 125 mg sprinkle capsule (Depakote Sprinkle);
125 mg, 250 mg, 500 mg delayed-release tablets (Depakote);
250 mg, 500 mg extended-release tablets (Depakote ER)
Available in generic: Yes, except Depakote ER, Depakote Sprinkle,
and Stavzor
Drug class: Anticonvulsant/mood stabilizer

General Information

Valproic acid (Depakene and Stavzor) and **divalproex sodium (Depakote and Depakote ER)** are similar medicines. Divalproex sodium is produced by modification of valproic acid. Although these medicines are commonly known for their use as anticonvulsants (i.e., for seizures), they are effective for treating other conditions as well. Besides treatment of seizures, Stavzor, Depakote, and Depakote ER are approved by the U.S. Food and Drug Administration (FDA) for treatment of manic episodes associated with bipolar disorder; Stavzor and Depakote ER also have indications for prophylaxis of migraine headaches. When Depakote, Stavzor, and Depakote ER are used for treating bipolar disorder, they are known as *mood stabilizers*.

Although divalproex sodium comes in many dosage forms, valproic acid is the active medication. All the different preparations are converted in the body to valproic acid. Depakene is the brand of immediate-release valproic acid, which is available in generic, and comes only in a 250 mg gel capsule and in liquid. Stavzor is the delayed-release formulation of valproic acid. Depakote and Depakote ER are formulations of valproic acid that give delayed and extended action, respectively.

Depakote tablets may be administered twice daily. Divalproex sodium is also available in a Depakote Sprinkle capsule, which can be opened and sprinkled over food. Depakote ER tablets are extended-release tablets for once-a-day dosing.

Clinical studies have shown that valproic acid and lithium are equally effective in treating acute mania and preventing relapse of bipolar disorder. Valproic acid is more effective in treating mixed episodes (characterized by both mania and depression coexisting in the same episode) and rapid-cycling types of bipolar disorder (when the person experiences four or more manic or major depressive episodes in 1 year). Because Depakote, Depakote ER, and Stavzor are better tolerated and less toxic than lithium, they are generally preferred for treating bipolar disorder.

When all the valproic acid formulations are being referred to, the brand name Depakote is used for convenience in this handout, but the discussion applies to the other derivatives of valproic acid as well.

Dosing Information

For treatment of acute mania, the usual starting dosage of Depakote is 500 mg twice a day, with the dosage increasing by 250 mg/day every 3–4 days until a therapeutic level is reached. Generally, the required dosage for treating acute mania is between 1,000 and 3,000 mg/day. Depakote may be switched to once-a-day dosing with Depakote ER.

The dosing of Stavzor for acute mania is similar to that of Depakote. The recommended starting dosage is 750 mg daily taken in divided doses. The dosage is increased as rapidly as needed to manage symptoms.

Common Side Effects

The most common side effects from Depakote are sedation, tiredness, and gastrointestinal symptoms, including nausea, cramping, and diarrhea. Shifting all or most of the dosage close to bedtime may decrease daytime sedation. The enteric-coated tablets of Depakote and Depakote ER are associated with fewer gastrointestinal side effects than with Depakene capsule or syrup.

Patients taking Depakote may experience tremor, impaired coordination, and clumsiness when walking (**ataxia**). Generally, these side effects are temporary and subside as tolerance to the medication develops. Some patients may experience hair loss (**alopecia**) while taking Depakote, which may be due to the medication's interference with zinc and selenium absorption. Taking a daily multivitamin with minerals containing zinc and selenium may stop and prevent hair loss. Depakote may induce significant weight gain. Patients taking Depakote should follow a sensible diet and exercise routinely to control their weight.

Adverse Reactions and Precautions

Depakote may cause drowsiness and impair alertness, especially at the start of therapy. Patients should use caution when driving or performing tasks that require alertness.

Due to reported cases of liver failure in patients taking Depakote, the FDA required manufacturers to issue a stern warning of potential liver toxicity in its labeling requirements. It appears that the risk is greatest in children younger than 2 years of age, and the risk declines significantly in adults. Because it is impossible to predict when liver toxicity will occur, liver function tests are recommended before treatment and every 6 months thereafter. Although liver toxicity is rare, patients should be aware of the potential risk and should be encouraged to report early symptoms of possible liver disease to their physician, including loss of appetite, tiredness, nausea, and yellowing of skin and eyes (**jaundice**).

Another potentially rare adverse reaction to Depakote is pancreatitis. Cases of life-threatening pancreatitis, which may occur shortly after starting therapy or after several years of use, have been reported in children and adults who were taking Depakote. Early warning symptoms of pancreatitis include severe abdominal pain, loss of appetite, nausea, and vomiting. The patient should seek immediate medical attention if these symptoms occur.

Depakote may cause a decrease in platelets (**thrombocytopenia**), which are routinely measured when the physician orders a complete blood count. If this condition occurs, generally the decrease in platelets is mild and has little or no clinical consequence. In rare instances, Depakote may significantly lower platelets and result in clotting dysfunction and bleeding.

Use in Pregnancy and Breastfeeding: Pregnancy Category D

Among women who took Depakote during the first trimester of pregnancy, a higher incidence of spinal cord defect (**spina bifida**) and abnormal brain development in their children has been found. Women should not receive Depakote if they are pregnant, or the medication should be discontinued if they plan to become pregnant. However, if the woman is prone to relapse, which may pose greater harm to the mother and unborn child if Depakote is discontinued, the physician may consider maintaining the medication with the patient's consent. The risk of birth defects from Depakote may be reduced if the mother takes 1 mg of folic acid, a B vitamin, daily during pregnancy. Use of Depakote should be restricted whenever possible to the second and third trimesters.

Nursing mothers should not take Depakote or other valproic acid preparations, because it is excreted in breast milk and may be harmful to the baby when ingested. If stopping the drug is not an alternative, breastfeeding should not be started or should be discontinued.

Possible Drug Interactions

Depakote can affect the liver enzymes that metabolize different medications and may reduce their metabolism, thus increasing their concentrations—and their adverse effects. Conversely, other medications can inhibit the metabolism of Depakote and increase its concentration in the blood. The clinically significant drug interactions reported with Depakote are summarized in the table below.

Tagamet (cimetidine), erythromycin, Prozac (fluoxetine), Luvox (fluvoxamine), phenothiazine antipsychotics (e.g., chlorpromazine and thioridazine), nonsteroidal anti-inflammatory medications (e.g., Motrin, aspirin)	When any of these medications are combined with Depakote, the medication may inhibit the metabolism of Depakote and increase Depakote levels.
Tegretol (carbamazepine), phenobarbital, Dilantin (phenytoin), Zarontin (ethosuximide), and rifampin	When any of these medications are combined with Depakote, Depakote levels may be decreased, leading to decreased effectiveness of Depakote.
Lamictal (lamotrigine)	Depakote may increase the blood levels of Lamictal, which can increase the risk of a potentially severe rash. When these two medications are used together, Lamictal dosages are increased very gradually.
Coumadin (warfarin)	The effects of Coumadin, an anticoagulant, may be increased when combined with Depakote, which may increase the risk of bleeding.

Patients taking Depakote should not consume alcohol because the combination may increase sedation and drowsiness. Moreover, the sedative effects of alcohol may act as a depressant, obscuring the therapeutic effects of Depakote and complicating treatment.

Overdose

Overdose with Depakote may be fatal, depending on the amount ingested and the age and size of the person. In seniors, for example, the lethal dose is lower than that for younger adults. Symptoms include somnolence, confusion, seizures, heart block, and coma. Depakote overdose may cause significant respiratory depression, which is often fatal if medical treatment is not immediate.

Any suspected overdose should be treated as an emergency. The person should be taken to the emergency room for observation and treatment. The prescription bottle of medication (and any other medication suspected in the overdose) should be brought as well, because the information on the prescription label can be helpful to the treating physician in determining the number of pills ingested.

Special Considerations

- If you miss a dose, take it as soon as possible, within 2–3 hours of the scheduled dose. If it is close to the next scheduled dose, skip the missed dose and continue on your regular dosing schedule. Do not take double doses.
- Depakote ER, the extended-release form, is intended for once-a-day dosing. Swallow the tablets whole and do not crush or chew them. If stomach upset occurs, take Depakote after meals or with food.
- Contact your physician if you have persistent abdominal symptoms, including pain, loss of appetite, nausea, vomiting, and jaundice.
- Depakote may cause sedation and drowsiness, especially during initiation of therapy, and impair your alertness. Use caution when driving or performing tasks that require alertness.
- Store the medication in its originally labeled, light-resistant container, away from heat and moisture. Heat and moisture may precipitate breakdown of your medication, and the medication may lose its therapeutic effects.
- Keep your medication out of reach of children, because overdose in small children is very dangerous.

If you have any questions about your medication, consult your physician or pharmacist.

Notes

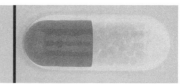

Equetro, Tegretol, and Tegretol-XR (carbamazepine)

Generic name: Carbamazepine
Available strengths: 100 mg (chewable), 200 mg tablets;
    100 mg/5 mL oral suspension;
    100 mg, 200 mg, 400 mg extended-release tablets
    (Tegretol-XR); 100 mg, 200 mg, 300 mg extended-release
    capsules (Equetro)
Available in generic: Yes, except Equetro and Tegretol-XR
Drug class: Anticonvulsant/mood stabilizer

General Information

Carbamazepine is better known for its use as an anticonvulsant—a medication for treating epilepsy. This may present some confusion for patients, as well as their families, when they are prescribed carbamazepine without a history of seizures. Although carbamazepine is approved by the U.S. Food and Drug Administration (FDA) for the treatment of epilepsy and nerve pain (trigeminal neuralgia), only the brand Equetro, an extended-release capsule form of carbamazepine, has been given an official approval for treatment of acute mania associated with bipolar disorder. However, carbamazepine has many uses other than its approved indications. The use of a medication for its approved indications is called its *labeled use*. In clinical practice, however, physicians often prescribe medications for *unlabeled* ("off-label") uses when published clinical studies, case reports, or their own clinical experiences support the efficacy and safety of those treatments. Carbamazepine, for example, may be used off-label for treating alcohol withdrawal, bipolar depression, certain symptoms associated with personality disorder, and other conditions. Physicians frequently use Tegretol, Tegretol-XR, and generic carbamazepine interchangeably for treatment of bipolar disorder.

Clinical studies have shown the effectiveness of carbamazepine for treating acute mania. Carbamazepine may also be effective in maintenance therapy to prevent relapse of mania. In treatment-resistant bipolar disorder, patients usually do better when carbamazepine is used in combination with another mood stabilizer, such as lithium. For some patients with rapid-cycling bipolar illness (those with four or more manic or major depressive episodes a year), carbamazepine alone or in combination with another mood stabilizer may be more effective for stabilizing from frequent cycling.

Dosing Information

The starting dosage of carbamazepine in treatment of bipolar disorder is 200 mg twice a day. The dosage is normally increased by 200 mg/day every 3–5 days. The therapeutic dosage depends on attaining a therapeutic blood level. Generally, the dosage range is 400–1,200 mg/day. Blood levels of carbamazepine should be monitored weekly for the first 4 weeks to ensure that adequate levels are achieved to produce the therapeutic response. Although therapeutic levels are attained with a given dosage, in about 2–4 weeks the levels may drop off significantly. This is due to carbamazepine's ability to speed up its own metabolism. The patient's dosage may need to be increased again to achieve the desired therapeutic level.

Carbamazepine is also available in extended-release capsule (Equetro) and tablet (Tegretol-XR) preparations, which require only once-a-day dosing. Carbamazepine also comes in a liquid preparation in a concentration of 100 mg/5 mL.

Common Side Effects

The most common side effects from carbamazepine are sedation, tiredness, nausea, and dizziness. At higher dosages, patients may experience jerky eye movements (**nystagmus**) or double vision (**diplopia**) and impaired coordination or clumsiness. Generally, these side effects are temporary and subside as tolerance to the medication develops.

Adverse Reactions and Precautions

Carbamazepine may cause drowsiness and impair alertness, especially at the start of therapy. Patients should use caution when driving or performing tasks that require alertness.

Agranulocytosis and **aplastic anemia** are very rare but serious—potentially fatal—adverse reactions from carbamazepine. Agranulocytosis presents with a sudden drop in the concentration of white blood cells (**leukopenia**). When a particular type of white blood cells (**granulocytes**), which are important for fighting infections, are severely decreased (**agranulocytosis,** or without granulocytes), the individual is susceptible to life-threatening infections. The risk of carbamazepine-induced agranulocytosis is very low. When detected early and with carbamazepine discontinued, patients recover completely. Early warning signs of infection, including sore throat, fever, and malaise, should be brought to the attention of the physician.

The risk of agranulocytosis may increase when carbamazepine is taken in combination with other medications that potentiate this risk. For example, carbamazepine should not be taken with Clozaril (clozapine), because the combination may increase the risk of agranulocytosis.

Another rare and potentially fatal adverse reaction is aplastic anemia, a condition in which the bone marrow stops producing blood cells, including platelets (important for clotting), white blood cells, and red blood cells. The risk of aplastic anemia from carbamazepine, however, is very rare. If it occurs, the individual may develop infections because of low white cells, anemia because of low red blood cells, and bleeding abnormalities because of low platelets. Some physicians may order a pretreatment complete blood count and repeat the test periodically, but many do not because carbamazepine-induced aplastic anemia is so rare. Instead, the physician will instruct the patient to report intractable infections, frequent bruising, frequent bleeding tendencies (e.g., bleeding of the gums from brushing teeth), and prolonged bleeding time.

Occasionally, carbamazepine causes mild elevation in liver enzyme levels, but there is rarely liver damage. The liver enzyme elevation is usually transient, and levels eventually return to normal. However, closer monitoring of liver function is warranted when liver enzyme levels are elevated. Discontinuation of carbamazepine may be necessary if liver enzyme levels increase to three times normal.

Use in Pregnancy and Breastfeeding: Pregnancy Category D

Carbamazepine crosses the placenta and may cause harm to the fetus. Cases of newborns with head and facial abnormalities, developmental delays, and spinal cord defects (**spina bifida**) have been reported in women who took carbamazepine during pregnancy. The risk appears to be highest when carbamazepine is taken in the first trimester. The use of carbamazepine should therefore be avoided in pregnancy whenever possible, especially in the first trimester. However, when carbamazepine is stopped and reoccurrence of mania occurs, the physician may discuss the need to restart carbamazepine after the first trimester or seek an alternative medication or treatment.

Nursing mothers should not take carbamazepine, because it is excreted in breast milk and may be harmful to the baby when ingested. If stopping the drug is not an alternative, breastfeeding should not be started or should be discontinued.

Possible Drug Interactions

Carbamazepine can affect the liver enzymes that metabolize many different medications, including carbamazepine itself, thus lowering the medications' concentration and diminishing their effectiveness. Conversely, other medications can also hinder the metabolism of carbamazepine and increase its levels. The clinically significant drug interactions reported with carbamazepine are summarized in the table below.

Tagamet (cimetidine), Prozac (fluoxetine), Luvox (fluvoxamine), Depakote (divalproex), erythromycin, Biaxin (clarithromycin), Calan (verapamil), Cardizem (diltiazem), Nizoral (ketoconazole), Diflucan (fluconazole), Sporanox (itraconazole), Darvon (propoxyphene), isoniazid (e.g., INH), and grapefruit juice	These medications, when combined with carbamazepine, can increase the blood levels of carbamazepine to toxic levels. Dosages of these medications may need to be lowered when the medications are used in combination with carbamazepine.
Oral contraceptives, Coumadin (warfarin), Dilantin (phenytoin), theophylline, Plendil (felodipine), benzodiazepines (e.g., Valium), Doryx (doxycycline), Haldol (haloperidol), phenothiazines (e.g., thioridazine), Wellbutrin (bupropion), and cyclosporine	When carbamazepine is combined with these medications, it can lower their blood levels and decrease their effectiveness. For example, decreased effectiveness of an oral contraceptive may lead to an unintended pregnancy.

Patients taking carbamazepine should not consume alcohol because the combination may increase sedation and drowsiness. Moreover, the sedative effects of alcohol may act as a depressant, obscuring the therapeutic effects of carbamazepine and complicating treatment.

Overdose

Carbamazepine overdose is extremely hazardous, and the severity of toxic symptoms depends on the amount ingested. In small children the lethal dose is much lower than for adults. Early symptoms of carbamazepine toxicity include neuromuscular disturbances, such as jerky eye movements (**nystagmus**), muscle jerks (**myoclonus**), increased reflex reactions (**hyperreflexia**), and severe nausea and vomiting. Symptoms of higher overdose, including respiratory depression, convulsions, cardiac arrhythmia, shock, and coma, may result in death, especially in small children.

Any suspected overdose should be treated as an emergency. The person should be taken to the emergency room for observation and treatment. The prescription bottle of medication (and any other medication suspected in the overdose) should be brought as well, because the information on the prescription label can be helpful to the treating physician in determining the number of pills ingested.

Special Considerations

- If you miss a dose, take it as soon as possible, within 2–3 hours of the scheduled dose. If it is close to the next scheduled dose, skip the missed dose and continue on your regular dosing schedule. Do not take double doses.
- Take carbamazepine immediately after meals or with food to decrease stomach upset.
- Contact your physician if you have persistent symptoms of infection, including fever, sore throat, or malaise, and unusual signs of bleeding or bruising.
- Carbamazepine may cause sedation and drowsiness, especially during initiation of therapy, and impair your alertness. Use caution when driving or performing tasks that require alertness.
- Store the medication in its originally labeled, light-resistant container, away from heat and moisture. Heat and moisture may precipitate breakdown of your medication, and the medication may lose its therapeutic effects.
- Keep your medication out of reach of children, because overdose in small children is very dangerous.

If you have any questions about your medication, consult your physician or pharmacist.

Notes

_____

_____

_____

_____

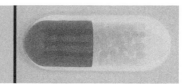

Lithium Carbonate and Lithium Citrate

Available strengths: 150 mg, 300 mg, 600 mg capsules;
   300 mg tablet; 300 mg extended-release tablet (Lithobid)
   and 450 mg extended-release tablet;
   300 mg/5 mL syrup (Lithium citrate)
Available in generic: Yes
Drug class: Mood stabilizer

General Information

Lithium has been the standard treatment for bipolar disorder for a number of years and was one of the first mood stabilizers used in the treatment of mood disorders. Over several decades of clinical experience, it has become evident that lithium is effective not only in treating mania but also in preventing relapse of mania and depression in bipolar disorder. Lithium is also used to augment antidepressant therapy when treatment of depression is unsuccessful with antidepressants alone. This augmentation of an antidepressant with lithium is often effective for treating refractory depression as well as preventing depressive relapse.

Lithium is a simple ion, not unlike sodium found in table salt (sodium chloride). It is available in the salt form as lithium carbonate and in a liquid preparation as lithium citrate. Lithium carbonate is also available in a controlled-release preparation (Lithobid), which may help reduce many of the gastrointestinal side effects associated with lithium.

It is interesting how a simple ion like lithium has such complex action in the brain. Lithium's actions in mood stabilization are probably the result of complex actions on different neurotransmitter systems in the brain. Lithium appears to stabilize the balance between excitatory and inhibitory effects of different neurons and their neurotransmitters. Bipolar disorder may be conceptualized as overactivation of neurons and neuronal systems. Mania may be the result of the excitatory neuronal system being overactivated, and conversely, overactivation of the inhibitory neural system may result in depression. Lithium's ability to dampen these neural systems may explain its effectiveness in mania and depression.

Dosing Information

Lithium therapy must be carefully monitored with laboratory tests because of its potential for toxicity. Before starting therapy, it is important for the patient's renal function to be determined, because the kidneys primarily eliminate lithium. The dosage must be adjusted for individuals with reduced renal function. Lithium levels are measured routinely to determine if adequate plasma levels are achieved with the specific dosage. When clinical response is achieved, lithium levels are generally in the range of 0.7–1.2 mEq/L (milliequivalents per liter). However, lithium has a narrow therapeutic window, and when serum levels exceed 1.5 mEq/L, lithium toxicity is a concern.

In acute mania, higher dosages are usually necessary for optimal response. One strategy is starting with 300 mg twice a day and increasing by 300 mg/day every 3–5 days until manic symptoms abate and if lithium has not reached toxic levels. Dosages may vary from 600 to 1,800 mg/day depending on the patient's size, age, and kidney function. Once the patient's mania is in remission, the goal is to prevent relapse with maintenance therapy. The maintenance dosage may be lowered so that the patient may better tolerate the medication and continue to take lithium on a long-term basis.

Common Side Effects

Gastrointestinal side effects are the most frequent side effects associated with taking lithium, including dry mouth, nausea, diarrhea, vomiting, abdominal cramping, indigestion, bloated feeling, and excessive salivation. Stomach upset may be avoided by taking lithium immediately after meals or with food. Other side effects related to lithium therapy include drowsiness and mental sluggishness, fine tremors of fingers, drying and thinning of hair, skin rash, exacerbation of acne and psoriasis, frequent urination, thirst, and weight gain. Generally, many of these side effects subside as the patient develops tolerance to lithium, or the side effect may be managed by lowering the dosage.

Adverse Reactions and Precautions

Lithium may cause drowsiness and impair alertness, especially at the start of therapy. Patients should use caution when driving or performing tasks that require alertness.

Lithium Toxicity

There is a narrow margin between the therapeutic and toxic levels of lithium. Close monitoring of lithium levels is important. Early symptoms of lithium toxicity include drowsiness, diarrhea, nausea, vomiting, dizziness, muscle weakness, and impaired coordination. At higher lithium levels, toxic symptoms include dizziness, ringing in the ears (**tinnitus**), slurred speech, increasing confusion, blurred vision, inability to coordinate movements (**ataxia**), twitching of facial muscles and limbs, and urinary and fecal incontinence. At very toxic levels, there is danger of death resulting from seizures, acute renal failure, cardiac arrhythmias, low blood pressure, cardiovascular collapse, and delirum. Thus, early recognition and intervention are important to reverse lithium toxicity. When the aforementioned symptoms develop, the patient should interrupt lithium therapy and contact his or her physician as soon as possible.

It is important to keep in mind that the kidneys excrete lithium, and interference with its elimination may increase lithium to toxic levels. In patients with renal disease, excretion of lithium may be significantly compromised. The dosage must be adjusted lower to compensate for reduced renal function. With dehydration, a low-salt diet, or taking lithium with thiazide diuretics, the kidneys reabsorb lithium back into the body more intensely, which results in high lithium levels and frequently causes toxicity. Dehydration can result from inadequate fluid intake, especially on hot days with excessive physical exertion and from fever and diarrhea.

Hypothyroidism

Long-term lithium therapy may affect the thyroid glands and diminish thyroid function (**hypothyroidism**). A common laboratory test used to measure thyroid function is to obtain a **thyroid-stimulating hormone (TSH)** level. TSH is a hormone that stimulates the function of the thyroid glands. An elevated TSH level in the presence of clinical symptoms is indicative of hypothyroidism. Clinical signs and symptoms of hypothyroidism may include enlarged thyroid glands, tiredness, intolerance to cold, low energy, and depression. Lithium-induced hypothyroidism may be reversed when the medication is discontinued or if the patient receives supplemental thyroid hormone.

Abnormal Electrocardiogram

Lithium may affect the electrical conduction in the heart and thus the rhythm of the heart. It may induce changes that show up on the electrocardiogram. Although most people taking lithium experience no change in cardiac function, the physician may order a pretreatment electrocardiogram for seniors or for those who have a history of cardiovascular disease.

Impairment of Kidneys to Concentrate Urine

Infrequently, chronic lithium administration is associated with impairment of the concentrating ability of the kidneys (**nephrogenic diabetes insipidus**). As a result, the individual is unusually thirsty and must drink copious amounts of water, which is lost through frequent urination because the kidneys cannot reabsorb and conserve the body's water. Fortunately, this disorder can be reversed when lithium is decreased or discontinued.

Use in Pregnancy and Breastfeeding: Pregnancy Category D

Lithium crosses the placenta and may cause harm to the fetus. Cases of newborns with cardiac abnormalities have been reported in women who took lithium during pregnancy. The risk appears to be highest when lithium is taken in the first trimester. The use of lithium should be avoided in pregnancy whenever possible, especially in the first trimester. However, when lithium is stopped, reoccurrence of mania may be harmful for the mother and unborn child. In these circumstances, the physician may discuss the need to restart lithium after the first trimester or seek an alternative medication or treatment.

Nursing mothers should not take lithium, because it is excreted in breast milk and may be harmful to the baby when ingested. If stopping the drug is not an alternative, breastfeeding should not be started or should be discontinued.

Possible Drug Interactions

Some medications when taken concomitantly with lithium may result in drug interactions that alter their levels, which may produce undesired reactions. The clinically significant drug interactions reported with lithium are summarized in the table on the next page.

Patients taking lithium should not consume alcohol because the combination may make some side effects worse. For example, drinking excessive alcohol can cause dehydration, and this may increase lithium to toxic blood levels. Moreover, the sedative effects of alcohol may act as a depressant, obscuring the therapeutic effects of lithium and complicating treatment.

Thiazide diuretics	Thiazide diuretics (e.g., hydrochlorothiazide, Zaroxolyn) may increase lithium serum levels and induce toxicity.
Haldol (haloperidol)	The combination of Haldol and lithium may increase neurotoxic effects despite normal lithium and Haldol levels.
Loop diuretics (e.g., Lasix)	Loop diuretics such as Lasix (furosemide) may increase levels of lithium and induce toxicity. This interaction is less likely with loop diuretics than with thiazide diuretics.
Potassium iodide	Concurrent use of potassium iodide (used as an expectorant) and lithium may increase the risk of hypothyroidism.

Overdose

Lithium overdose is extremely hazardous, and the severity of toxic symptoms increases with increasing lithium levels. When serum lithium levels are between 1.5 and 2.0 mEq/L, common symptoms include diarrhea, nausea, vomiting, dizziness, muscle weakness, and impaired coordination. As the levels increase greater than 2.0 mEq/L, symptoms may include dizziness, ringing in the ears, slurred speech, increasing confusion and disorientation, blurred vision, inability to coordinate movements, twitching of facial muscles and limbs, and urinary and fecal incontinence. When levels reach 3.0 mEq/L and higher, complications may include seizures, acute renal failure, cardiac arrhythmias, low blood pressure, cardiovascular collapse, and delirum, with a high risk of mortality.

Any suspected overdose should be treated as an emergency. The person should be taken to the emergency room for observation and treatment. In severe cases, hemodialysis may be indicated. The prescription bottle of medication (and any other medication suspected in the overdose) should be brought as well, because the information on the prescription label can be helpful to the treating physician in determining the number of pills ingested.

Special Considerations

- It is important to understand that after your manic symptoms abate, you will need to continue taking your medication to prevent relapse.
- If you miss a dose, take it as soon as possible, within 2–3 hours of the scheduled dose. If it is close to the next scheduled dose, skip the missed dose and continue on your regular dosing schedule. Do not take double doses.
- Take lithium immediately after meals or with food to decrease stomach upset.
- Drink plenty of water or liquid to prevent dehydration, especially from prolonged exposure to hot weather.
- Contact your physician if you have fever or diarrhea.
- Lithium may cause drowsiness and impair alertness, especially at the start of therapy. Patients should use caution when driving or performing tasks that require alertness.
- Store the medication in its originally labeled, light-resistant container, away from heat and moisture. Heat and moisture may precipitate breakdown of your medication, and the medication may lose its therapeutic effects.
- Keep your medication out of reach of children.

If you have any questions about your medication, consult your physician or pharmacist.

Notes

_____

_____

_____

_____

_____

_____

_____

_____

_____

_____

From Chew RH, Hales RE, Yudofsky SC: *What Your Patients Need to Know About Psychiatric Medications*, Second Edition. Washington, DC, American Psychiatric Publishing, 2009

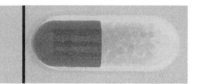

Lamictal (lamotrigine)

Generic name: Lamotrigine
Available strengths: 25 mg, 100 mg, 150 mg, 200 mg tablets;
   2 mg, 5 mg, 25 mg chewable tablets
Available in generic: Yes
Drug class: Anticonvulsant/mood stabilizer

General Information

Lamictal (lamotrigine) is better known for its use as an anticonvulsant—a medication for treating epilepsy. This may present some confusion for patients, as well as their families, when they are prescribed Lamictal without a history of seizures. Lamictal was first approved by the U.S. Food and Drug Administration (FDA) for the treatment of epilepsy, and it was later approved for the treatment of acute mania associated with bipolar disorder. The use of a medication for its approved indications is called its *labeled use*. In clinical practice, however, physicians often prescribe medications for *unlabeled* ("off-label") uses when published clinical studies, case reports, or their own clinical experiences support the efficacy and safety of those treatments. Unlabeled uses of Lamictal include treatment of cyclothymia (a milder form of bipolar disorder), treatment-resistant depression, schizoaffective disorder, and, in some cases, borderline personality disorder. When Lamictal is used to treat mood disorders, it is considered a **mood stabilizer.**

Clinical studies have shown that Lamictal is effective in treating depressed and rapid-cycling bipolar disorder, especially in patients who had incomplete or no response to lithium. Lamictal can be used alone or in combination with another mood stabilizer, such as lithium. If it is used with Depakote, however, there are certain precautions that must be followed to minimize the risk of developing a potentially severe rash (see "Adverse Reactions and Precautions"). Lamictal may be especially effective in treating people who are "rapid cyclers" (those with four or more manic or major depressive episodes a year). Patients whose mania is accompanied by irritability rather than euphoria may benefit from Lamictal. Moreover, Lamictal may be especially effective for treating or preventing bipolar depression. Patients receiving Lamictal alone for treatment of bipolar depression showed marked improvement in depressive symptoms.

Dosing Information

Lamictal is usually started at a low dosage of 25 mg/day, and the dosage is gradually increased by 25–50 mg every 2 weeks. By week 6, most patients are taking a target dosage of 100–200 mg/day. When Lamictal is administered in combination with Depakote (or shortly after discontinuation of the medication), it should be introduced even more slowly (e.g., 25 mg every other day for the first 2 weeks), and the target dosage should not exceed 100 mg/day. On the other hand, when Lamictal is administered with Tegretol (carbamazepine), the Lamictal dosage may need to be adjusted higher because Tegretol increases its metabolism.

Common Side Effects

The most common side effects associated with Lamictal are rash, dizziness, headache, somnolence, impaired coordination, difficulty with walking (**ataxia**), and gastrointestinal symptoms, including nausea, vomiting, and abdominal cramping. The incidence of rash associated with Lamictal is approximately 10%, but the risk may significantly increase when Lamictal is dosed too rapidly or administered in combination with Depakote or other valproate derivatives. Of greater concern is the rare occasion in which the patient receiving Lamictal develops a rash that progresses to life-threatening systemic symptoms (see "Adverse Reactions and Precautions").

Adverse Reactions and Precautions

Lamictal may cause drowsiness and impair alertness, especially at the start of therapy. Patients should use caution when driving or performing tasks that require alertness.

Because of the risk of serious rashes associated with Lamictal, the FDA required the manufacturer to issue a "black box" warning in its labeling. The risk of a serious skin reaction occurs in about 1 in 1,000 patients among adults but in 1 in 100 patients among children younger than 16 years of age. Life-threatening skin rashes include a form called **Stevens-Johnson syndrome,** which is characterized by painful blistering of the skin and mucous membranes and is often fatal. The skin reaction is based on individual susceptibility, and other than age, there are no factors that can predict one's susceptibility to the rash or the severity of rash associated with Lamictal. Patients should stop taking Lamictal at the first sign of rash, and if the rash is accompanied by malaise, sore throat, and fever, they should seek immediate medical attention at an emergency room for evaluation.

Use in Pregnancy and Breastfeeding: Pregnancy Category C

There are no adequate controlled studies of Lamictal in pregnant women to determine the medication's risk to the woman and fetus. However, animal studies suggest that Lamictal may have a potential risk because it has been shown to decrease the concentration of folic acid, a B vitamin, in rats. Decreased fetal concentrations of folic acid are known to have harmful effects in animals and humans. The use of Lamictal should be avoided in pregnancy whenever possible, especially during the first trimester. However, if Lamictal is required because stopping the medication may result in relapse and present a greater danger to the mother and unborn child, the patient may continue to take Lamictal, after giving informed consent to the physician, or an alternative medication or treatment may be used.

Nursing mothers should not take Lamictal, because it is excreted in breast milk and may be harmful to the baby when ingested. If stopping the drug is not an alternative, breastfeeding should not be started or should be discontinued.

Possible Drug Interactions

When Lamictal is combined with another medication, the combination may alter its metabolism and thus affect the blood levels of the other medication or of Lamictal. If the level of the other medication is significantly reduced, the person's responsiveness to that medication may be compromised. If the level is significantly elevated, the person has a greater susceptibility to the toxic effects of the other medication. The clinically significant drug interactions reported with Lamictal are summarized in the table below.

Tegretol (carbamazepine)	When Lamictal is administered in combination with Tegretol, the blood levels of Lamictal may be significantly reduced. Under these conditions, the Lamictal dosage should be increased to 300–400 mg/day.
Depakote (divalproex) and valproic acid	Depakote and other valproic acid preparations may significantly increase Lamictal levels, which may increase the risk of developing a rash. Under these conditions, Lamictal should be started slowly and the maximum daily dosage generally should not exceed 100 mg/day.
Dilantin (phenytoin), phenobarbital, and Mysoline (primidone)	Dilantin, phenobarbital, and Mysoline are anticonvulsants that, when combined with Lamictal, may decrease its blood levels. Under these conditions, a higher Lamictal dosage may be needed.
Estrogens in oral contraceptives and hormone replacements (e.g., Premarin)	Blood levels of Lamictal may be significantly reduced when the medication is administered with estrogens or oral contraceptives with estrogen, thus reducing the effectiveness of Lamictal.

Patients taking Lamictal should not consume alcohol because the combination may increase sedation and drowsiness. Moreover, the sedative effects of alcohol may act as a depressant, obscuring the therapeutic effects of Lamictal and complicating treatment.

Overdose

Depending on the amount ingested, overdose with Lamictal can be serious. Non-life-threatening symptoms of overdose include dizziness, ataxia (impaired coordination while walking), headache, and somnolence. In severe cases, overdose may result in delirium, liver and renal failure, severe rash, and coma. In small children the lethal dosage may be lower than for an adult of average size.

Any suspected overdose should be treated as an emergency. The person should be taken to the emergency room for observation and treatment. The prescription bottle of medication (and any other medication suspected in the overdose) should be brought as well, because the information on the prescription label can be helpful to the treating physician in determining the number of pills ingested.

Special Considerations

- If you miss a dose, take it as soon as possible, within 2–3 hours of the scheduled dose. If it is close to the next scheduled dose, skip the missed dose and continue on your regular dosing schedule. Do not take double doses.
- Take Lamictal immediately after meals or with food to decrease stomach upset.
- Contact your physician immediately if you develop a rash.
- Lamictal may cause sedation and drowsiness, especially during initiation of therapy, and impair your alertness. Use caution when driving or performing tasks that require alertness.
- Store the medication in its originally labeled, light-resistant container, away from heat and moisture. Heat and moisture may precipitate breakdown of your medication, and the medication may lose its therapeutic effects.
- Keep your medication out of reach of children, because overdose in small children is very dangerous.

If you have any questions about your medication, consult your physician or pharmacist.

Notes

_____

_____

_____

_____

_____

_____

_____

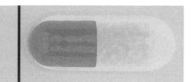

Lyrica (pregabalin)

Generic name: Pregabalin
Available strengths: 25 mg, 50 mg, 75 mg, 100 mg,
   150 mg, 200 mg, 225 mg, 300 mg capsules
Available in generic: No
Drug class: Analgesic/anticonvulsant/mood stabilizer

General Information

Lyrica (pregabalin) was introduced in the United States in 2004. The U.S. Food and Drug Administration approved Lyrica for the treatment of epilepsy and the management of pain caused by herpes infection (**shingles**) or associated with diabetes mellitus, known as **diabetic peripheral neuropathy** (DPN). Lyrica also received an indication for the treatment of fibromyalgia, a disorder defined by chronic, widespread pain and sensitivity to touch. The use of medication for its approved indications is called its *labeled use*. However, physicians often prescribe medications for *unlabeled* ("off-label") uses when published clinical studies, case reports, or their own clinical experiences support the efficacy and safety of those treatments. Lyrica's off-label uses in psychiatry may include treatment of bipolar disorder and anxiety disorders. When Lyrica is used for treating mood disorders, it is considered a **mood stabilizer.**

Dosing Information

For treatment of fibromyalgia and diabetic peripheral neuropathy, the starting dose of Lyrica is increased slowly to reach a target dosage of 300–450 mg/day, given in divided doses. In management of pain due to herpes infection, the dosage range is 150–300 mg/day, in divided doses. For treating seizures (partial-onset), the maintenance dosage ranges from 150 to 600 mg/day, given in two or three divided doses. For treatment of generalized anxiety disorder, a starting dosage of 50 mg three times a day (150 mg/day), titrated up to a target dosage of 100–200 mg three times a day (300–600 mg/day), was found to be effective in reducing symptoms and well tolerated by most patients. The use of Lyrica for treatment of bipolar disorder is limited.

Common Side Effects

The major complaints from patients taking Lyrica are drowsiness and dizziness. These side effects generally are most pronounced when Lyrica is started and occur more frequently at higher doses. As the patient develops better tolerance to the medication, these side effects usually subside. Other side effects associated with Lyrica include dry mouth, blurred vision, incoordination (**ataxia**), and weight gain.

Adverse Reactions and Precautions

Lyrica may cause sedation and dizziness, which may impair an individual's ability to perform tasks such as driving or operating machinery. Elderly patients may be susceptible to falling from dizziness and incoordination.

Patients may experience blurred vision from Lyrica. If changes in vision occur, patients should notify their physician. Taking Lyrica may induce weight gain. Patients should watch their weight while taking Lyrica, especially when starting therapy. In some patients the weight gain may be attributed to the retention of fluid, which may cause swelling of tissues, particularly in the lower limbs (**peripheral edema**). The retention of fluid caused by Lyrica was not found to be associated with any cardiovascular complications such as high blood pressure or heart problems. It is advised that patients notify their physician when they retain fluid while taking Lyrica, especially if there is a history of cardiovascular disease.

Some patients who abruptly or rapidly discontinued Lyrica reported symptoms of insomnia, headaches, and diarrhea. Patients should notify their physician before stopping Lyrica so that the dosage can be gradually tapered before discontinuation.

Use in Pregnancy and Breastfeeding: Pregnancy Category C

There are no adequately controlled studies of Lyrica in pregnant women to determine the medication's risk to the woman and fetus. It is not recommended for use during pregnancy, especially during the first trimester.

It is not known whether Lyrica is excreted in breast milk. Nursing mothers should avoid taking Lyrica. If stopping the drug is not an alternative, breastfeeding should not be started or should be discontinued.

Possible Drug Interactions

Because Lyrica is not extensively metabolized in the liver like many of the other mood stabilizers, it exerts little influence on the hepatic enzymes. Therefore, Lyrica has very few drug interactions that are of any clinical importance. However, patients should be aware that when Lyrica is taken with other medications that cause central nervous system side effects, the drowsiness and dizziness can be worse.

Patients taking Lyrica should not consume alcohol because the combination may increase sedation and drowsiness. Moreover, the sedative effects of alcohol may act as a depressant, obscuring the therapeutic effects of Lyrica and complicating treatment.

Overdose

In the few cases of overdose reported with Lyrica, there were no serious clinical consequences. In the reported cases of an acute overdose, all patients recovered with supportive care. Symptoms of an acute overdose of Lyrica include somnolence, double vision, incoordination, slurred speech, lethargy, and diarrhea. Any suspected overdose should be treated as an emergency. The person should be taken to the emergency room for observation and treatment. The prescription bottle of medication (and any other medication suspected in the overdose) should be brought as well, because the information on the prescription label can be helpful to the treating physician in determining the number of pills ingested.

Special Considerations

- If you miss a dose, take it as soon as possible within 2–3 hours of the scheduled dose. If it is close to the next scheduled dose, skip the missed dose and continue on your regular dosing schedule. Do not take double doses.
- Lyrica may cause dizziness and drowsiness, especially during initiation of therapy, and impair your alertness. Use caution when driving or performing tasks that require alertness.
- Do not discontinue Lyrica abruptly. The medication should be tapered gradually before completely stopping it.
- Store the medication in its originally labeled, light-resistant container, away from heat and moisture. Heat and moisture may precipitate breakdown of your medication, and the medication may lose its therapeutic effects.
- Keep your medication out of reach of children.

If you have any questions about your medication, consult your physician or pharmacist.

Notes

_____

_____

_____

_____

_____

_____

_____

_____

From Chew RH, Hales RE, Yudofsky SC: *What Your Patients Need to Know About Psychiatric Medications*, Second Edition. Washington, DC, American Psychiatric Publishing, 2009

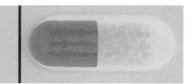

Neurontin (gabapentin)

Generic name: Gabapentin
Available strengths: 100 mg, 300 mg, 400 mg,
   600 mg, 800 mg tablets;
   100 mg, 300 mg, 400 mg capsules
Available in generic: Yes
Drug class: Anticonvulsant/mood stabilizer

General Information

Neurontin (gabapentin) is better known for its use as an anticonvulsant—a medication for treating epilepsy. This may present some confusion for patients, as well as their families, when they are prescribed Neurontin without a history of seizures. Although Neurontin is approved by the U.S. Food and Drug Administration for the treatment of epilepsy and late-stage nerve pain from herpes zoster (*shingles*), this medicine has many uses other than its approved indications. The use of a medication for its approved indications is called its *labeled use*. In clinical practice, however, physicians often prescribe medications for *unlabeled* ("off-label") uses when published clinical studies, case reports, or their own clinical experiences support the efficacy and safety of those treatments. The use of Neurontin for treatment of bipolar disorder, particularly in acute mania, is an example of its off-label use. Other conditions for which Neurontin is commonly used off-label include nerve pain (neuropathy and neuralgia) from complications of diabetes and other causes, migraine headaches, and fibromyalgia.

Dosing Information

Neurontin is usually started at a dosage of 300 mg two or three times a day, and the dosage is increased by 300 mg every 3–4 days as clinically indicated. The usual maximum daily dosage for treatment of bipolar disorder is 1,800–2,400 mg. Because Neurontin is eliminated primarily by the kidneys, patients with significant renal impairment may require lower dosages.

Common Side Effects

Neurontin is generally well tolerated and has very few adverse effects. The common side effects associated with Neurontin are sedation, dizziness, impaired coordination, difficulty with walking (**ataxia**), tiredness, jerky eye movements (**nystagmus**), double vision (**diplopia**), and tremor. Daytime sedation may be reduced by taking a larger proportion of the divided dosage at bedtime. The side effects are generally temporary and subside as tolerance to the medication develops.

Adverse Reactions and Precautions

Neurontin is generally a well-tolerated medication and is infrequently discontinued because of adverse events. Sedation and dizziness are the most frequent side effects that may become troubling, especially for seniors and those taking other sedating medications. Seniors may be susceptible to falling from the effects of vertigo or dizziness. Sedation becomes hazardous when driving or operating machinery. For individuals who are sensitive to these side effects, increasing the dosage slowly or using lower dosages may be necessary.

Use in Pregnancy and Breastfeeding: Pregnancy Category C

There are no adequately controlled studies of Neurontin in pregnant women to determine the medication's risk to the woman and fetus. Compared with lithium, Tegretol, and Depakote, Neurontin is safer for use in pregnancy. However, it is not recommend for use during pregnancy, especially during the first trimester. If Neurontin is required because stopping the medication may result in relapse and present a greater danger to the mother and unborn child, the patient may continue to take Neurontin, after giving informed consent to the physician, or an alternative medication or treatment may be used.

Nursing mothers should not take Neurontin, because it is excreted in breast milk and may be harmful to the baby when ingested. If stopping the drug is not an alternative, breastfeeding should not be started or should be discontinued.

Possible Drug Interactions

Because Neurontin is not extensively metabolized in the liver like many of the other mood stabilizers, it exerts little influence on the hepatic enzymes. Therefore, Neurontin has very few drug interactions of any clinical importance. Patients, however, should be aware that when Neurontin is taken with other medications that have central nervous system side effects, it may make sedation, fatigue, dizziness, and ataxia worse.

Patients taking Neurontin should not consume alcohol because the combination may increase sedation and drowsiness. Moreover, the sedative effects of alcohol may act as a depressant, obscuring the therapeutic effects of Neurontin and complicating treatment.

Overdose

Symptoms of acute overdose with Neurontin include somnolence, double vision, ataxia, slurred speech, lethargy, and diarrhea. In the reported cases of acute overdose, all patients recovered with supportive care.

Any suspected overdose should be treated as an emergency. The person should be taken to the emergency room for observation and treatment. The prescription bottle of medication (and any other medication suspected in the overdose) should be brought as well, because the information on the prescription label can be helpful to the treating physician in determining the number of pills ingested.

Special Considerations

- If you miss a dose, take it as soon as possible, within 2–3 hours of the scheduled dose. If it is close to the next scheduled dose, skip the missed dose and continue on your regular dosing schedule. Do not take double doses.
- Take Neurontin immediately after meals or with food to decrease stomach upset.
- Sedation and dizziness are the most frequent side effects that may become troubling, especially for seniors and those taking other sedating medications. Seniors may be susceptible to falling from the effects of vertigo or dizziness. Sedation becomes hazardous when driving or operating machinery. For individuals who are sensitive to these side effects, increasing the dosage slowly or using lower dosages may be necessary.
- Store the medication in its originally labeled, light-resistant container, away from heat and moisture. Heat and moisture may precipitate breakdown of your medication, and the medication may lose its therapeutic effects.
- Keep your medication out of reach of children.

If you have any questions about your medication, consult your physician or pharmacist.

Notes

_____

_____

_____

_____

_____

From Chew RH, Hales RE, Yudofsky SC: *What Your Patients Need to Know About Psychiatric Medications*, Second Edition. Washington, DC, American Psychiatric Publishing, 2009

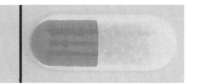

Topamax (topiramate)

Generic name: Topiramate
Available strengths: 25 mg, 50 mg, 100 mg,
   200 mg capsules and tablets;
    15 mg, 25 mg sprinkle capsules (Topamax Sprinkle)
Available in generic: Yes, except Topamax Sprinkle
Drug class: Anticonvulsant/mood stabilizer

General Information

Topamax (topiramate) is better known for its use as an anticonvulsant—a medication for treating epilepsy. This may present some confusion for patients, as well as their families, when they are prescribed Topamax without a history of seizures. Topamax was first approved by the U.S. Food and Drug Administration for the treatment of epilepsy and, recently, for prophylaxis of migraine headache. The use of a medication for its approved indications is called its *labeled use*. In clinical practice, however, physicians often prescribe medications for *unlabeled* ("off-label") uses when published clinical studies, case reports, or their own clinical experiences support the efficacy and safety of those treatments. The use of Topamax for treatment of bipolar disorder, particularly in acute mania, is an example of its off-label use. Other conditions for which Topamax is commonly used off-label include eating disorders (e.g., binge eating and bulimia) and alcohol and cocaine withdrawal.

Preliminary clinical studies suggest that Topamax may be effective when used in conjunction with another mood stabilizer for treatment of bipolar disorder in both the manic and depressive phases. The advantage of Topamax over some other mood stabilizers, such as Depakote, is that it does not induce weight gain but rather can produce mild weight loss. When Topamax is used in combination therapy, it can counteract the side effect of weight gain of another mood stabilizer and provide mood stabilization as well.

Dosing Information

Topamax is usually started at a dosage of 12.5–25 mg/day, and the dosage is increased by 25 mg a week. Average dosages for mood stabilization are usually 100–200 mg/day given in divided doses. Dosage should not exceed the usual maximum of 400 mg/day.

Common Side Effects

The most common side effects associated with Topamax are somnolence, fatigue, impaired coordination, difficulty with walking (**ataxia**), difficulty with concentration and attention, and gastrointestinal symptoms, including nausea, vomiting, and abdominal cramping. Generally, these side effects are more frequent and intense at higher dosages.

Adverse Reactions and Precautions

Topamax may cause drowsiness and impair alertness, especially at the start of therapy. Patients should use caution when driving or performing tasks that require alertness.

Kidney Stones

A total of 1.5% of patients treated with Topamax experienced kidney stones. The risk of kidney stones appeared to be higher in men treated with Topamax. By increasing fluid intake to promote urine output, the risk of kidney stone formation may be decreased.

Central Nervous System

Central nervous system–related adverse reactions with Topamax include mental and physical slowing, difficulty with concentration, dizziness or imbalance, confusion, and irritability. Seniors may be particularly susceptible to losing their balance and falling.

Metabolic Acidosis

Topamax can induce an electrolyte imbalace and cause a condition called **metabolic acidosis.** This adverse reaction is generally rare, but patients with renal disease, severe respiratory disease, chronic diarrhea, or other medical conditions may be more susceptible to Topamax. The clinical signs of metabolic acidosis include rapid respiration on resting, nonspecific symptoms such as tiredness and loss of appetite, and rapid heart rate. Patients should report any of these symptoms to their physician. A laboratory test to measure the serum bicarbonate level can help diagnose metabolic acidosis.

Use in Pregnancy and Breastfeeding: Pregnancy Category C

There are no adequate controlled studies of Topamax in pregnant women to determine the medication's risk to the woman and fetus. However, Topamax may have potential risks in humans because it has been associated with fetal malformations in animal studies. The use of Topamax should be avoided in pregnancy whenever possible, especially in the first trimester. However, if Topamax is required because stopping the medication may result in relapse and present a greater danger to the mother and unborn child, the patient may continue to take Topamax, after giving informed consent to the physician, or an alternative medication or treatment may be used.

It is not known if Topamax is excreted in human breast milk. However, nursing mothers should not take Topamax. If stopping the medication is not an alternative, breastfeeding should not be started or should be discontinued.

Possible Drug Interactions

When Topamax is combined with other medications, it may alter their metabolism and the blood levels of these medications. When the levels are lowered, it may decrease the medication's effectiveness; conversely, when levels are elevated, the person may become susceptible to the medication's toxic effects. Other medications may similarly affect the blood levels of Topamax. The clinically significant drug interactions reported with Topamax are summarized in the table below.

Estrogens in oral contraceptives	When Topamax is taken in combination with oral contraceptives containing estrogen, the level of estrogen may be lowered, decreasing the effectiveness of the contraceptive and perhaps resulting in an unplanned pregnancy.
Tegretol (carbamazepine)	Topamax concentrations may be decreased significantly if it is used with Tegretol, decreasing Topamax's effectiveness.
Dilantin (phenytoin)	Topamax concentrations may be decreased significantly if it is used with Dilantin, decreasing Topamax's effectiveness.
Diamox (acetazolamide) and other carbonic anhydrase inhibitors	Combination of Topamax with medications known as carbonic anhydrase inhibitors, such as Diamox, may increase the risk of renal stones and should be avoided.

Patients taking Topamax should not consume alcohol because the combination may increase sedation and drowsiness. Moreover, the sedative effects of alcohol may act as a depressant, obscuring the therapeutic effects of Topamax and complicating treatment.

Overdose

Depending on the amount ingested, overdose with Topamax can be serious. Non-life-threatening symptoms of overdose include dizziness, ataxia (impaired coordination while walking), headache, and somnolence. In severe cases, overdose may result in delirium, liver and renal failure, and coma.

Any suspected overdose should be treated as an emergency. The person should be taken to the emergency room for observation and treatment. The prescription bottle of medication (and any other medication suspected in the overdose) should be brought as well, because the information on the prescription label can be helpful to the treating physician in determining the number of pills ingested.

Special Considerations

- If you miss a dose, take it as soon as possible, within 2–3 hours of the scheduled dose. If it is close to the next scheduled dose, skip the missed dose and continue on your regular dosing schedule. Do not take double doses.

- Take Topamax immediately after meals or with food to decrease stomach upset.
- Maintain an adequate fluid intake to minimize the risk of kidney stone formation, especially if you are predisposed to kidney stones.
- Topamax may cause sedation and drowsiness, especially during initiation of therapy, and impair your alertness. Use caution when driving or performing tasks that require alertness.
- Store the medication in its originally labeled, light-resistant container, away from heat and moisture. Heat and moisture may precipitate breakdown of your medication, and the medication may lose its therapeutic effects.
- Keep your medication out of reach of children.

If you have any questions about your medication, consult your physician or pharmacist.

Notes

_____

_____

_____

_____

_____

_____

_____

_____

From Chew RH, Hales RE, Yudofsky SC: *What Your Patients Need to Know About Psychiatric Medications*, Second Edition. Washington, DC, American Psychiatric Publishing, 2009

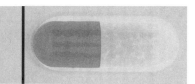

Trileptal (oxcarbazepine)

Generic name: Oxcarbazepine
Available strengths: 150 mg, 300 mg, 600 mg tablets;
   300 mg/5 mL oral suspension
Available in generic: Yes, but only the tablets
Drug class: Anticonvulsant/mood stabilizer

General Information

Trileptal (oxcarbazepine) is better known for its use as an anticonvulsant—a medication for treating epilepsy. This may present some confusion for patients, as well as their families, when they are prescribed Trileptal without a history of seizures. Trileptal was approved by the U.S. Food and Drug Administration for the treatment of epilepsy. The use of a medication for its approved indications is called its *labeled use*. In clinical practice, however, physicians often prescribe medications for *unlabeled* ("off-label") uses when published clinical studies, case reports, or their own clinical experiences support the efficacy and safety of those treatments. The use of Trileptal for treatment of bipolar disorder, particularly in acute mania, is an example of its off-label use. Other off-label uses for Trileptal include use as an alternative medication for neuropathies (degeneration of nerves) and neuralgias (nerve pain).

Trileptal's chemical structure is very similar to that of Tegretol (carbamazepine), another anticonvulsant commonly used as a mood stabilizer. Trileptal, however, is better tolerated and has fewer significant drug interactions than Tegretol. Trileptal has been available in the United States only since 2000, but it has been used to treat bipolar disorder in Europe for many years. In limited clinical studies, it was shown to be effective in managing acute mania. Trileptal's effectiveness in preventing relapse in bipolar disorder remains equivocal. Because it is structurally similar to Tegretol, which is an effective mood stabilizer in maintenance therapy, Trileptal is expected to offer similar treatment benefits.

Trileptal is not associated with any significant risk of **agranulocytosis** and **aplastic anemia,** which are potentially fatal conditions associated with Tegretol. Agranulocytosis is a condition in which the level of a particular type of white blood cells (**granulocytes**) is dramatically and dangerously low. Aplastic anemia is a condition in which the bone marrow stops producing blood cells, including platelets (important for clotting), white blood cells, and red blood cells. Because Trileptal has an improved safety profile and fewer drug interactions than Tegretol, physicians generally prefer to use it over the older anticonvulsant. One disadvantage of Trileptal had been cost, but it is now available in a generic form.

Dosing Information

The starting dosage of Trileptal is usually 300 mg twice a day. The dosage is then increased gradually, by approximately 300 mg every 3 days, to 2,400 mg/day in a twice-daily regimen. Seniors and individuals with renal impairment may require lower dosages.

Common Side Effects

The most common side effects from Trileptal are somnolence, tiredness, dizziness, and gastrointestinal symptoms, including nausea, vomiting, constipation, and abdominal pain. When starting Trileptal, patients may experience mental sluggishness and difficulty in concentration and may feel tired and sleepy. Other common side effects, usually at higher dosages, include problems with double vision (**diplopia**), jerky eye movements (**nystagmus**), and impaired coordination or clumsiness when walking (**ataxia**). These side effects are generally temporary and subside as tolerance to the medication develops, but if they persist, the dosage may be lowered to make it more tolerable.

Adverse Reactions and Precautions

Trileptal may cause drowsiness and impair alertness, especially at the start of therapy. Patients should use caution when driving or performing tasks that require alertness.

In patients with significant renal impairment, the dosage of Trileptal should be reduced to prevent toxic levels. The active metabolite of Trileptal is excreted primarily by the kidneys, and in the presence of renal impairment the medication may accumulate significantly in the body and result in a toxic reaction.

Trileptal may induce some bothersome central nervous system effects such as disturbance of cognition, difficulty with concentration, impaired coordination, and clumsiness in walking. The risks of falling and accidents may be especially hazardous for seniors.

Trileptal may lower serum sodium levels (**hyponatremia**), and symptoms of hyponatremia may develop if the sodium level is not normalized. The body's sodium concentration is regulated by the mechanisms of thirst, hormones (e.g., antidiuretic hormone), and the kidneys. Disturbance of sodium balance can disrupt many of the body's physiological functions, with serious clinical consequences. Usually, Trileptal-induced hyponatremia is mild and produces no symptoms (asymptomatic), but in clinically significant hyponatremia, symptoms may include loss of appetite, nausea and vomiting, confusion, lethargy, headache, and agitation. Individuals who are also receiving medications known to decrease serum sodium levels (e.g., thiazide diuretics) or those with a medical condition that disrupts sodium balance may be particularly susceptible to hyponatremia during treatment with Trileptal. The serum sodium levels of patients who are taking Trileptal should be monitored routinely, especially during the first 3 months of treatment, when hyponatremia generally occurs.

Use in Pregnancy and Breastfeeding: Pregnancy Category C

There are no adequate clinical studies of Trileptal in pregnant women to determine the medication's risk to the woman and fetus. However, because Trileptal is structurally similar to Tegretol, which is known to cause birth defects, it may carry similar risk and should not be used during pregnancy. Trileptal and its metabolite can cross the placenta and cause harmful effects to the fetus. The use of Trileptal should therefore be avoided in pregnancy whenever possible, especially in the first trimester. However, if Trileptal is stopped and mania reoccurs, the physician may discuss the need to restart Trileptal after the first trimester or seek an alternative medication or treatment.

Nursing mothers should not take Trileptal, because it is excreted in breast milk and may be harmful to the baby when ingested. If stopping the drug is not an alternative, breastfeeding should not be started or should be discontinued.

Possible Drug Interactions

Trileptal can affect the liver enzymes that metabolize other medications, lowering their blood levels and diminishing their effectiveness. Conversely, other medications can affect the metabolism of Trileptal and decrease its blood levels. The clinically significant drug interactions reported with Trileptal are summarized in the table below.

Oral contraceptives containing ethinyl estradiol and levonorgestrel (e.g., Demulen, Nordette, Alesse)	When Trileptal is taken in combination with oral contraceptives that contain ethinyl estradiol and levonorgestrel, it can decrease the levels of these hormones and their effectiveness, which may result in unintended pregnancy.
Tegretol, Calan (verapamil), and Depakote	Any of these medications, when taken in combination with Trileptal, can lower the blood levels of Trileptal and decrease its effectiveness.
Dilantin and phenobarbital	Trileptal may inhibit the metabolism of these medications and increase their blood levels, which may potentially result in toxicity. Conversely, these medications can lower the blood levels of Trileptal and decrease its effectiveness.
Plendil (felodipine)	Blood levels of Plendil, a calcium channel blocker, may be decreased by Trileptal, decreasing Plendil's effectiveness.

Patients taking Trileptal should not consume alcohol because the combination may increase sedation and drowsiness. Moreover, the sedative effects of alcohol may act as a depressant, obscuring the therapeutic effects of Trileptal and complicating treatment.

Overdose

In the reported cases of Trileptal overdose, all of the patients recovered with supportive treatment. The extent of danger from overdose depends on the amount ingested and the size and age of the person. In small children, for example, the lethal dosage may be much lower than for an average adult. Symptoms of Trileptal toxicity include neuromuscular disturbances such as nystagmus, muscle jerks (**myoclonus**), increased reflex reactions (**hyperreflexia**), and severe nausea and vomiting. Higher overdose may lead to respiratory depression, convulsions, cardiac arrhythmia, shock, coma, and death.

Any suspected overdose should be treated as an emergency. The person should be taken to the emergency room for observation and treatment. The prescription bottle of medication (and any other medication suspected in the overdose) should be brought as well, because the information on the prescription label can be helpful to the treating physician in determining the number of pills ingested.

Special Considerations

- If you miss a dose, take it as soon as possible, within 2–3 hours of the scheduled dose. If it is close to the next scheduled dose, skip the missed dose and continue on your regular dosing schedule. Do not take double doses.
- Take Trileptal immediately after meals or with food to decrease stomach upset.
- Contact your physician if you have excessive thirst, loss of appetite, nausea and vomiting, difficulty in concentrating, confusion, lethargy, headache, and agitation. These may be signs and symptoms of hyponatremia.
- Trileptal may cause sedation and drowsiness, especially during initiation of therapy, and impair your alertness. Use caution when driving or performing tasks that require alertness.
- Store the medication in its originally labeled, light-resistant container, away from heat and moisture. Heat and moisture may precipitate breakdown of your medication, and the medication may lose its therapeutic effects.
- Keep your medication out of reach of children, because overdose in small children is very dangerous.

If you have any questions about your medication, consult your physician or pharmacist.

Notes

_____

_____

_____

_____

_____

_____

_____

From Chew RH, Hales RE, Yudofsky SC: *What Your Patients Need to Know About Psychiatric Medications*, Second Edition. Washington, DC, American Psychiatric Publishing, 2009

First-Generation Antipsychotics

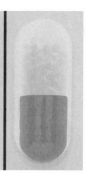

Chlorpromazine (Thorazine)
Fluphenazine HCl and fluphenazine decanoate (Prolixin)
Haldol and Haldol Decanoate (haloperidol)
Loxitane (loxapine)
Navane (thiothixene)
Orap (pimozide)
Perphenazine (Trilafon)
Thioridazine (Mellaril)
Trifluoperazine (Stelazine)

The **first-generation antipsychotics** represent an older class of antipsychotics that have been the standard for treating psychotic disorders for many decades. These earlier antipsychotics are often called **typical** or **conventional antipsychotics** because, when compared with a newer class of **second-generation antipsychotics,** they lack a wider spectrum of therapeutic activity. Moreover, the conventional antipsychotics are associated with many side effects and lack the tolerability of the newer antipsychotics. Yet for patients in whom conventional antipsychotics are effective and tolerable, these medications continue to have a place in the treatment of mental disorders.

How Antipsychotics Work

The actions of antipsychotic medications may be explained by the *dopamine receptor antagonist hypothesis.* **Dopamine** is a neurotransmitter, a chemical produced by brain cells called **neurons** that enables neurons to communicate with each other. Dopamine is released by one neuron into the space between that neuron and the next neuron and then binds to specific sites on the other neuron called **receptors.** The interaction of the neurotransmitter with the receptor results in very specialized activities coded in the neuron, and it ultimately generates an electrical impulse that is transmitted down the nerve cell. At the end of the nerve, the nerve terminal, the electrical impulse causes further release of dopamine. This form of communication between neurons is called **neurotransmission.** In specific areas of the brain, excessive dopamine neurotransmission may produce the psychotic symptoms (e.g., hallucinations, delusions, bizarre behavior) characteristic of schizophrenia and more severe cases of bipolar disorder. Drugs such as amphetamine and cocaine, for example, are known to increase dopamine release. In excessive amounts, these drugs induce psychotic symptoms not unlike schizophrenia.

Psychotic symptoms commonly seen in schizophrenia and other mental disorders, such as bipolar disorder, dementia, and drug-induced psychosis, include delusions, hallucinations, disorganized speech, and bizarre, agitated, or catatonic behavior. These symptoms are also called the **positive symptoms** of psychosis because of the excessive and overt nature of their clinical presentation.

Antipsychotics work principally by blocking, or antagonizing, the action of dopamine at its receptors, decreasing the chemical signals that drive psychotic behavior. That is, antipsychotics decrease neurotransmission by blocking dopamine from binding to the receptors. Excessive dopamine activity in selected areas of the brain may be the underlying cause of psychosis. Both conventional and second-generation antipsychotics are dopamine antagonists and are therefore effective in treating the positive symptoms of psychosis. In areas of the brain where antipsychotics have no therapeutic benefits, they may produce side effects.

Common Side Effects

The side effects commonly seen with conventional antipsychotics include sedation, extrapyramidal symptoms (EPS), elevated prolactin levels, weight gain, anticholinergic effects, and orthostatic hypotension.

Sedation and the feeling of tiredness are common with all antipsychotics, but the low-potency conventional antipsychotics, such as chlorpromazine and thioridazine, are generally more sedating than the higher-potency agents, such as fluphenazine and Haldol (haloperidol). Sometimes sedation may be useful to decrease agitation and help the patient sleep, but too often patients experience daytime sedation and fatigue that is not well tolerated.

Extrapyramidal symptoms are neurological disturbances caused by antipsychotics (or a neurological disorder) in the area of the brain that controls motor coordination. High-potency first-generation antipsychotics, such as fluphenazine and Haldol, are more likely to induce EPS than the lower-potency agents. The antipsychotics can produce symptoms that mimic Parkinson's disease. They cause Parkinson-like symptoms (**parkinsonism**) that include muscle stiffness, rigidity, tremor, drooling, and a "mask-like" facial expression. However, unlike Parkinson's disease, which is a progressive neurological disease, parkinsonism from antipsychotic medications is reversible. It may be treated, and prevented, by using antiparkinson agents (also called anticholinergic agents), such as Cogentin (benztropine), Benadryl (diphenhydramine), Artane (trihexyphenidyl), and Kemadrin (procyclidine).

Akathisia is another form of EPS characterized as a subjective sense of restlessness accompanied by fidgeting, inability to sit still, nervousness, muscle discomfort, and agitation. Generally, antiparkinson agents are not effective in managing akathisia. Use of Inderal (propranolol), a beta-blocker, may be helpful.

Dystonia is a type of EPS with acute onset. It is manifested by a sudden spasm of muscles involving the tongue, jaw, and neck. **This is not an allergic reaction to the antipsychotic medication.** Although a dystonic reaction may be painful and frightening, it can be rapidly reversed with an intramuscular injection of an anticholinergic medication, such as Cogentin or Benadryl. With a dystonic reaction, the patient should seek immediate medical attention and receive treatment.

Elevation of **prolactin levels** is common with conventional antipsychotics. Prolactin is a hormone produced in the area of the brain called the pituitary gland. It is normally elevated in women following childbirth, stimulating lactation, or milk production. The elevation of prolactin caused by antipsychotic medications may cause breast enlargement and milk production (**galactorrhea**) in both women and men. Elevated prolactin is also associated with impotence in men and irregular menstrual cycles or absence of menstruation in women. When side effects from elevated prolactin levels become bothersome, the alternative is to switch to one of the second-generation antipsychotic agents, which do not elevate prolactin.

Weight gain is a frequent side effect of all antipsychotic medications. Certain antipsychotics are associated with greater weight gain than others. It is unclear whether this is due to an underlying metabolic change caused by the antipsychotic or to increased appetite. Weight should be monitored closely during therapy, and if weight gain occurs, an intervention program of diet and exercise should be started.

When antipsychotics interfere with the action of **cholinergic neurons** in the nervous system, they produce bothersome **anticholinergic** side effects. When an organ system is affected by cholinergic inhibition, it causes side effects particular to that organ. For example, when the gastrointestinal tract is affected, dry mouth, cramping, and constipation result. Other anticholinergic side effects include blurred vision (when muscles of the eyes are affected) and difficulty urinating (when the bladder is affected). The low-potency first-generation antipsychotics have more anticholinergic activity than the high-potency agents. When antipsychotics are combined with other medications with significant anticholinergic activity, such as tricyclic antidepressants and antiparkinson agents, the anticholinergic action of the medications are additive. Seniors and individuals with a medical condition may be especially sensitive to anticholinergic side effects. Excessive anticholinergic activity may induce delirium, a toxic reaction that impairs consciousness, causes confusion, and makes it difficult for the person to sustain attention.

Antipsychotic medications may block a compensatory response—the narrowing of blood vessels—that counterbalances postural change, resulting in a momentary drop in blood pressure when the person rises too rapidly, which may cause dizziness and lightheadedness. This reaction is known as **orthostatic hypotension.** Patients, especially seniors and those taking antihypertensive medications, need to be cautious and rise slowly to allow the body to adjust to the change in position, avoiding a sudden drop in blood pressure.

Adverse Reactions and Precautions

Adverse reactions may be defined as those reactions from the medication that are usually rare but may have serious consequences. Some medications may enhance ultraviolet light absorption—a reaction known as **photosensitivity**—in the skin. The conventional antipsychotics, such as chlorpromazine, fluphenazine, perphenazine, Serentil (mesoridazine), thioridazine, and trifluoperazine, are notorious for inducing photosensitivity. Patients taking these medications should use sunscreen and protective clothing to prevent sunburn. In addition, all antipsychotics are associated with neuroleptic malignant syndrome (NMS), heatstroke, tardive dyskinesia (TD), seizures, and arrhythmias.

Neuroleptic Malignant Syndrome

Neuroleptic malignant syndrome is a rare, toxic reaction to all antipsychotics. The symptoms are severe muscle stiffness, rigidity, elevated body temperature, increased heart rate and blood pressure, irregular pulse, and profuse sweating. NMS may lead to delirium and coma. It can be fatal if medical intervention is not immediately provided. There is no test to predict whether an individual may develop NMS when exposed to an antipsychotic. Thus NMS must be recognized early because it is a medical emergency that requires immediate discontinuation of the antipsychotic, hospitalization, and intensive medical treatment.

Heatstroke

Antipsychotics may disrupt the area of the brain that regulates temperature, and individuals taking antipsychotics may be especially sensitive to heat. Their body temperature may rise to dangerous levels when they are exposed to hot weather, resulting in a condition commonly known as **heatstroke.** Conventional antipsychotics appear to have a higher occurrence of causing heat-regulating disturbances. Individuals taking antipsychotics must take precautions to protect themselves from prolonged exposure to hot, humid weather.

Tardive Dyskinesia

Tardive dyskinesia is a potential adverse reaction from antipsychotic medications. It is a late-onset abnormal involuntary movement disorder. It is a potentially irreversible condition with symptoms that commonly include "pill-rolling" movements of the fingers, darting and writhing movements of the tongue, lip puckering, facial grimacing, and other irregular movements. The risk of TD is increased the longer the person has been taking the antipsychotic, and this risk also increases with age.

With several decades of experience, scientists now have a better understanding of the relative risk of TD with conventional antipsychotics than with the second-generation antipsychotics. However, because the second-generation antipsychotics have a very low incidence of EPS, these newer antipsychotics may also have very low risk of inducing TD. For example, the oldest second-generation antipsychotic, Clozaril, rarely causes TD according to more than 30 years of clinical experience. When early signs of TD are detected in the patient taking a conventional antipsychotic, an option is to switch to a second-generation antipsychotic, which may reverse the symptoms or decrease any further progression of TD.

Seizures

Antipsychotics can lower the seizure threshold and induce **seizures** in susceptible individuals, especially those with a history of seizure disorder. Of the conventional antipsychotics, chlorpromazine and Loxitane (loxapine) have a higher incidence of seizures than other conventional agents. Patients with a seizure disorder who are taking anticonvulsants often take antipsychotics without any increase in seizures.

Arrhythmia

Antipsychotics may slow electrical conduction in heart tissues (**myocardium**). Some patients taking antipsychotics show on their electrocardiogram (ECG) a prolongation of the electrical impulse as it travels in the myocardium. This abnormal ECG finding, called **QTc prolongation,** may signal a potential for developing an irregular heartbeat (**arrhythmia**). Orap (pimozide) and thioridazine are associated with a greater tendency to alter the electrical impulse, and therefore these antipsychotics have a higher risk of causing arrhythmias, especially in individuals with cardiac disease. Patients who have a history of arrhythmia should have an ECG before starting an antipsychotic and periodically during treatment.

Elderly Patients With Dementia

After warning that elderly patients with dementia treated with second-generation antipsychotic medicines (atypical antipsychotics) may be associated with risk of death, the FDA determined that the first-generation antipsychotics may be also associated with this risk. The FDA now deems that all antipsychotic medications are not indicated for treating elderly patients with dementia-related psychosis. Physicians who prescribe antipsychotics to elderly patients for dementia-related psychosis should discuss this fatal risk with the patient, the patient's family, or the patient's caretaker.

For more information about a particular first-generation antipsychotic medication, refer to the handout for that medication.

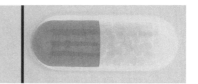

Chlorpromazine (Thorazine)

Generic name: Chlorpromazine
Available strengths: 10 mg, 25 mg, 50 mg,
    100 mg, 200 mg tablets; 25 mg/mL injection
Available in generic: Yes
Drug class: First-generation (conventional) antipsychotic

General Information

Chlorpromazine (Thorazine), the first antipsychotic used for the treatment of psychosis, belongs to the class of antipsychotics known as the **first-generation antipsychotics,** sometimes referred to as *conventional* or *typical* antipsychotics. Chlorpromazine was sold under the brand Thorazine, but Thorazine has since been discontinued. Currently, only generic chlorpromazine is available. The first-generation antipsychotics represent an older class of antipsychotics that have been the standard for treating psychotic disorders for many decades. When compared with a newer class of **second-generation antipsychotics,** these earlier antipsychotics are referred to as *typical* or *conventional* because they lack the wider spectrum of therapeutic activity. The first-generation antipsychotics are also more likely to induce side effects that cause movement disorders, such as **extrapyramidal symptoms** (EPS) and **tardive dyskinesia** (TD), than the newer antipsychotics.

Chlorpromazine is a relatively low-potency agent, compared with other first-generation antipsychotics such as fluphenazine and Haldol (haloperidol). The low-potency antipsychotics are generally sedating and more likely to induce **anticholinergic side effects** but are less likely to cause EPS than are high-potency agents.

Chlorpromazine is approved by the U.S. Food and Drug Administration for the treatment of psychotic disorders, such as schizophrenia, schizoaffective disorder, acute mania, and psychotic depression. In children, chlorpromazine is indicated for short-term treatment of severe behavioral problems marked by combativeness and explosive anger and behavior. In addition, chlorpromazine is indicated in treatment of nausea and vomiting and intractable hiccups. The use of a medication for its approved indications is called its *labeled use*. In clinical practice, however, physicians often prescribe medications for *unlabeled* ("off-label") uses when published clinical studies, case reports, or their own clinical experiences support the efficacy and safety of those treatments. For instance, chlorpromazine may be prescribed with a mood stabilizer to treat acute mania, since the mood stabilizer has a slower onset of action. After the symptoms of mania abate, chlorpromazine is discontinued and the mood stabilizer is continued alone.

Dosing Information

The starting dosage of chlorpromazine for acute psychosis may range from 400 mg/day to 1,000 mg/day, taken in divided doses, depending on whether the patient is being treated in an outpatient or inpatient setting. Chlorpromazine is infrequently used as the single agent in treatment of schizophrenia or schizoaffective disorder. It has been replaced by better-tolerated medications. Usually, chlorpromazine is used in combination as an adjunct with another antipsychotic to treat acute psychosis. Chlorpromazine's sedating properties may be useful to decrease agitation and to help the patient sleep. When chlorpromazine is combined with another antipsychotic, lower dosages of 100–400 mg/day are used and are often taken at bedtime or on an as-needed schedule.

Common Side Effects

When starting chlorpromazine, patients may experience sedation and fatigue. Taking a larger portion of the total dosage at bedtime may minimize daytime sedation. Tolerance to the sedation generally develops after about 1 week.

With higher dosages, chlorpromazine may induce **extrapyramidal symptoms.** These are neurological disturbances caused by antipsychotics (or a neurological disorder) in the area of the brain that controls motor coordination. When disruption occurs in a particular area of the brain, it can produce symptoms that mimic Parkinson's disease (**parkinsonism**), including muscle stiffness, rigidity, tremor, drooling, and a "mask-like" facial expression. However, unlike Parkinson's disease, which is a progressive neurological disease, parkinsonism from treatment with an antipsychotic is reversible. The Parkinson-like symptoms may be treated, and prevented, by using antiparkinson agents (also called anticholinergic agents) such as Cogentin (benztropine), Benadryl (diphenhydramine), Artane (trihexyphenidyl), and Kemadrin (procyclidine).

Akathisia is another form of EPS characterized by a subjective sense of restlessness accompanied by fidgeting, inability to sit still, nervousness, muscle discomfort, and agitation. Generally, antiparkinson agents are not effective in managing akathisia. Use of Inderal (propranolol), a beta-blocker, may be helpful and is sometimes prescribed by physicians.

Dystonia is a type of EPS with acute onset. The patient may develop a sudden spasm of the muscles of the tongue, jaw, and neck. **This is not an allergic reaction to the antipsychotic medication.** Although a dystonic reaction may be painful and frightening, it can be rapidly reversed with an intramuscular injection of an anticholinergic medication such as Cogentin or Benadryl. With a dystonic reaction, the patient should seek immediate medical attention and receive treatment.

Elevation of **prolactin levels** is common with conventional antipsychotics. Prolactin is a hormone produced in the area of the brain called the pituitary gland. It is normally elevated in women following childbirth, stimulating lactation, or milk production. The effects of elevated prolactin include breast enlargement and milk production (**galactorrhea**) in both women and men. Elevated prolactin is also associated with impotence in men and irregular menstrual cycles or absence of menstruation in women. When side effects from elevated prolactin levels become bothersome, the alternative is to switch to one of the second-generation antipsychotic agents with no propensity to elevate this hormone.

Chlorpromazine may induce weight gain. It is unclear whether this is due to an underlying metabolic change caused by the antipsychotic or to increased appetite. Weight should be monitored closely during therapy, and if weight gain occurs, an intervention program of diet and exercise should be started.

When a medication inhibits the action of **cholinergic neurons** in the nervous system, it produces an **anticholinergic reaction,** which may produce bothersome symptoms. Because many of the antipsychotics block the normal function of cholinergic neurons, they frequently produce anticholinergic side effects. When an organ system is affected by cholinergic inhibition, it causes side effects particular to that organ. For example, when the gastrointestinal tract is affected, it may result in dry mouth, cramping, and constipation. Other anticholinergic side effects include blurred vision (when muscles of the eyes are affected) and difficulty urinating (when the bladder is affected). Chlorpromazine has more anticholinergic activity than the high-potency antipsychotics. When chlorpromazine is combined with other medications with significant anticholinergic activity, such as tricyclic antidepressants (TCAs) and antiparkinson agents, the total anticholinergic action of all the medications may produce severe symptoms because the effects are additive. Seniors and individuals with a medical condition may be particularly sensitive to anticholinergic side effects. Excessive anticholinergic activity may induce delirium, a toxic reaction characterized by impaired consciousness, confusion, and inability to sustain attention.

Chlorpromazine may block a compensatory response—the narrowing of blood vessels—that counterbalances postural change, resulting in a momentary drop in blood pressure when the person rises too rapidly, which may cause dizziness and lightheadedness. This reaction is known as **orthostatic hypotension.** Patients, especially seniors and those taking antihypertensive medications, need to be cautious and rise slowly to allow the body to adjust to the change in position, avoiding a sudden drop in blood pressure.

Adverse Reactions and Precautions

Chlorpromazine may cause drowsiness and sedation and impair physical coordination and mental alertness. Patients should avoid potentially dangerous activities, such as driving a car or operating machinery, until they are sure that these side effects will not affect their ability to perform these tasks.

Chlorpromazine may enhance ultraviolet light absorption in the skin—a reaction known as **photosensitivity**—and predispose the person to sunburn. Patients should avoid prolonged exposure to sunlight, use sunscreen, and wear protective clothing until tolerance is developed to the medication.

Under very hot conditions, patients may be predisposed to heat-related illness and **heatstroke** because antipsychotics may disrupt the body's ability to regulate temperature. Patients should take precautions to protect themselves from prolonged exposure to hot, humid weather. It is important that patients maintain adequate ventilation and stay indoors.

Tardive dyskinesia is a potential adverse reaction from antipsychotic medications. It is characterized by late-onset abnormal involuntary movements. TD is a potentially irreversible condition with symptoms that commonly include "pill-rolling" movements of the fingers, darting and writhing movements of the tongue, lip puckering, facial grimacing, and other irregular movements. The risk of TD is associated with the duration of exposure to antipsychotic medication, and this risk increases with age. The conventional antipsychotics are associated with a greater risk of TD than the more recent second-generation antipsychotics.

Neuroleptic malignant syndrome (NMS) is a rare, toxic reaction to antipsychotics. The symptoms are severe muscle stiffness, rigidity, elevated body temperature, increased heart rate and blood pressure, irregular pulse, and profuse sweating. NMS may lead to delirium and coma. It can be fatal if medical intervention is not immediately provided. There are no tests to predict whether an individual is susceptible to developing NMS when exposed to an antipsychotic. Thus NMS must be recognized early because it is a medical emergency that requires immediate discontinuation of the antipsychotic, hospitalization, and intensive medical treatment.

Antipsychotics can lower the seizure threshold and induce **seizures** in susceptible individuals, especially those with a history of seizure disorder. Patients with a seizure disorder who are receiving anticonvulsants often receive antipsychotics without any increase in seizures.

The FDA found that the first-generation antipsychotic medicines may be associated with an increased risk of death when used in treating elderly patients with dementia-related psychosis. The FDA now deems that all antipsychotic medications, including chlorpromazine, are not indicated for treating elderly patients with dementia. Physicians who prescribe antipsychotic medications to elderly patients for dementia-related psychosis should discuss this fatal risk with the patient, the patient's family, or the patient's caretaker.

Use in Pregnancy and Breastfeeding: Pregnancy Category C

Chlorpromazine has not been tested in women to determine its safety in pregnancy. The effects of the medication on the developing fetus in pregnant women are unknown. In animal studies, there was no evidence of harm to the fetus when exposed to chlorpromazine. Animal studies, however, are not always predictive of effects in humans. Women who are pregnant or may become pregnant should discuss this with their physician. Some women may experience a recurrence of their psychosis when they stop chlorpromazine. In these circumstances, the physician may discuss the need to restart the medication or seek an alternative medication or treatment.

Nursing mothers should not take chlorpromazine, because small amounts will pass into breast milk and be ingested by the baby. If stopping the antipsychotic is not an alternative, breastfeeding should not be started or should be discontinued.

Possible Drug Interactions

Some medications when taken with chlorpromazine may result in drug interactions that alter their levels, which may produce undesired reactions. Medications that may prolong cardiac conduction should not be taken together with chlorpromazine because the combination may increase the risk of arrhythmias. The possible drug interactions with chlorpromazine are summarized in the table below.

Tricyclic antidepressants (TCAs)	Chlorpromazine may increase the blood levels of TCAs, which may increase the risk of arrhythmia.
Demerol (meperidine)	The combination of chlorpromazine and Demerol may result in excessive sedation and hypotension.
Orap (pimozide)	Chlorpromazine and Orap should never be combined. The two medications may have an additive effect on prolongation of cardiac conduction, increasing the risk of arrhythmia.
Antiparkinson agents (e.g., Cogentin, Artane, Benadryl)	The combination of chlorpromazine with an antiparkinson agent may increase side effects from excessive anticholinergic activity such as dry mouth, blurred vision, constipation, and confusion.
Seroquel (quetiapine)	Chlorpromazine may significantly decrease the blood levels of Seroquel, reducing its effectiveness.

Patients taking chlorpromazine should not consume alcohol because the combination may impair thinking, judgment, and coordination.

Overdose

Depression of the central nervous system (CNS) with deep somnolence, low blood pressure, and EPS, and abnormal electrocardiograms are frequent signs of chlorpromazine overdose. More serious complications may include agitation, restlessness, convulsions, fever, arrhythmias, and coma. The risk of death from the overdose depends on the amount of chlorpromazine ingested and whether it was combined with other medications, especially CNS depressants.

Any suspected overdose should be treated as an emergency. The person should be taken to the emergency room for observation and treatment. The prescription bottle of medication (and any other medication suspected in the overdose) should be brought as well, because the information on the prescription label can be helpful to the treating physician in determining the number of pills ingested.

Special Considerations

- Do not discontinue chlorpromazine without consulting your physician.
- If you miss a dose, take it as soon as possible. If it is close to the next scheduled dose, skip the missed dose and continue on your regular dosing schedule. Do not take double doses.
- Chlorpromazine may be taken with or without food.
- Chlorpromazine may cause sedation and drowsiness, especially during initiation of therapy, and may impair your alertness. Use caution when driving or performing tasks that require alertness.
- Chlorpromazine may enhance ultraviolet light absorption and increase the risk of sunburn. Use a sunscreen, and avoid excessive exposure to sunlight.
- Store the medication in its originally labeled, light-resistant container, away from heat and moisture. Heat and moisture may precipitate breakdown of your medication, and the medication may lose its therapeutic effects.
- Keep your medication out of reach of children.

If you have any questions about your medication, consult your physician or pharmacist.

Notes

_____

_____

_____

_____

_____

From Chew RH, Hales RE, Yudofsky SC: *What Your Patients Need to Know About Psychiatric Medications*, Second Edition. Washington, DC, American Psychiatric Publishing, 2009

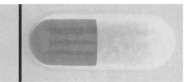

Fluphenazine HCl and Fluphenazine Decanoate (Prolixin)

Generic names: Fluphenazine and fluphenazine decanoate
Available strengths: 1 mg, 2.5 mg, 5 mg, 10 mg tablets;
 2.5 mg/mL, 5 mg/mL oral solution;
 2.5 mg/mL injection; 25 mg/mL injection (Prolixin Decanoate)
Available in generic: Yes
Drug class: First-generation (conventional) antipsychotic

General Information

Fluphenazine (Prolixin) belongs to the class of antipsychotics known as the **first-generation antipsychotics,** sometimes referred to as *conventional* or *typical* antipsychotics. Fluphenazine was sold under the brand Prolixin, but Prolixin has since been discontinued. Currently, only generic fluphenazine is available. The first-generation antipsychotics represent an older class of antipsychotics that have been the standard for treating psychotic disorders for many decades. When compared with a newer class of **second-generation antipsychotics,** these earlier antipsychotics are referred to as *typical* or *conventional* because they lack the wider spectrum of therapeutic activity. The first-generation antipsychotics are also more likely to induce side effects that cause movement disorders, such as **extrapyramidal symptoms** (EPS) and **tardive dyskinesia** (TD), than the newer antipsychotics.

Fluphenazine is a relatively high-potency agent, compared with other first-generation antipsychotics such as chlorpromazine and thioridazine. The high-potency antipsychotics are less sedating, less likely to lower blood pressure with postural changes, and have fewer **anticholinergic side effects,** but they are associated with more neurological disturbances that cause EPS than the lower-potency antipsychotics.

Fluphenazine was approved by the U.S. Food and Drug Administration for treatment of psychotic disorders, including schizophrenia, schizoaffective disorder, and drug-induced psychosis. The use of a medication for its approved indications is called its *labeled use*. In clinical practice, however, physicians often prescribe medications for *unlabeled* ("off-label") uses when published clinical studies, case reports, or their own clinical experiences support the efficacy and safety of those treatments. For instance, fluphenazine may be prescribed with a mood stabilizer to treat acute mania, since the mood stabilizer has a slower onset of action. After the symptoms of mania abate, fluphenazine is discontinued and the mood stabilizer is continued alone.

Fluphenazine is available in generic form in all preparations from various generic manufacturers. Fluphenazine also comes in a long-acting preparation, fluphenazine decanoate, for intramuscular injection. Given by deep intramuscular injection, the drug is deposited into muscle tissues and is absorbed slowly into circulation from its depot site. For patients who may have difficulty taking their medication as scheduled, fluphenazine decanoate offers the convenience of an injectable form that can be given every 2–3 weeks without the need for oral medication.

Dosing Information

The recommended starting oral dosage of fluphenazine in treating schizophrenia is 2–5 mg/day, taken in divided doses twice daily. It may be taken without regard to meals. The dosage may be increased weekly in increments of 2.5 mg/day. The dosage usually ranges between 5 mg/day and 10 mg/day but should not exceed 20 mg/day. Dosages above 20 mg/day may be needed for some patients but may be associated with more frequent EPS.

Fluphenazine decanoate is administered by deep intramuscular injection. Patients' symptoms should be stabilized while they are taking oral fluphenazine before switching to the decanoate injection. The initial dosage of fluphenazine decanoate should not exceed 50 mg, and the patient may need to continue taking oral fluphenazine until the effective decanoate dosage is established. The usual maintenance dosage for fluphenazine decanoate is in the range of 25–50 mg every 2–3 weeks.

Common Side Effects

Fluphenazine is less sedating than the low-potency, conventional antipsychotics, but it often induces bothersome side effects called **extrapyramidal symptoms.** These are neurological disturbances caused by antipsychotics (or a neurological disorder) in the area of the brain that controls motor coordination. When disruption occurs in a particular area of the brain, it can produce symptoms that mimic Parkinson's disease (**parkinsonism**), including muscle stiffness, rigidity, tremor, drooling, and a "mask-like" facial expression. However, unlike Parkinson's disease, which is a progressive neurological disease, parkinsonism from treatment with an antipsychotic is reversible. The Parkinson-like symptoms may be treated, and prevented, by using antiparkinson agents (also called anticholinergic agents) such as Cogentin (benztropine), Benadryl (diphenhydramine), Artane (trihexyphenidyl), and Kemadrin (procyclidine).

Akathisia is another form of EPS characterized by a subjective sense of restlessness accompanied by fidgeting, inability to sit still, nervousness, muscle discomfort, and agitation. Generally, antiparkinson agents are not effective in managing akathisia. Use of Inderal (propranolol), a beta-blocker, may be helpful and is sometimes prescribed by physicians.

Dystonia is a type of EPS with acute onset. The patient may develop a sudden spasm of the muscles of the tongue, jaw, and neck. **This is not an allergic reaction to the antipsychotic medication.** Although a dystonic reaction may be painful and frightening, it can be rapidly reversed with an intramuscular injection of an anticholinergic medication such as Cogentin or Benadryl. With a dystonic reaction, the patient should seek immediate medical attention and receive treatment.

Elevation of **prolactin levels** is common with conventional antipsychotics. Prolactin is a hormone produced in the area of the brain called the pituitary gland. It is normally elevated in women following childbirth, stimulating lactation, or milk production. The effects of elevated prolactin include breast enlargement and milk production (**galactorrhea**) in both women and men. Elevated prolactin is also associated with impotence in men and irregular menstrual cycles or absence of menstruation in women. When side effects from elevated prolactin levels become bothersome, the alternative is to switch to one of the second-generation antipsychotic agents with no propensity to elevate this hormone.

Fluphenazine has a moderate effect on weight gain. It is unclear whether this is due to an underlying metabolic change caused by the antipsychotic or to increased appetite. Weight should be monitored closely during therapy, and if weight gain occurs, an intervention program of diet and exercise should be started.

232

Orthostatic hypotension and anticholinergic side effects are usually not as troubling with fluphenazine as they are with the low-potency antipsychotics.

Adverse Reactions and Precautions

Fluphenazine may cause drowsiness and sedation and impair physical coordination and mental alertness. Patients should avoid potentially dangerous activities, such as driving a car or operating machinery, until they are sure that these side effects will not affect their ability to perform these tasks.

Tardive dyskinesia is a potential adverse reaction from antipsychotic medications. It is characterized by late-onset abnormal involuntary movements. TD is a potentially irreversible condition with symptoms that commonly include "pill-rolling" movements of the fingers, darting and writhing movements of the tongue, lip puckering, facial grimacing, and other irregular movements. The risk of TD is associated with the duration of exposure to antipsychotic medication, and this risk increases with age. The conventional antipsychotics are associated with a greater risk of TD than the more recent second-generation antipsychotics.

Neuroleptic malignant syndrome (NMS) is a rare, toxic reaction to antipsychotics. The symptoms are severe muscle stiffness, rigidity, elevated body temperature, increased heart rate and blood pressure, irregular pulse, and profuse sweating. NMS may lead to delirium and coma. It can be fatal if medical intervention is not immediately provided. There are no tests to predict whether an individual is susceptible to developing NMS when exposed to an antipsychotic. Thus NMS must be recognized early because it is a medical emergency that requires immediate discontinuation of the antipsychotic, hospitalization, and intensive medical treatment.

Antipsychotics can lower the seizure threshold and induce **seizures** in susceptible individuals, especially those with a history of seizure disorder. Patients with a seizure disorder who are receiving anticonvulsants often receive antipsychotics without any increase in seizures.

The FDA found that the first-generation antipsychotic medications may be associated with an increased risk of death when used in treating elderly patients with dementia-related psychosis. The FDA now deems that all antipsychotic medications, including fluphenazine, are not indicated for treating elderly patients with dementia. Physicians who prescribe antipsychotic medications to elderly patients for dementia-related psychosis should discuss this fatal risk with the patient, the patient's family, or the patient's caretaker.

Use in Pregnancy and Breastfeeding: Pregnancy Category C

Fluphenazine has not been tested in women to determine its safety in pregnancy. The effects of the medication on the developing fetus in pregnant women are unknown. In animal studies, there was no evidence of harm to the fetus when exposed to fluphenazine. Animal studies, however, are not always predictive of effects in humans. Women who are pregnant or may become pregnant should discuss this with their physician. Some women may experience a recurrence of their psychosis when they stop fluphenazine. In these circumstances, the physician may discuss the need to restart the medication or seek an alternative medication or treatment.

Nursing mothers should not take fluphenazine, because small amounts will pass into breast milk and be ingested by the baby. If stopping the antipsychotic is not an alternative, breastfeeding should not be started or should be discontinued.

Possible Drug Interactions

Some medications when taken with fluphenazine may result in drug interactions that alter their levels, which may produce undesired reactions. The possible drug interactions with fluphenazine are summarized in the table on the next page.

Patients taking fluphenazine should not consume alcohol because the combination may impair thinking, judgment, and coordination.

Prozac (fluoxetine)	Prozac may inhibit the metabolism of fluphenazine and increase fluphenazine's blood levels, which may increase the side effects and risk for toxicity from fluphenazine.
Paxil (paroxetine)	Paxil may inhibit the metabolism of fluphenazine and increase fluphenazine's blood levels, which may increase the side effects and risk for toxicity from fluphenazine.
Barbiturates	Barbiturates such as phenobarbital may reduce the blood levels of fluphenazine and lower its therapeutic effectiveness.
Tricyclic antidepressants (TCAs)	Fluphenazine may increase the blood levels of TCAs such as Elavil and Sinequan and increase the side effects and risk for toxicity from these antidepressants.
Antacids with aluminum	Antacids containing aluminum salts (e.g., aluminum hydroxide) may impair the gastrointestinal absorption of fluphenazine, reducing its therapeutic effectiveness. Take the antacid 1 hour before or 2 hours after fluphenazine.
Orap (pimozide)	The coadministration of fluphenazine and Orap, another antipsychotic, may produce an additive effect of prolonging cardiac conduction (QT interval) and increase the risk of arrhythmias. Concomitant administration of these two antipsychotics should be avoided.

Overdose

Depression of the central nervous system (CNS) with deep somnolence, low blood pressure, and EPS are common signs of fluphenazine overdose. More serious complications may include agitation, restlessness, convulsions, fever, arrhythmias, and coma. The risk of death from the overdose depends on the amount of fluphenazine ingested and whether it was combined with other medications, especially CNS depressants.

Any suspected overdose should be treated as an emergency. The person should be taken to the emergency room for observation and treatment. The prescription bottle of medication (and any other medication suspected in the overdose) should be brought as well, because the information on the prescription label can be helpful to the treating physician in determining the number of pills ingested.

Special Considerations

- Do not discontinue fluphenazine without consulting your physician.
- If you miss a dose, take it as soon as possible. If it is close to the next scheduled dose, skip the missed dose and continue on your regular dosing schedule. Do not take double doses.
- Fluphenazine may be taken with or without food.
- Fluphenazine may cause sedation and drowsiness, especially during initiation of therapy, and may impair your alertness. Use caution when driving or performing tasks that require alertness.
- Store the medication in its originally labeled, light-resistant container, away from heat and moisture. Heat and moisture may precipitate breakdown of your medication, and the medication may lose its therapeutic effects.
- Keep your medication out of reach of children.

If you have any questions about your medication, consult your physician or pharmacist.

Notes

From Chew RH, Hales RE, Yudofsky SC: *What Your Patients Need to Know About Psychiatric Medications*, Second Edition. Washington, DC, American Psychiatric Publishing, 2009

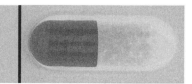

Haldol and Haldol Decanoate (haloperidol)

Generic name: Haloperidol and haloperidol decanoate
Available strengths: 0.5 mg, 1 mg, 2 mg, 5 mg,
   10 mg, 20 mg tablets; 2 mg/mL oral concentrate;
   5 mg/mL injection; 50 mg/mL, 100 mg/mL injection
   (Haldol Decanoate)
Available in generic: Yes
Drug class: First-generation (conventional) antipsychotic

General Information

Haldol (haloperidol) belongs to the class of antipsychotics known as the **first-generation antipsychotics,** sometimes referred to as *conventional* or *typical* antipsychotics. The first-generation antipsychotics represent an older class of antipsychotics that have been the standard for treating psychotic disorders for many decades. When compared with a newer class of **second-generation antipsychotics,** these earlier antipsychotics are referred to as *typical* or *conventional* because they lack the wider spectrum of therapeutic activity. The first-generation antipsychotics are also more likely to induce side effects that cause movement disorders, such as **extrapyramidal symptoms** (EPS) and **tardive dyskinesia** (TD), than the newer antipsychotics.

Haldol is a relatively high-potency agent, compared with other first-generation antipsychotics such as chlorpromazine and thioridazine. The high-potency antipsychotics are less sedating, less likely to lower blood pressure with postural changes, and have fewer **anticholinergic side effects,** but they are associated with more neurological disturbances that cause EPS than are the lower-potency antipsychotics.

Haldol was approved by the U.S. Food and Drug Administration for treatment of psychotic disorders, including schizophrenia, schizoaffective disorder, drug-induced psychosis, Tourette's syndrome, and behavioral problems in children with combative and explosive disorders. The use of a medication for its approved indications is called its *labeled use.* In clinical practice, however, physicians often prescribe medications for *unlabeled* ("off-label") uses when published clinical studies, case reports, or their own clinical experiences support the efficacy and safety of those treatments. For instance, Haldol may be prescribed with a mood stabilizer to treat acute mania, since the mood stabilizer has a slower onset of action. After the symptoms of mania abate, Haldol is discontinued and the mood stabilizer is continued alone.

Haloperidol tablets, oral solution, and decanoate are available in generic preparations from various manufacturers. Haldol, the brand, however, comes only in injectable forms: Haldol Injection and Haldol Decanoate. Haldol Decanoate is a long-acting preparation. Given by deep intramuscular injection, Haldol Decanoate is deposited into muscle tissues and is absorbed slowly into circulation from its depot site. For patients who may have difficulty taking their medications as scheduled, Haldol Decanoate offers the convenience of a long-acting injection, which can be given every 3–4 weeks without the need for oral medication.

Dosing Information

The recommended starting dose of oral Haldol for treatment of schizophrenia is 2–10 mg, taken once daily, preferably in the evening or at bedtime. It may be taken without regard to meals. The dosage may be increased in increments of 5 mg/day on a weekly basis. The dosage range is usually between 10 mg/day and 20 mg/day and may be taken twice a day if the patient cannot tolerate once-a-day dosing. Dosages greater than 20 mg/day may be needed for some patients.

Haldol Decanoate is administered by deep intramuscular injection. Patients' symptoms should be stabilized while they are taking the oral form before converting to the injection. The initial dosage of Haldol Decanoate should not exceed 100 mg, and the patient may need to continue taking oral Haldol until the effective decanoate dosage is established. The usual maintenance dosage for Haldol Decanoate is 100–200 mg every 3–4 weeks. From the intramuscular site of injection, Haldol is split from the decanoate chain and is slowly absorbed into the bloodstream.

Common Side Effects

Haldol is less sedating than the lower-potency antipsychotics, but it induces bothersome side effects called **extrapyramidal symptoms.** These are neurological disturbances caused by antipsychotics (or a neurological disorder) in the area of the brain that controls motor coordination. Haldol is more likely to induce EPS than are lower-potency agents. When disruption occurs in a particular area of the brain, it can produce symptoms that mimic Parkinson's disease, **parkinsonism,** including muscle stiffness, rigidity, tremor, drooling, and a "mask-like" facial expression. However, unlike Parkinson's disease, which is a progressive neurological disease, parkinsonism from treatment with an antipsychotic is reversible. The Parkinson-like symptoms may be treated, and prevented, by using antiparkinson agents (also called anticholinergic agents) such as Cogentin (benztropine), Benadryl (diphenhydramine), Artane (trihexyphenidyl), and Kemadrin (procyclidine).

Akathisia is another form of EPS characterized by a subjective sense of restlessness accompanied by fidgeting, inability to sit still, nervousness, muscle discomfort, and agitation. Generally, antiparkinson agents are not effective in managing akathisia. Use of Inderal (propranolol), a beta-blocker, may be helpful and is sometimes prescribed by physicians.

Dystonia is a type of EPS with acute onset. The patient may develop a sudden spasm of the muscles of the tongue, jaw, and neck. **This is not an allergic reaction to the antipsychotic medication.** Although a dystonic reaction may be painful and frightening, it can be rapidly reversed with an intramuscular injection of an anticholinergic medication such as Cogentin or Benadryl. With a dystonic reaction, the patient should seek immediate medical attention and receive treatment.

Elevation of **prolactin levels** is common with conventional antipsychotics. Prolactin is a hormone produced in the area of the brain called the pituitary gland. It is normally elevated in women following childbirth, stimulating lactation, or milk production. The effects of elevated prolactin include breast enlargement and milk production (**galactorrhea**) in both women and men. Elevated prolactin is also associated with impotence in men and irregular menstrual cycles or absence of menstruation in women. When side effects from elevated prolactin levels become bothersome, the alternative is to switch to one of the second-generation antipsychotic agents with no propensity to elevate this hormone.

Haldol has a moderate effect on weight gain. It is unclear whether this is due to an underlying metabolic change caused by the antipsychotic or to increased appetite. Weight should be monitored closely during therapy, and if weight gain occurs, an intervention program of diet and exercise should be started.

Orthostatic hypotension and anticholinergic side effects are usually not as troubling with Haldol as they are with the low-potency antipsychotics.

Adverse Reactions and Precautions

Haldol may cause drowsiness and sedation and impair physical coordination and mental alertness. Patients should avoid potentially dangerous activities, such as driving a car or operating machinery, until they are sure that these side effects will not affect their ability to perform these tasks.

Tardive dyskinesia is a potential adverse reaction from antipsychotic medications. It is characterized by late-onset abnormal involuntary movements. TD is a potentially irreversible condition with symptoms that commonly include "pill-rolling" movements of the fingers, darting and writhing movements of the tongue, lip puckering, facial grimacing, and other irregular movements. The risk of TD is associated with the duration of exposure to antipsychotic medication, and this risk increases with age. The conventional antipsychotics are associated with a greater risk of TD than the more recent second-generation antipsychotics.

Neuroleptic malignant syndrome (NMS) is a rare, toxic reaction to antipsychotics. The symptoms are severe muscle stiffness, rigidity, elevated body temperature, increased heart rate and blood pressure, irregular pulse, and profuse sweating. NMS may lead to delirium and coma. It can be fatal if medical intervention is not immediately provided. There are no tests to predict whether an individual is susceptible to developing NMS when exposed to an antipsychotic. Thus NMS must be recognized early because it is a medical emergency that requires immediate discontinuation of the antipsychotic, hospitalization, and intensive medical treatment.

Antipsychotics can lower the seizure threshold and induce **seizures** in susceptible individuals, especially those with a history of seizure disorder. Patients with a seizure disorder who are receiving anticonvulsants often receive antipsychotics without any increase in seizures.

The FDA found that the first-generation antipsychotic medicines may be associated with an increased risk of death when used in treating elderly patients with dementia-related psychosis. The FDA now deems that all antipsychotic medications, including haloperidol, are not indicated for treating elderly patients with dementia. Physicians who prescribe antipsychotic medications to elderly patients for dementia-related psychosis should discuss this fatal risk with the patient, the patient's family, or the patient's caretaker.

Use in Pregnancy and Breastfeeding: Pregnancy Category C

Haldol has not been tested in women to determine its safety in pregnancy. The effects of the medication on the developing fetus in pregnant women are unknown. In animal studies, there was no evidence of harm to the fetus when exposed to Haldol. Animal studies, however, are not always predictive of effects in humans. Women who are pregnant or may become pregnant should discuss this with their physician. Some women may experience a recurrence of their psychosis when they stop Haldol. In these circumstances, the physician may discuss the need to restart the medication or seek an alternative medication or treatment.

Nursing mothers should not take Haldol, because small amounts will pass into breast milk and be ingested by the baby. If stopping the antipsychotic is not an alternative, breastfeeding should not be started or should be discontinued.

Possible Drug Interactions

Some medications when taken with Haldol may result in drug interactions that alter their levels, which may produce undesired reactions. The possible drug interactions with Haldol are summarized in the table below.

Tricyclic antidepressants (TCAs) (e.g., Elavil)	Haldol may increase the blood levels of TCAs, which may increase the side effects and toxicity of these types of antidepressants.
Tegretol (carbamazepine)	Tegretol may decrease the blood levels of Haldol, reducing its effectiveness.
Barbiturates	Barbiturates such as phenobarbital may reduce the blood levels of Haldol and its therapeutic effectiveness.
Lithium carbonate	The combination of lithium and Haldol may be associated with higher incidence of adverse reactions such as neurotoxicity. Although the two medications are often coadministered and appear to be safe and effective, they should be closely monitored.
Prozac (fluoxetine)	Prozac may inhibit the metabolism of Haldol and increase the blood levels, which may increase the side effects and toxicity of Haldol.
Effexor (venlafaxine)	Effexor may decrease the clearance of Haldol and increase Haldol's blood levels, potentially increasing adverse side effects of the antipsychotic medication.

Patients taking Haldol should not consume alcohol because the combination may impair thinking, judgment, and coordination.

Overdose

Depression of the central nervous system (CNS) with deep somnolence, low blood pressure, and EPS are common signs of Haldol overdose. More serious complications may include agitation, restlessness, convulsions, fever, arrhythmias, and coma. The risk of death from the overdose depends on the amount of Haldol ingested and whether it was combined with other medications, especially CNS depressants.

Any suspected overdose should be treated as an emergency. The person should be taken to the emergency room for observation and treatment. The prescription bottle of medication (and any other medication suspected in the overdose) should be brought as well, because the information on the prescription label can be helpful to the treating physician in determining the number of pills ingested.

Special Considerations

- Do not discontinue Haldol without consulting your physician.
- If you miss a dose, take it as soon as possible. If it is close to the next scheduled dose, skip the missed dose and continue on your regular dosing schedule. Do not take double doses.
- Haldol may be taken with or without food.
- Haldol may cause sedation and drowsiness, especially during initiation of therapy, and may impair your alertness. Use caution when driving or performing tasks that require alertness.
- Store the medication in its originally labeled, light-resistant container, away from heat and moisture. Heat and moisture may precipitate breakdown of your medication, and the medication may lose its therapeutic effects.
- Keep your medication out of reach of children.

   If you have any questions about your medication, consult your physician or pharmacist.

Notes

   From Chew RH, Hales RE, Yudofsky SC: *What Your Patients Need to Know About Psychiatric Medications*, Second Edition. Washington, DC, American Psychiatric Publishing, 2009

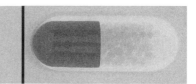

Loxitane (loxapine)

Generic name: Loxapine
Available strengths: 5 mg, 10 mg, 25 mg, 50 mg capsules
Available in generic: Yes
Drug class: First-generation (conventional) antipsychotic

General Information

Loxitane (loxapine) belongs to the class of antipsychotics known as the **first-generation antipsychotics,** sometimes referred to as *conventional* or *typical* antipsychotics. The first-generation antipsychotics represent an older class of antipsychotics that have been the standard for treating psychotic disorders for many decades. When compared with a newer class of **second-generation antipsychotics,** these earlier antipsychotics are referred to as *typical* or *conventional* because they lack the wider spectrum of therapeutic activity. The first-generation antipsychotics are also more likely to induce side effects that cause movement disorders, such as **extrapyramidal symptoms** (EPS) and **tardive dyskinesia** (TD), than the newer antipsychotics.

Loxitane is an intermediate-potency antipsychotic relative to other first-generation antipsychotics such as chlorpromazine and thioridazine, which are low-potency agents, and fluphenazine and Haldol (haloperidol), which are high-potency antipsychotics. Unlike low-potency first-generation antipsychotics, Loxitane is only mildly sedating and is less likely to lower blood pressure. Loxitane produces fewer EPS than the high-potency antipsychotics.

Although loxapine is better known by its brand name, Loxitane, it is dispensed by pharmacies primarily in generic form. Loxitane was approved by the U.S. Food and Drug Administration for treatment of psychotic disorders, including schizophrenia, schizoaffective disorder, and drug-induced psychosis. The use of a medication for its approved indications is called its *labeled use*. In clinical practice, however, physicians often prescribe drugs for *unlabeled* ("off-label") uses when published clinical studies, case reports, or their own clinical experiences support the efficacy and safety of those treatments. For instance, Loxitane may be prescribed with a mood stabilizer to treat acute mania, since the mood stabilizer has a slower onset of action. After the symptoms of mania abate, Loxitane is discontinued and the mood stabilizer is continued alone.

Dosing Information

The usual starting dosage of Loxitane is 10 mg twice a day (20 mg/day). In patients with severe symptoms, the dosage is increased rapidly over 7–10 days to a therapeutic range of 60–100 mg/day administered in divided doses of two or three times daily. Some patients with chronic schizophrenia may require dosages of

100–200 mg/day, but the dosage should not exceed 250 mg/day. When acute symptoms are stabilized, the physician may attempt to reduce the patient's dosage.

Common Side Effects

Loxitane may induce bothersome side effects known as **extrapyramidal symptoms.** Loxitane is more likely to induce EPS than are lower-potency agents. EPS are neurological disturbances caused by antipsychotics (or a neurological disorder) in the area of the brain that controls motor coordination. When disruption occurs in a particular area of the brain, it can produce symptoms that mimic Parkinson's disease (**parkinsonism**), including muscle stiffness, rigidity, tremor, drooling, and a "mask-like" facial expression. However, unlike Parkinson's disease, which is a progressive neurological disease, parkinsonism from treatment with an antipsychotic is reversible. The Parkinson-like symptoms may be treated, and prevented, by using antiparkinson agents (also called anticholinergic agents) such as Cogentin (benztropine), Benadryl (diphenhydramine), Artane (trihexyphenidyl), and Kemadrin (procyclidine).

Akathisia is another form of EPS characterized by a subjective sense of restlessness accompanied by fidgeting, inability to sit still, nervousness, muscle discomfort, and agitation. Generally, antiparkinson agents are not effective in managing akathisia. Use of Inderal (propranolol), a beta-blocker, may be helpful and is sometimes prescribed by physicians.

Dystonia is a type of EPS with acute onset. The patient may develop a sudden spasm of the muscles of the tongue, jaw, and neck. **This is not an allergic reaction to the antipsychotic medication.** Although a dystonic reaction may be painful and frightening, it can be rapidly reversed with an intramuscular injection of an anticholinergic medication such as Cogentin or Benadryl. With a dystonic reaction, the patient should seek immediate medical attention and receive treatment.

Elevation of **prolactin levels** is common with conventional antipsychotics. Prolactin is a hormone produced in the area of the brain called the pituitary gland. It is normally elevated in women following childbirth, stimulating lactation, or milk production. The effects of elevated prolactin include breast enlargement and milk production (**galactorrhea**) in both women and men. Elevated prolactin is also associated with impotence in men and irregular menstrual cycles or absence of menstruation in women. When side effects from elevated prolactin levels become bothersome, the alternative is to switch to one of the second-generation antipsychotic agents with no propensity to elevate this hormone.

Loxitane has a moderate effect on weight gain. It is unclear whether this is due to an underlying metabolic change caused by the antipsychotic or to increased appetite. Weight should be monitored closely during therapy, and if weight gain occurs, an intervention program of diet and exercise should be started.

When a medication inhibits the action of **cholinergic neurons** in the nervous system, it produces an **anticholinergic reaction,** which may produce bothersome symptoms. Anticholinergic side effects from Loxitane may include blurred vision, dry mouth, constipation, and difficulty with urination. Seniors and individuals with a medical condition may be particularly sensitive to anticholinergic side effects.

Loxitane may block a compensatory response—the narrowing of blood vessels—that counterbalances postural change, resulting in a momentary drop in blood pressure when the person rises too rapidly, which may cause dizziness and lightheadedness. This reaction is known as **orthostatic hypotension.** Patients, especially seniors and those taking antihypertensive medications, need to be cautious and rise slowly to allow the body to adjust to the change in position, avoiding a sudden drop in blood pressure. Orthostatic hypotension and anticholinergic side effects, which occur more frequently with low-potency, first-generation antipsychotics, are usually not as troublesome with the intermediate- and higher-potency agents.

Adverse Reactions and Precautions

Loxitane may cause drowsiness and sedation and impair physical coordination and mental alertness. Patients should avoid potentially dangerous activities, such as driving a car or operating machinery, until they are sure that these side effects will not affect their ability to perform these tasks.

244

Loxitane may enhance ultraviolet light absorption in the skin—a reaction known as **photosensitivity**—and predispose the person to sunburn. Patients should avoid prolonged exposure to sunlight, use sunscreen, and wear protective clothing until tolerance is developed to the medication.

Under very hot conditions, patients may be predisposed to heat-related illness and **heatstroke** because antipsychotics may disrupt the body's ability to regulate temperature. Patients should take precautions to protect themselves from prolonged exposure to hot, humid weather. It is important that patients maintain adequate ventilation and stay indoors.

Tardive dyskinesia is a potential adverse reaction from antipsychotic medications. It is characterized by late-onset abnormal involuntary movements. TD is a potentially irreversible condition with symptoms that commonly include "pill-rolling" movements of the fingers, darting and writhing movements of the tongue, lip puckering, facial grimacing, and other irregular movements. The risk of TD is associated with the duration of exposure to antipsychotic medication, and this risk increases with age. The conventional antipsychotics are associated with a greater risk of TD than the more recent second-generation antipsychotics.

Neuroleptic malignant syndrome (NMS) is a rare, toxic reaction to antipsychotics. The symptoms are severe muscle stiffness, rigidity, elevated body temperature, increased heart rate and blood pressure, irregular pulse, and profuse sweating. NMS may lead to delirium and coma. It can be fatal if medical intervention is not immediately provided. There are no tests to predict whether an individual is susceptible to developing NMS when exposed to an antipsychotic. Thus NMS must be recognized early because it is a medical emergency that requires immediate discontinuation of the antipsychotic, hospitalization, and intensive medical treatment.

Antipsychotics can lower the seizure threshold and induce **seizures** in susceptible individuals, especially those with a history of seizure disorder. Patients with a seizure disorder who are receiving anticonvulsants often receive antipsychotics without any increase in seizures.

The FDA found that the first-generation antipsychotic medicines may be associated with an increased risk of death when used in treating elderly patients with dementia-related psychosis. The FDA now deems that all antipsychotic medications, including loxapine, are not indicated for treating elderly patients with dementia. Physicians who prescribe antipsychotic medications to elderly patients for dementia-related psychosis should discuss this fatal risk with the patient, the patient's family, or the patient's caretaker.

Use in Pregnancy and Breastfeeding: Pregnancy Category C

Loxitane has not been tested in women to determine its safety in pregnancy. The effects of the medication on the developing fetus in pregnant women are unknown. In animal studies, there was no evidence of harm to the fetus when exposed to Loxitane. Animal studies, however, are not always predictive of effects in humans. Women who are pregnant or may become pregnant should discuss this with their physician. Some women may experience a recurrence of their psychosis when they stop Loxitane. In these circumstances, the physician may discuss the need to restart the medication or seek an alternative medication or treatment.

Nursing mothers should not take Loxitane, because small amounts will pass into breast milk and be ingested by the baby. If stopping the antipsychotic is not an alternative, breastfeeding should not be started or should be discontinued.

Possible Drug Interactions

Some medications when taken with Loxitane may result in drug interactions that alter their levels, which may produce undesired reactions. Use of medications for lowering blood pressure (antihypertensive medications) should be monitored closely because Loxitane may lower blood pressure and produce an additive effect. Medications that act on the central nervous system (CNS), including benzodiazepines (e.g., Valium), antihistamines, and narcotic pain medications, may possibly increase the risk and severity of CNS-related side effects, including somnolence, drowsiness, dizziness, and fatigue.

Patients taking Loxitane should not consume alcohol because the combination may increase drowsiness and sedation and impair thinking, judgment, and coordination.

Overdose

Depression of the CNS with deep somnolence, low blood pressure, and EPS are common signs of Loxitane overdose. More serious complications may include agitation, restlessness, convulsions, fever, arrhythmias, and coma. The risk of death from the overdose depends on the amount of Loxitane ingested and whether it was combined with other medications, especially CNS depressants.

Any suspected overdose should be treated as an emergency. The person should be taken to the emergency room for observation and treatment. The prescription bottle of medication (and any other medication suspected in the overdose) should be brought as well, because the information on the prescription label can be helpful to the treating physician in determining the number of pills ingested.

Special Considerations

- Do not discontinue Loxitane without consulting your physician.
- If you miss a dose, take it as soon as possible. If it is close to the next scheduled dose, skip the missed dose and continue on your regular dosing schedule. Do not take double doses.
- Loxitane may be taken with or without food.
- Loxitane may cause sedation and drowsiness, especially during initiation of therapy, and may impair your alertness. Use caution when driving or performing tasks that require alertness.
- Loxitane may enhance ultraviolet light absorption and increase the risk of sunburn. Use a sunscreen, and avoid excessive exposure to sunlight.
- Store the medication in its originally labeled, light-resistant container, away from heat and moisture. Heat and moisture may precipitate breakdown of your medication, and the medication may lose its therapeutic effects.
- Keep your medication out of reach of children.

If you have any questions about your medication, consult your physician or pharmacist.

Notes

From Chew RH, Hales RE, Yudofsky SC: *What Your Patients Need to Know About Psychiatric Medications,* Second Edition. Washington, DC, American Psychiatric Publishing, 2009.

Navane (thiothixene)

Generic name: Thiothixene
Available strengths: 1 mg, 2 mg, 5 mg, 10 mg,
   20 mg capsules; 5 mg/mL oral concentrate
Available in generic: Yes
Drug class: First-generation (conventional) antipsychotic

General Information

Navane (thiothixene) belongs to the class of antipsychotics known as the **first-generation antipsychotics,** sometimes referred to as *conventional* or *typical* antipsychotics. The first-generation antipsychotics represent an older class of antipsychotics that have been the standard for treating psychotic disorders for many decades. When compared with a newer class of **second-generation antipsychotics,** these earlier antipsychotics are referred to as *typical* or *conventional* because they lack the wider spectrum of therapeutic activity. The first-generation antipsychotics are also more likely to induce side effects that cause movement disorders, such as **extrapyramidal symptoms** (EPS) and **tardive dyskinesia** (TD), than the newer antipsychotics.

Navane is a relatively high-potency agent, compared with other first-generation antipsychotics such as chlorpromazine and thioridazine. The high-potency antipsychotics are less sedating, less likely to lower blood pressure with postural changes, and have fewer **anticholinergic side effects,** but they are associated with more neurological disturbances that cause EPS than are the lower-potency antipsychotics.

Navane was approved by the U.S. Food and Drug Administration for treatment of psychotic disorders, including schizophrenia, schizoaffective disorder, and drug-induced psychosis. It is available generically from various manufacturers, although it is better known by its brand name, Navane. The use of a medication for its approved indications is called its *labeled use.* In clinical practice, however, physicians often prescribe medication for *unlabeled* ("off-label") uses when published clinical studies, case reports, or their own clinical experiences support the efficacy and safety of those treatments. For instance, Navane may be prescribed with a mood stabilizer to treat acute mania, since the mood stabilizer has a slower onset of action. After the symptoms of mania abate, Navane is discontinued and the mood stabilizer is continued alone.

Dosing Information

For treatment of acute psychosis, the usual starting dosage of Navane is 5 mg twice daily. The dosage is increased as needed to an optimal range of 20–30 mg/day, given in divided doses. The maximum dosage is 60 mg/day. For outpatient treatment when the symptoms are less severe, for example, the starting dosage may be 2 mg two to three times a day and, if indicated, increased to 15 mg/day, given in divided doses.

Common Side Effects

Navane is less sedating than the lower-potency antipsychotics, but it induces bothersome side effects called **extrapyramidal symptoms.** These are neurological disturbances caused by antipsychotics (or a neurological disorder) in the area of the brain that controls motor coordination. Navane is more likely to induce EPS than are lower-potency agents. When disruption occurs in a particular area of the brain, it can produce symptoms that mimic Parkinson's disease (**parkinsonism**), including muscle stiffness, rigidity, tremor, drooling, and a "mask-like" facial expression. However, unlike Parkinson's disease, which is a progressive neurological disease, parkinsonism from treatment with an antipsychotic is reversible. The Parkinson-like symptoms may be treated, and prevented, by using antiparkinson agents (also called anticholinergic agents) such as Cogentin (benztropine), Benadryl (diphenhydramine), Artane (trihexyphenidyl), and Kemadrin (procyclidine).

Akathisia is another form of EPS characterized by a subjective sense of restlessness accompanied by fidgeting, inability to sit still, nervousness, muscle discomfort, and agitation. Generally, antiparkinson agents are not effective in managing akathisia. Use of Inderal (propranolol), a beta-blocker, may be helpful and is sometimes prescribed by physicians.

Dystonia is a type of EPS with acute onset. The patient may develop a sudden spasm of the muscles of the tongue, jaw, and neck. **This is not an allergic reaction to the antipsychotic medication.** Although a dystonic reaction may be painful and frightening, it can be rapidly reversed with an intramuscular injection of an anticholinergic medication such as Cogentin or Benadryl. With a dystonic reaction, the patient should seek immediate medical attention and receive treatment.

Elevation of **prolactin levels** is common with conventional antipsychotics. Prolactin is a hormone produced in the area of the brain called the pituitary gland. It is normally elevated in women following childbirth, stimulating lactation, or milk production. The effects of elevated prolactin include breast enlargement and milk production (**galactorrhea**) in both women and men. Elevated prolactin is also associated with impotence in men and irregular menstrual cycles or absence of menstruation in women. When side effects from elevated prolactin levels become bothersome, the alternative is to switch to one of the second-generation antipsychotic agents with no propensity to elevate this hormone.

Navane has a moderate effect on weight gain. It is unclear whether this is due to an underlying metabolic change caused by the antipsychotic or to increased appetite. Weight should be monitored closely during therapy, and if weight gain occurs, an intervention program of diet and exercise should be started.

When a medication inhibits the action of **cholinergic neurons** in the nervous system, it produces an **anticholinergic reaction,** which may produce bothersome symptoms. Anticholinergic side effects from Navane may include blurred vision, dry mouth, constipation, and difficulty with urination. Seniors and individuals with a medical condition may be particularly sensitive to anticholinergic side effects.

Navane may block a compensatory response—the narrowing of blood vessels—that counterbalances postural change, resulting in a momentary drop in blood pressure when the person rises too rapidly, which may cause dizziness and lightheadedness. This reaction is known as **orthostatic hypotension.** Patients, especially seniors and those taking antihypertensive medications, need to be cautious and rise slowly to allow the body to adjust to the change in position, avoiding a sudden drop in blood pressure. Orthostatic hypotension and anticholinergic side effects, which occur more frequently with low-potency, first-generation antipsychotics, are usually not as troublesome with the intermediate- and higher-potency agents.

Adverse Reactions and Precautions

Navane may cause drowsiness and sedation and impair physical coordination and mental alertness. Patients should avoid potentially dangerous activities, such as driving a car or operating machinery, until they are sure that these side effects will not affect their ability to perform these tasks.

Navane may enhance ultraviolet light absorption in the skin—a reaction known as **photosensitivity**—and predispose the person to sunburn. Patients should avoid prolonged exposure to sunlight, use sunscreen, and wear protective clothing until tolerance is developed to the medication.

Under very hot conditions, patients may be predisposed to heat-related illness and **heatstroke** because antipsychotics may disrupt the body's ability to regulate temperature. Patients should take precautions to protect themselves from prolonged exposure to hot, humid weather. It is important that patients maintain adequate ventilation and stay indoors.

Tardive dyskinesia is a potential adverse reaction from antipsychotic medications. It is characterized by late-onset abnormal involuntary movements. TD is a potentially irreversible condition with symptoms that commonly include "pill-rolling" movements of the fingers, darting and writhing movements of the tongue, lip puckering, facial grimacing, and other irregular movements. The risk of TD is associated with the duration of exposure to antipsychotic medication, and this risk increases with age. The conventional antipsychotics are associated with a greater risk of TD than the more recent second-generation antipsychotics.

Neuroleptic malignant syndrome (NMS) is a rare, toxic reaction to antipsychotics. The symptoms are severe muscle stiffness, rigidity, elevated body temperature, increased heart rate and blood pressure, irregular pulse, and profuse sweating. NMS may lead to delirium and coma. It can be fatal if medical intervention is not immediately provided. There are no tests to predict whether an individual is susceptible to developing NMS when exposed to an antipsychotic. Thus NMS must be recognized early because it is a medical emergency that requires immediate discontinuation of the antipsychotic, hospitalization, and intensive medical treatment.

Antipsychotics can lower the seizure threshold and induce **seizures** in susceptible individuals, especially those with a history of seizure disorder. Patients with a seizure disorder who are receiving anticonvulsants often receive antipsychotics without any increase in seizures.

The FDA found that the first-generation antipsychotic medicines may be associated with an increased risk of death when used in treating elderly patients with dementia-related psychosis. The FDA now deems that all antipsychotic medications, including thioxthixene, are not indicated for treating elderly patients with dementia. Physicians who prescribe antipsychotic medications to elderly patients for dementia-related psychosis should discuss this fatal risk with the patient, the patient's family, or the patient's caretaker.

Use in Pregnancy and Breastfeeding: Pregnancy Category C

Navane has not been tested in women to determine its safety in pregnancy. The effects of the medication on the developing fetus in pregnant women are unknown. In animal studies, there was no evidence of harm to the fetus when exposed to Navane. Animal studies, however, are not always predictive of effects in humans. Women who are pregnant or may become pregnant should discuss this with their physician. Some women may experience a recurrence of their psychosis when they stop Navane. In these circumstances, the physician may discuss the need to restart the medication or seek an alternative medication or treatment.

Nursing mothers should not take Navane, because small amounts will pass into breast milk and be ingested by the baby. If stopping the antipsychotic is not an alternative, breastfeeding should not be started or should be discontinued.

Possible Drug Interactions

Some medications when taken with Navane may result in drug interactions that alter their levels, which may produce undesired reactions. Use of medications for lowering blood pressure (antihypertensive medications), when Navane is also being taken, should be monitored closely because the high-potency antipsychotics may also lower blood pressure. Medications that act on the central nervous system (CNS), including benzodiazepines (e.g., Valium), antihistamines, and narcotic pain medications, may possibly increase the risk and severity of CNS-related side effects of antipsychotics, including somnolence, drowsiness, dizziness, and fatigue.

Patients taking Navane should not consume alcohol because the combination may impair thinking, judgment, and coordination.

Overdose

Depression of the CNS with deep somnolence, low blood pressure, and EPS are common signs of Navane overdose. More serious complications may include agitation, restlessness, convulsions, fever, arrhythmias, and coma. The risk of death from the overdose depends on the amount of Navane ingested and whether it was combined with other medications, especially CNS depressants.

Any suspected overdose should be treated as an emergency. The person should be taken to the emergency room for observation and treatment. The prescription bottle of medication (and any other medication suspected in the overdose) should be brought as well, because the information on the prescription label can be helpful to the treating physician in determining the number of pills ingested.

Special Considerations

- Do not discontinue Navane without consulting your physician.
- If you miss a dose, take it as soon as possible. If it is close to the next scheduled dose, skip the missed dose and continue on your regular dosing schedule. Do not take double doses.
- Navane may be taken with or without food.
- Navane may cause sedation and drowsiness, especially during initiation of therapy, and may impair your alertness. Use caution when driving or performing tasks that require alertness.
- Navane may enhance ultraviolet light absorption and increase the risk of sunburn. Use a sunscreen, and avoid excessive exposure to sunlight.
- Store the medication in its originally labeled, light-resistant container, away from heat and moisture. Heat and moisture may precipitate breakdown of your medication, and the medication may lose its therapeutic effects.
- Keep your medication out of reach of children.

If you have any questions about your medication, consult your physician or pharmacist.

Notes

From Chew RH, Hales RE, Yudofsky SC: *What Your Patients Need to Know About Psychiatric Medications,* Second Edition. Washington, DC, American Psychiatric Publishing, 2009

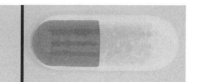

Orap (pimozide)

Generic name: Pimozide
Available strengths: 1 mg, 2 mg tablets
Available in generic: No
Drug class: First-generation (conventional) antipsychotic

General Information

Orap (pimozide) belongs to the class of antipsychotics known as the **first-generation antipsychotics,** sometimes referred to as *conventional* or *typical* antipsychotics. The first-generation antipsychotics represent an older class of antipsychotics that have been the standard for treating psychotic disorders for many decades. When compared with a newer class of **second-generation antipsychotics,** these earlier antipsychotics are "typical" or "conventional" because they lack the wider spectrum of therapeutic activity. The first-generation antipsychotics are also more likely to induce side effects that cause movement disorders, such as **extrapyramidal symptoms** (EPS) and **tardive dyskinesia** (TD), than the newer antipsychotics.

Orap is a relatively high-potency agent, compared with other first-generation antipsychotics such as chlorpromazine and thioridazine. The high-potency antipsychotics are less sedating, less likely to lower blood pressure with postural changes, and have fewer **anticholinergic side effects,** but are associated with more neurological disturbances that cause EPS than are the lower-potency antipsychotics.

Orap was approved by the U.S. Food and Drug Administration for treatment of Tourette's disorder, an inherited tic disorder that begins with simple facial tics and may progress to more complex tics, including grunting and compulsive utterances that can be publicly embarrassing and disabling for the individual. Generally, Orap is reserved for treatment of more severe cases of Tourette's disorder that do not respond to standard treatments. The use of a medication for its approved indications is called its *labeled* use. In clinical practice, however, physicians often prescribe medications for *unlabeled* ("off-label") uses when published clinical studies, case reports, or their own clinical experiences support the efficacy and safety of those treatments. Orap has limited unlabeled use and is prescribed only rarely for treatment of psychotic disorders, even though it is very similar to Haldol (haloperidol), another antipsychotic agent.

Dosing Information

The recommended starting dosage of Orap in treatment of Tourette's disorder is 1–2 mg/day, administered in divided doses and increased slowly up to 6–10 mg/day as needed.

Common Side Effects

Orap is less sedating than the lower-potency antipsychotics, but it may induce bothersome side effects called **extrapyramidal symptoms.** These are neurological disturbances caused by antipsychotics (or a neurological disorder) in the area of the brain that controls motor coordination. When disruption occurs in a particular area of the brain, it can produce symptoms that mimic Parkinson's disease (**parkinsonism**), including muscle stiffness, rigidity, tremor, drooling, and a "mask-like" facial expression. However, unlike Parkinson's disease, which is a progressive neurological disease, parkinsonism from treatment with an antipsychotic is reversible. The Parkinson-like symptoms may be treated, and prevented, by using antiparkinson agents (also called anticholinergic agents) such as Cogentin (benztropine), Benadryl (diphenhydramine), Artane (trihexyphenidyl), and Kemadrin (procyclidine).

Akathisia is another form of EPS characterized by a subjective sense of restlessness accompanied by fidgeting, inability to sit still, nervousness, muscle discomfort, and agitation. Generally, antiparkinson agents are not effective in managing akathisia. Use of Inderal (propranolol), a beta-blocker, may be helpful and is sometimes prescribed by physicians.

Dystonia is a type of EPS with acute onset. The patient may develop a sudden spasm of the muscles of the tongue, jaw, and neck. **This is not an allergic reaction to the antipsychotic medication.** Although a dystonic reaction may be painful and frightening, it can be rapidly reversed with an intramuscular injection of an anticholinergic medication such as Cogentin or Benadryl. With a dystonic reaction, the patient should seek immediate medical attention and receive treatment.

Elevation of **prolactin levels** is common with conventional antipsychotics. Prolactin is a hormone produced in the area of the brain called the pituitary gland. It is normally elevated in women following childbirth, stimulating lactation, or milk production. The effects of elevated prolactin include breast enlargement and milk production (**galactorrhea**) in both women and men. Elevated prolactin is also associated with impotence in men and irregular menstrual cycles or absence of menstruation in women. When side effects from elevated prolactin levels become bothersome, the alternative is to switch to one of the second-generation antipsychotic agents with no propensity to elevate this hormone.

Orap has a moderate effect on weight gain. It is unclear whether this is due to an underlying metabolic change caused by the antipsychotic or to increased appetite. Weight should be monitored closely during therapy, and if weight gain occurs, an intervention program of diet and exercise should be started.

Orthostatic hypotension and anticholinergic side effects are usually not as troubling with Orap as they are with low-potency antipsychotics.

Adverse Reactions and Precautions

Orap may cause drowsiness and sedation and impair physical coordination and mental alertness. Patients should avoid potentially dangerous activities, such as driving a car or operating machinery, until they are sure that these side effects will not affect their ability to perform these tasks.

Orap may enhance ultraviolet light absorption in the skin—a reaction known as **photosensitivity**—and predispose the person to sunburn. Patients should avoid prolonged exposure to sunlight, use sunscreen, and wear protective clothing until tolerance is developed to the medication.

Under very hot conditions, patients may be predisposed to heat-related illness and **heatstroke** because antipsychotics may disrupt the body's ability to regulate temperature. Patients should take precautions to protect themselves from prolonged exposure to hot, humid weather. It is important that patients maintain adequate ventilation and stay indoors.

Tardive dyskinesia is a potential adverse reaction from antipsychotic medications. It is characterized by late-onset abnormal involuntary movements. TD is a potentially irreversible condition with symptoms that commonly include "pill-rolling" movements of the fingers, darting and writhing movements of the tongue, lip puckering, facial grimacing, and other irregular movements. The risk of TD is associated with the duration of exposure to antipsychotic medication, and this risk increases with age. The conventional antipsychotics are associated with a greater risk of TD than the more recent second-generation antipsychotics.

Neuroleptic malignant syndrome (NMS) is a rare, toxic reaction to antipsychotics. The symptoms are severe muscle stiffness, rigidity, elevated body temperature, increased heart rate and blood pressure, irregular pulse, and profuse sweating. NMS may lead to delirium and coma. It can be fatal if medical intervention is not immediately provided. There are no tests to predict whether an individual is susceptible to developing NMS when exposed to an antipsychotic. Thus NMS must be recognized early because it is a medical emergency that requires immediate discontinuation of the antipsychotic, hospitalization, and intensive medical treatment.

Antipsychotics may slow electrical conduction in heart tissues (**myocardium**). Some patients taking antipsychotics show on their electrocardiogram (ECG) a prolongation of the electrical impulse as it travels in the myocardium. This abnormal ECG finding, called **QTc prolongation,** may signal a potential for developing an irregular heartbeat (**arrhythmia**). Orap is associated with a greater tendency to alter the electrical impulse, and therefore it has a higher risk of causing arrhythmias, especially in individuals with cardiac disease. Patients should have ECGs before and during Orap treatment. Moreover, medications that increase this potential for cardiac risk should not be taken with Orap (see "Possible Drug Interactions").

Antipsychotics can lower the seizure threshold and induce **seizures** in susceptible individuals, especially those with a history of seizure disorder. Patients with a seizure disorder who are receiving anticonvulsants often receive antipsychotics without any increase in seizures.

The FDA found that the first-generation antipsychotic medicines may be associated with an increased risk of death when used in treating elderly patients with dementia-related psychosis. The FDA now deems that all antipsychotic medications, including pimozide, are not indicated for treating elderly patients with dementia. Physicians who prescribe antipsychotic medications to elderly patients for dementia-related psychosis should discuss this fatal risk with the patient, the patient's family, or the patient's caretaker.

Use in Pregnancy and Breastfeeding: Pregnancy Category C

Orap has not been tested in women to determine its safety in pregnancy. The effects of the medication on the developing fetus in pregnant women are unknown. In animal studies, there was no evidence of harm to the fetus when exposed to Orap. Animal studies, however, are not always predictive of effects in humans. Women who are pregnant or may become pregnant should discuss this with their physician. Some women may experience a recurrence of their psychosis when they stop Orap. In these circumstances, the physician may discuss the need to restart the medication or seek an alternative medication or treatment.

Nursing mothers should not take Orap, because small amounts will pass into breast milk and be ingested by the baby. If stopping the antipsychotic is not an alternative, breastfeeding should not be started or should be discontinued.

Possible Drug Interactions

Some medications when taken with Orap may result in drug interactions that alter their levels, which may produce undesired reactions. Medications that may prolong cardiac conduction should not be taken together with Orap because the combination may increase the risk of arrhythmias. The possible drug interactions with Orap are summarized in the table on the next page.

Patients taking Orap should not consume alcohol because the combination may impair thinking, judgment, and coordination.

Tricyclic antidepressants (TCAs)	TCAs, which may prolong cardiac conduction, in combination with Orap can have an additive effect that increases the risk for arrhythmias.
Phenothiazine antipsychotics (e.g., Thorazine)	These medications should never be combined with Orap. This combination may have an additive effect of prolonging cardiac conduction, increasing the risk for arrhythmias.
Antiarrhythmic agents	Orap must be avoided if medications for treating arrhythmias are being taken, because the combination may further depress cardiac conduction.
Prozac (fluoxetine)	Prozac may inhibit the metabolism of Orap and increase its blood levels, which may increase the cardiac side effects and toxicity of Orap.
Macrolide antibiotics (e.g., erythromycin, Biaxin [clarithromycin], Zithromax [azithromycin])	These antibiotics may inhibit the metabolism of Orap and increase cardiac side effects and the risk for arrhythmias.
Nizoral (ketoconazole) and Sporanox (itraconazole)	These two antifungal agents may inhibit the metabolism of Orap and increase cardiac side effects and the risk for arrhythmias.
Cipro (ciprofloxacin) and Noroxin (norfloxacin)	These antibiotics, as well as others in this group (fluoroquinolones), may inhibit the metabolism of Orap and increase cardiac side effects and the risk for arrhythmias.

Overdose

Depression of the central nervous system (CNS) with deep somnolence, low blood pressure, EPS, and abnormal ECG results are signs of Orap overdose. More serious complications may include agitation, restlessness, convulsions, fever, arrhythmias, and coma. The risk of death from the overdose depends on the amount of Orap ingested and whether it was combined with other medications, especially CNS depressants.

Any suspected overdose should be treated as an emergency. The person should be taken to the emergency room for observation and treatment. The prescription bottle of medication (and any other medication suspected in the overdose) should be brought as well, because the information on the prescription label can be helpful to the treating physician in determining the number of pills ingested.

Special Considerations

- Do not discontinue Orap without consulting your physician.
- If you miss a dose, take it as soon as possible. If it is close to the next scheduled dose, skip the missed dose and continue on your regular dosing schedule. Do not take double doses.
- Orap may be taken with or without food.
- Orap may cause sedation and drowsiness, especially during initiation of therapy, and may impair your alertness. Use caution when driving or performing tasks that require alertness.

- Orap may enhance ultraviolet light absorption and increase the risk of sunburn. Use a sunscreen, and avoid excessive exposure to sunlight.
- Store the medication in its originally labeled, light-resistant container, away from heat and moisture. Heat and moisture may precipitate breakdown of your medication, and the medication may lose its therapeutic effects.
- Keep your medication out of reach of children.

If you have any questions about your medication, consult your physician or pharmacist.

Notes

From Chew RH, Hales RE, Yudofsky SC: *What Your Patients Need to Know About Psychiatric Medications*, Second Edition. Washington, DC, American Psychiatric Publishing, 2009

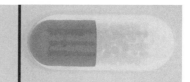

Perphenazine (Trilafon)

Generic name: Perphenazine
Available strengths: 2 mg, 4 mg, 8 mg, 16 mg tablets;
  16 mg/5 mL oral concentrate
Available in generic: Yes
Drug class: First-generation (conventional) antipsychotic

General Information

Perphenazine (Trilafon) belongs to the class of antipsychotics known as the **first-generation antipsychotics,** sometimes referred to as *conventional* or *typical* antipsychotics. Perphenazine was sold under the brand Trilafon, but Trilafon has since been discontinued. Currently, only generic perphenazine is available. The first-generation antipsychotics represent an older class of antipsychotics that have been the standard for treating psychotic disorders for many decades. When compared with a newer class of **second-generation antipsychotics,** these earlier antipsychotics are referred to as *typical* or *conventional* because they lack the wider spectrum of therapeutic activity. The first-generation antipsychotics are also more likely to induce side effects that cause movement disorders, such as **extrapyramidal symptoms** (EPS) and **tardive dyskinesia** (TD), than the newer antipsychotics.

Perphenazine is an intermediate-potency antipsychotic relative to other first-generation antipsychotics such as chlorpromazine and thioridazine, which are low-potency agents, and fluphenazine and Haldol (haloperidol), which are high-potency antipsychotics. Perphenazine is moderately sedating and less likely to lower blood pressure than the lower-potency agents. Perphenazine produces fewer EPS than the high-potency antipsychotics.

Perphenazine was approved by the U.S. Food and Drug Administration for treatment of psychotic disorders, including schizophrenia, schizoaffective disorder, and drug-induced psychosis. The use of a medication for its approved indications is called its *labeled use*. In clinical practice, however, physicians often prescribe medications for *unlabeled* ("off-label") uses when published clinical studies, case reports, or their own clinical experiences support the efficacy and safety of those treatments. For instance, perphenazine may be prescribed with a mood stabilizer to treat acute mania, since the mood stabilizer has a slower onset of action. After the symptoms of mania abate, perphenazine is discontinued and the mood stabilizer is continued alone.

Dosing Information

For treatment of acute psychosis, the hospitalized patient's starting dosage of perphenazine may be as high as 16–64 mg/day, given in divided doses. The maximum dosage should not exceed 64 mg/day. As symptoms abate, the dosage is reduced as soon as possible to a minimum effective dosage, which is usually in the range of 12–24 mg/day, given in divided doses. The dosage for seniors may be in the 8–16 mg/day range.

Common Side Effects

Perphenazine may induce bothersome side effects known as **extrapyramidal symptoms.** These are neurological disturbances caused by antipsychotics (or a neurological disorder) in the area of the brain that controls motor coordination. When disruption occurs in a particular area of the brain, it can produce symptoms that mimic Parkinson's disease (**parkinsonism**), including muscle stiffness, rigidity, tremor, drooling, and a "mask-like" facial expression. However, unlike Parkinson's disease, which is a progressive neurological disease, parkinsonism from treatment with an antipsychotic is reversible. The Parkinson-like symptoms may be treated, and prevented, by using antiparkinson agents (also called anticholinergic agents) such as Cogentin (benztropine), Benadryl (diphenhydramine), Artane (trihexyphenidyl), and Kemadrin (procyclidine).

Akathisia is another form of EPS characterized by a subjective sense of restlessness accompanied by fidgeting, inability to sit still, nervousness, muscle discomfort, and agitation. Generally, antiparkinson agents are not effective in managing akathisia. Use of Inderal (propranolol), a beta-blocker, may be helpful and is sometimes prescribed by physicians.

Dystonia is a type of EPS with acute onset. The patient may develop a sudden spasm of the muscles of the tongue, jaw, and neck. **This is not an allergic reaction to the antipsychotic medication.** Although a dystonic reaction may be painful and frightening, it can be rapidly reversed with an intramuscular injection of an anticholinergic medication such as Cogentin or Benadryl. With a dystonic reaction, the patient should seek immediate medical attention and receive treatment.

Elevation of **prolactin levels** is common with conventional antipsychotics. Prolactin is a hormone produced in the area of the brain called the pituitary gland. It is normally elevated in women following childbirth, stimulating lactation, or milk production. The effects of elevated prolactin include breast enlargement and milk production (**galactorrhea**) in both women and men. Elevated prolactin is also associated with impotence in men and irregular menstrual cycles or absence of menstruation in women. When side effects from elevated prolactin levels become bothersome, the alternative is to switch to one of the second-generation antipsychotic agents with no propensity to elevate this hormone.

Perphenazine has a moderate effect on weight gain. It is unclear whether this is due to an underlying metabolic change caused by the antipsychotic or to increased appetite. Weight should be monitored closely during therapy, and if weight gain occurs, an intervention program of diet and exercise should be started.

When a medication inhibits the action of **cholinergic neurons** in the nervous system, it produces an **anticholinergic reaction,** which may produce bothersome symptoms. Anticholinergic side effects from Perphenazine may include blurred vision, dry mouth, constipation, and difficulty with urination. Seniors and individuals with a medical condition may be particularly sensitive to anticholinergic side effects.

Perphenazine may block a compensatory response—the narrowing of blood vessels—that counterbalances postural change, resulting in a momentary drop in blood pressure when the person rises too rapidly, which may cause dizziness and lightheadedness. This reaction is known as **orthostatic hypotension.** Patients, especially seniors and those taking antihypertensive medications, need to be cautious and rise slowly to allow the body to adjust to the change in position, avoiding a sudden drop in blood pressure. Orthostatic hypotension and anticholinergic side effects, which occur more frequently with low-potency, first-generation antipsychotics, are usually not as troublesome with the intermediate- and higher-potency agents.

Adverse Reactions and Precautions

Perphenazine may cause sedation and drowsiness, but generally these effects are not as troublesome as with the lower-potency antipsychotics like chlorpromazine and thioridazine. Patients should avoid potentially dangerous activities, such as driving a car or operating machinery, until they are sure that these side effects will not affect their ability to perform these tasks.

Perphenazine may enhance ultraviolet light absorption in the skin—a reaction known as **photosensitivity**—and predispose the person to sunburn. Patients should avoid prolonged exposure to sunlight, use sunscreen, and wear protective clothing until tolerance is developed to the medication.

Under very hot conditions, patients may be predisposed to heat-related illness and **heatstroke** because antipsychotics may disrupt the body's ability to regulate temperature. Patients should take precautions to protect themselves from prolonged exposure to hot, humid weather. It is important that patients maintain adequate ventilation and stay indoors.

Tardive dyskinesia is a potential adverse reaction from antipsychotic medications. It is characterized by late-onset abnormal involuntary movements. TD is a potentially irreversible condition with symptoms that commonly include "pill-rolling" movements of the fingers, darting and writhing movements of the tongue, lip puckering, facial grimacing, and other irregular movements. The risk of TD is associated with the duration of exposure to antipsychotic medication, and this risk increases with age. The conventional antipsychotics are associated with a greater risk of TD than the more recent second-generation antipsychotics.

Neuroleptic malignant syndrome (NMS) is a rare, toxic reaction to antipsychotics. The symptoms are severe muscle stiffness, rigidity, elevated body temperature, increased heart rate and blood pressure, irregular pulse, and profuse sweating. NMS may lead to delirium and coma. It can be fatal if medical intervention is not immediately provided. There are no tests to predict whether an individual is susceptible to developing NMS when exposed to an antipsychotic. Thus NMS must be recognized early because it is a medical emergency that requires immediate discontinuation of the antipsychotic, hospitalization, and intensive medical treatment.

Antipsychotics can lower the seizure threshold and induce **seizures** in susceptible individuals, especially those with a history of seizure disorder. Patients with a seizure disorder who are receiving anticonvulsants often receive antipsychotics without any increase in seizures.

The FDA found that the first-generation antipsychotic medicines may be associated with an increased risk of death when used in treating elderly patients with dementia-related psychosis. The FDA now deems that all antipsychotic medications, including perphenazine, are not indicated for treating elderly patients with dementia. Physicians who prescribe antipsychotic medications to elderly patients for dementia-related psychosis should discuss this fatal risk with the patient, the patient's family, or the patient's caretaker.

Use in Pregnancy and Breastfeeding: Pregnancy Category C

Perphenazine has not been tested in women to determine its safety in pregnancy. The effects of the medication on the developing fetus in pregnant women are unknown. In animal studies, there was no evidence of harm to the fetus when exposed to perphenazine. Animal studies, however, are not always predictive of effects in humans. Women who are pregnant or may become pregnant should discuss this with their physician. Some women may experience a recurrence of their psychosis when they stop perphenazine. In these circumstances, the physician may discuss the need to restart the medication or seek an alternative medication or treatment.

Nursing mothers should not take perphenazine, because small amounts will pass into breast milk and be ingested by the baby. If stopping the antipsychotic is not an alternative, breastfeeding should not be started or should be discontinued.

Possible Drug Interactions

Some medications when taken with perphenazine may result in drug interactions that alter their levels, which may produce undesired reactions. Use of medications for lowering blood pressure (antihypertensive medications), when perphenazine is also being taken, should be monitored closely because the antipsychotic medication may lower blood pressure and produce an additive effect with the antihypertensive medication.

Medications that act on the central nervous system (CNS), including benzodiazepines (e.g., Valium), antihistamines, and narcotic pain medications, may possibly increase the risk and severity of CNS-related side effects of antipsychotics, including somnolence, drowsiness, dizziness, and fatigue.

Patients taking perphenazine should not consume alcohol because the combination may worsen drowsiness and sedation and impair thinking, judgment, and coordination.

Overdose

Depression of the CNS with deep somnolence, low blood pressure, and EPS are common signs of perphenazine overdose. More serious complications may include agitation, restlessness, convulsions, fever, arrhythmias, and coma. The risk of death from the overdose depends on the amount of perphenazine ingested and whether it was combined with other medications, especially CNS depressants.

Any suspected overdose should be treated as an emergency. The person should be taken to the emergency room for observation and treatment. The prescription bottle of medication (and any other medication suspected in the overdose) should be brought as well, because the information on the prescription label can be helpful to the treating physician in determining the number of pills ingested.

Special Considerations

- Do not discontinue perphenazine without consulting your physician.
- If you miss a dose, take it as soon as possible. If it is close to the next scheduled dose, skip the missed dose and continue on your regular dosing schedule. Do not take double doses.
- Perphenazine may be taken with or without food.
- Perphenazine may cause sedation and drowsiness, especially during initiation of therapy, and may impair your alertness. Use caution when driving or performing tasks that require alertness.
- Perphenazine may enhance ultraviolet light absorption and predispose to sunburn. Use a sunscreen, and avoid excessive exposure to sunlight.
- Store the medication in its originally labeled, light-resistant container, away from heat and moisture. Heat and moisture may precipitate breakdown of the medication, and the medication may lose its therapeutic effects.
- Keep your medication out of reach of children.

If you have any questions about your medication, consult your physician or pharmacist.

Notes

From Chew RH, Hales RE, Yudofsky SC: *What Your Patients Need to Know About Psychiatric Medications*, Second Edition. Washington, DC, American Psychiatric Publishing, 2009

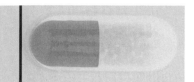

Thioridazine (Mellaril)

Generic name: Thioridazine
Available strengths: 10 mg, 15 mg, 25 mg, 50 mg, 100 mg,
   150 mg, 200 mg tablets
Available in generic: Yes
Drug class: First-generation (conventional) antipsychotic

General Information

Thioridazine (Mellaril) belongs to the class of antipsychotics known as the **first-generation antipsychotics,** sometimes referred to as *conventional* or *typical* antipsychotics. Thioridazine was sold under the brand Mellaril, but Mellaril has since been discontinued. Currently, only generic thioridazine is available in the United States. The first-generation antipsychotics represent an older class of antipsychotics that have been the standard for treating psychotic disorders for many decades. When compared with a newer class of **second-generation antipsychotics,** these earlier antipsychotics are referred to as *typical* or *conventional* because they lack the wider spectrum of therapeutic activity. The first-generation antipsychotics are also more likely to induce side effects that cause movement disorders, such as **extrapyramidal symptoms** (EPS) and **tardive dyskinesia** (TD), than the newer antipsychotics.

Thioridazine is a relatively low-potency agent, compared with other first-generation antipsychotics such as fluphenazine and Haldol (haloperidol). The low-potency antipsychotics are generally sedating and more likely to induce **anticholinergic side effects** but are less likely to cause EPS than are high-potency agents.

Thioridazine is approved by the U.S. Food and Drug Administration for the treatment of psychotic disorders such as schizophrenia, schizoaffective disorder, acute mania, and psychotic depression. In children, thioridazine is indicated for short-term treatment of severe behavioral problems marked by combativeness and explosive anger and behavior. The use of a medication for its approved indications is called its *labeled use.* In clinical practice, however, physicians often prescribe medications for *unlabeled* ("off-label") uses when published clinical studies, case reports, or their own clinical experiences support the efficacy and safety of those treatments. For instance, thioridazine may be prescribed with a mood stabilizer to treat acute mania, since the mood stabilizer has a slower onset of action. After the symptoms of mania abate, thioridazine is discontinued and the mood stabilizer is continued alone.

Dosing Information

The usual starting dosage of thioridazine for psychotic disorders is 50–100 mg three times a day, and the dosage is gradually increased as needed to a maximum of 800 mg/day. The total daily dose ranges from 200 mg to 800 mg taken in divided doses, but in seniors and those with a medical condition, the daily dosage is significantly lower and may range from 20 mg/day to 200 mg/day.

Common Side Effects

When starting thioridazine, patients may experience sedation and fatigue. Taking a larger portion of the total dosage at bedtime may minimize daytime sedation. Tolerance to the sedation usually develops after about 1 week.

With higher dosages, thioridazine may induce **extrapyramidal symptoms.** These are neurological disturbances caused by antipsychotics (or a neurological disorder) in the area of the brain that controls motor coordination. Usually, thioridazine is unlikely to induce EPS at the lower dosage range; at higher dosages, it may produce these side effects in the susceptible individual. When disruption occurs in a particular area of the brain, it can produce symptoms that mimic Parkinson's disease (**parkinsonism**), including muscle stiffness, rigidity, tremor, drooling, and a "mask-like" facial expression. However, unlike Parkinson's disease, which is a progressive neurological disease, parkinsonism from treatment with an antipsychotic is reversible. The Parkinson-like symptoms may be treated, and prevented, by using antiparkinson agents (also called anticholinergic agents) such as Cogentin (benztropine), Benadryl (diphenhydramine), Artane (trihexyphenidyl), and Kemadrin (procyclidine).

Akathisia is another form of EPS characterized by a subjective sense of restlessness accompanied by fidgeting, inability to sit still, nervousness, muscle discomfort, and agitation. Generally, antiparkinson agents are not effective in managing akathisia. Use of Inderal (propranolol), a beta-blocker, may be helpful and is sometimes prescribed by physicians.

Dystonia is a type of EPS with acute onset. The patient may develop a sudden spasm of the muscles of the tongue, jaw, and neck. **This is not an allergic reaction to the antipsychotic medication.** Although a dystonic reaction may be painful and frightening, it can be rapidly reversed with an intramuscular injection of an anticholinergic medication such as Cogentin or Benadryl. With a dystonic reaction, the patient should seek immediate medical attention and receive treatment.

Elevation of **prolactin levels** is common with conventional antipsychotics. Prolactin is a hormone produced in the area of the brain called the pituitary gland. It is normally elevated in women following childbirth, stimulating lactation, or milk production. The effects of elevated prolactin include breast enlargement and milk production (**galactorrhea**) in both women and men. Elevated prolactin is also associated with impotence in men and irregular menstrual cycles or absence of menstruation in women. When side effects from elevated prolactin levels become bothersome, the alternative is to switch to one of the second-generation antipsychotic agents with no propensity to elevate this hormone.

Thioridazine may induce weight gain. It is unclear whether this is due to an underlying metabolic change caused by the antipsychotic or to increased appetite. Weight should be closely monitored during therapy, and if weight gain occurs, an intervention program of diet and exercise should be started.

When a medication inhibits the action of **cholinergic neurons** in the nervous system, it produces an **anticholinergic reaction,** which may produce bothersome symptoms. Because many of the antipsychotics block the normal function of cholinergic neurons, they frequently produce anticholinergic side effects. When an organ system is affected by cholinergic inhibition, it causes side effects particular to that organ. For example, when the gastrointestinal tract is affected, it may result in dry mouth, cramping, and constipation. Other anticholinergic side effects include blurred vision (when muscles of the eyes are affected) and difficulty urinating (when the bladder is affected). Low-potency first-generation antipsychotics like thioridazine have more anticholinergic activity than the high-potency agents. When thioridazine is combined with other medications with significant anticholinergic activity, such as tricyclic antidepressants (TCAs) and antiparkinson agents, the total anticholinergic action of all the medications may produce severe symptoms because the effects are additive. Seniors and individuals with a medical condition may be particularly sensitive to anticholinergic side effects. Excessive anticholinergic activity may induce delirium, a toxic reaction characterized by impaired consciousness, confusion, and inability to sustain attention.

Thioridazine may block a compensatory response—the narrowing of blood vessels—that counterbalances postural change, resulting in a momentary drop in blood pressure when the person rises too rapidly, which may cause dizziness and lightheadedness. This reaction is known as **orthostatic hypotension.** Patients, especially seniors and those taking antihypertensive medications, need to be cautious and rise slowly to allow the body to adjust to the change in position, avoiding a sudden drop in blood pressure.

Adverse Reactions and Precautions

Thioridazine may cause drowsiness and sedation and impair physical coordination and mental alertness. Patients should avoid potentially dangerous activities, such as driving a car or operating machinery, until they are sure that these side effects will not affect their ability to perform these tasks.

Thioridazine may enhance ultraviolet light absorption in the skin—a reaction known as **photosensitivity**—and predispose the person to sunburn. Patients should avoid prolonged exposure to sunlight, use sunscreen, and wear protective clothing until tolerance is developed to the medication.

Under very hot conditions, patients may be predisposed to heat-related illness and **heatstroke** because antipsychotics may disrupt the body's ability to regulate temperature. Patients should take precautions to protect themselves from exposure to hot, humid weather. It is important that patients maintain adequate ventilation and stay indoors.

The daily dosage of thioridazine should not exceed 800 mg/day. **Pigmentary retinopathy (retinitis pigmentosa)** occurs most frequently in patients taking more than 800 mg/day. The visual impairment is caused by pigment deposits in the inner surface of the eye opposite the pupil (fundus). Pigmentary retinopathy is characterized by diminished visual acuity, impaired night vision, and vision colored by a brownish tinge.

Tardive dyskinesia is a potential adverse reaction from antipsychotic medications. It is characterized by late-onset abnormal involuntary movements. TD is a potentially irreversible condition with symptoms that commonly include "pill-rolling" movements of the fingers, darting and writhing movements of the tongue, lip puckering, facial grimacing, and other irregular movements. The risk of TD is associated with the duration of exposure to antipsychotic medication, and this risk increases with age. The conventional antipsychotics are associated with a greater risk of TD than the more recent second-generation antipsychotics.

Neuroleptic malignant syndrome (NMS) is a rare, toxic reaction to antipsychotics. The symptoms are severe muscle stiffness, rigidity, elevated body temperature, increased heart rate and blood pressure, irregular pulse, and profuse sweating. NMS may lead to delirium and coma. It can be fatal if medical intervention is not immediately provided. There are no tests to predict whether an individual is susceptible to developing NMS when exposed to an antipsychotic. Thus NMS must be recognized early because it is a medical emergency that requires immediate discontinuation of the antipsychotic, hospitalization, and intensive medical treatment.

Thioridazine may slow electrical conduction in heart tissues (**myocardium**). The slowing of the electrical impulse may show up in an electrocardiogram (ECG) as it travels in the myocardium. This abnormal ECG finding, called **QTc prolongation,** may signal a potential for developing an irregular heartbeat (**arrhythmia**). Patients should have ECGs before and during thioridazine treatment. Moreover, medications that increase this potential for cardiac risk should not be taken with thioridazine (see "Possible Drug Interactions").

Antipsychotics can lower the seizure threshold and induce **seizures** in susceptible individuals, especially those with a history of seizure disorder. Patients with a seizure disorder who are receiving anticonvulsants often receive antipsychotics without any increase in seizures.

The FDA found that the first-generation antipsychotic medicines may be associated with an increased risk of death when used in treating elderly patients with dementia-related psychosis. The FDA now deems that all antipsychotic medications, including thioridazine, are not indicated for treating elderly patients with dementia. Physicians who prescribe antipsychotic medications to elderly patients for dementia-related psychosis should discuss this fatal risk with the patient, the patient's family, or the patient's caretaker.

Use in Pregnancy and Breastfeeding: Pregnancy Category C

Thioridazine has not been tested in women to determine its safety in pregnancy. The effects of the medication on the developing fetus in pregnant women are unknown. In animal studies, there was no evidence of harm to the fetus when exposed to thioridazine. Animal studies, however, are not always predictive of effects in humans. Women who are pregnant or may become pregnant should discuss this with their physician. Some women may experience a recurrence of their psychosis when they stop thioridazine. In these circumstances, the physician may discuss the need to restart the medication or seek an alternative medication or treatment.

Nursing mothers should not take thioridazine, because small amounts will pass into breast milk and be ingested by the baby. If stopping the antipsychotic is not an alternative, breastfeeding should not be started or should be discontinued.

Possible Drug Interactions

Some medications when taken with thioridazine may result in drug interactions that alter their levels, which may produce undesired reactions. Medications that may prolong cardiac conduction should not be taken together with thioridazine because the combination may increase the risk of arrhythmias. The possible drug interactions with thioridazine are summarized in the table below.

Tricyclic antidepressants (TCAs)	Thioridazine may increase the blood levels of TCAs, which may increase the risk of arrhythmia.
Demerol (meperidine)	The combination of thioridazine and Demerol may result in excessive sedation and hypotension.
Orap (pimozide)	Thioridazine and Orap should never be combined. The two medications may have an additive effect on prolongation of cardiac conduction, increasing the risk of arrhythmia.
Antiparkinson agents (e.g., Cogentin, Artane, Benadryl)	The combination of thioridazine with an antiparkinson agent may increase side effects from excessive anticholinergic activity.
Seroquel (quetiapine)	Thioridazine may significantly decrease the blood levels of Seroquel, reducing its effectiveness.

Patients taking thioridazine should not consume alcohol because the combination may impair thinking, judgment, and coordination.

Overdose

Depression of the central nervous system (CNS) with deep somnolence, low blood pressure, EPS, and abnormal electrocardiograms are frequent signs of thioridazine overdose. More serious complications may include agitation, restlessness, convulsions, fever, arrhythmias, and coma. The risk of death from the overdose depends on the amount of thioridazine ingested and whether it was combined with other medications, especially CNS depressants.

Any suspected overdose should be treated as an emergency. The person should be taken to the emergency room for observation and treatment. The prescription bottle of medication (and any other medication suspected in the overdose) should be brought as well, because the information on the prescription label can be helpful to the treating physician in determining the number of pills ingested.

Special Considerations

- Do not discontinue thioridazine without consulting your physician.
- If you miss a dose, take it as soon as possible. If it is close to the next scheduled dose, skip the missed dose and continue on your regular dosing schedule. But do not take double doses.
- Thioridazine may be taken with or without food.
- Thioridazine may cause sedation and drowsiness, especially during initiation of therapy, and may impair your alertness. Use caution when driving or performing tasks that require alertness.
- Thioridazine may enhance ultraviolet light absorption and increase the risk of sunburn. Use a sunscreen, and avoid excessive exposure to sunlight.
- Store the medication in its originally labeled, light-resistant container, away from heat and moisture. Heat and moisture may precipitate breakdown of your medication, and the medication may lose its therapeutic effects.
- Keep your medication out of reach of children.

If you have any questions about your medication, consult your physician or pharmacist.

Notes

From Chew RH, Hales RE, Yudofsky SC: *What Your Patients Need to Know About Psychiatric Medications*, Second Edition. Washington, DC, American Psychiatric Publishing, 2009

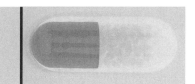

Trifluoperazine (Stelazine)

Generic name: Trifluoperazine
Available strengths: 1 mg, 2 mg, 5 mg, 10 mg tablets
Available in generic: Yes
Drug class: First-generation (conventional) antipsychotic

General Information

Trifluoperazine (Stelazine) belongs to the class of antipsychotics known as the **first-generation antipsychotics,** sometimes referred to as *conventional* or *typical* antipsychotics. Trifluoperazine was sold under the brand Stelazine, but Stelazine has since been discontinued. Currently, only generic trifluoperazine is available. The first-generation antipsychotics represent an older class of antipsychotics that have been the standard for treating psychotic disorders for many decades. When compared with a newer class of **second-generation antipsychotics,** these earlier antipsychotics are referred to as *typical* or *conventional* because they lack the wider spectrum of therapeutic activity. The first-generation antipsychotics are also more likely to induce side effects that cause movement disorders, such as **extrapyramidal symptoms** (EPS) and **tardive dyskinesia** (TD), than the newer antipsychotics.

Trifluoperazine is a high-potency antipsychotic, relative to low-potency first-generation antipsychotics such as chlorpromazine and thioridazine. Trifluoperazine is moderately sedating and less likely to lower blood pressure. Like other high-potency antipsychotics such as fluphenazine and Haldol (haloperidol), trifluoperazine frequently induces EPS.

Trifluoperazine was approved by the U.S. Food and Drug Administration for treatment of psychotic disorders, including schizophrenia, schizoaffective disorder, and drug-induced psychosis. The use of a medication for its approved indications is called its *labeled use*. In clinical practice, however, physicians often prescribe medications for *unlabeled* ("off-label") uses when published clinical studies, case reports, or their own clinical experiences support the efficacy and safety of those treatments. For instance, trifluoperazine may be prescribed with a mood stabilizer to treat acute mania, since the mood stabilizer has a slower onset of action. After the symptoms of mania abate, trifluoperazine is discontinued and the mood stabilizer is continued alone.

Dosing Information

For treatment of acute psychosis, the usual starting dosage of trifluoperazine is 2–5 mg two times a day. The dosage is increased as indicated until symptoms improve. Most patients have symptom relief with 15–20 mg/day, given in divided doses. The maximum dosage should not exceed 40 mg/day. As symptoms abate, the dosage is reduced to a minimum effective dosage, which is the maintenance dosage.

Common Side Effects

Patients taking trifluoperazine may experience sedation and drowsiness accompanied by fatigue. Sedation may be useful early on in therapy to lessen agitation and help the patient sleep, but as acute symptoms improve, this side effect may become bothersome, interfering with daily activities. Over time, most patients develop tolerance to the side effects of the medication. Daytime sedation may be minimized by taking a larger proportion of the divided dosage at bedtime and a small dose in the morning.

Trifluoperazine may induce side effects known as **extrapyramidal symptoms.** These are neurological disturbances caused by antipsychotics (or a neurological disorder) in the area of the brain that controls motor coordination. When disruption occurs in a particular area of the brain, it can produce symptoms that mimic Parkinson's disease (**parkinsonism**), including muscle stiffness, rigidity, tremor, drooling, and a "mask-like" facial expression. However, unlike Parkinson's disease, which is a progressive neurological disease, parkinsonism from treatment with an antipsychotic is reversible. The Parkinson-like symptoms may be treated, and prevented, by using antiparkinson agents (also called anticholinergic agents) such as Cogentin (benztropine), Benadryl (diphenhydramine), Artane (trihexyphenidyl), and Kemadrin (procyclidine).

Akathisia is another form of EPS characterized by a subjective sense of restlessness accompanied by fidgeting, inability to sit still, nervousness, muscle discomfort, and agitation. Generally, antiparkinson agents are not effective in managing akathisia. Use of Inderal (propranolol), a beta-blocker, may be helpful and is sometimes prescribed by physicians.

Dystonia is a type of EPS with acute onset. The patient may develop a sudden spasm of the muscles of the tongue, jaw, and neck. **This is not an allergic reaction to the antipsychotic medication.** Although a dystonic reaction may be painful and frightening, it can be rapidly reversed with an intramuscular injection of an anticholinergic medication such as Cogentin or Benadryl. With a dystonic reaction, the patient should seek immediate medical attention and receive treatment.

Elevation of **prolactin levels** is common with conventional antipsychotics. Prolactin is a hormone produced in the area of the brain called the pituitary gland. It is normally elevated in women following childbirth, stimulating lactation, or milk production. The effects of elevated prolactin include breast enlargement and milk production (**galactorrhea**) in both women and men. Elevated prolactin is also associated with impotence in men and irregular menstrual cycles or absence of menstruation in women. When side effects from elevated prolactin levels become bothersome, the alternative is to switch to one of the second-generation antipsychotic agents with no propensity to elevate this hormone.

Trifluoperazine may induce **weight gain.** It is unclear whether this is due to an underlying metabolic change caused by the antipsychotic or to increased appetite. Weight should be monitored closely during therapy, and if weight gain occurs, an intervention program of diet and exercise should be started.

When a medication inhibits the action of **cholinergic neurons** in the nervous system, it produces an **anticholinergic reaction,** which may produce bothersome symptoms. Anticholinergic side effects from trifluoperazine may include blurred vision, dry mouth, constipation, and difficulty with urination. Seniors and individuals with a medical condition may be particularly sensitive to anticholinergic side effects.

Trifluoperazine may block a compensatory response—the narrowing of blood vessels—that counterbalances postural change, resulting in a momentary drop in blood pressure when the person rises too rapidly, which may cause dizziness and lightheadedness. This reaction is known as **orthostatic hypotension.** Patients, especially seniors and those taking antihypertensive medications, need to be cautious and rise slowly to allow the body to adjust to the change in position, avoiding a sudden drop in blood pressure. Orthostatic hypotension and anticholinergic side effects, which occur more frequently with low-potency, first-generation antipsychotics, are usually not as troublesome with the intermediate- and higher-potency agents.

Adverse Reactions and Precautions

Trifluoperazine may cause drowsiness and sedation and impair physical coordination and mental alertness. Patients should avoid potentially dangerous activities, such as driving a car or operating machinery, until they are sure that these side effects will not affect their ability to perform these tasks.

Trifluoperazine may enhance ultraviolet light absorption in the skin—a reaction known as **photosensitivity**—and predispose the person to sunburn. Patients should avoid prolonged exposure to sunlight, use sunscreen, and wear protective clothing until tolerance is developed to the medication.

Under very hot conditions, patients may be predisposed to heat-related illness and **heatstroke** because antipsychotics may disrupt the body's ability to regulate temperature. Patients should take precautions to protect themselves from prolonged exposure to hot, humid weather. It is important that patients maintain adequate ventilation and stay indoors.

Tardive dyskinesia is a potential adverse reaction from antipsychotic medications. It is characterized by late-onset abnormal involuntary movements. TD is a potentially irreversible condition with symptoms that commonly include "pill-rolling" movements of the fingers, darting and writhing movements of the tongue, lip puckering, facial grimacing, and other irregular movements. The risk of TD is associated with the duration of exposure to antipsychotic medication, and this risk increases with age. The conventional antipsychotics are associated with a greater risk of TD than the more recent second-generation antipsychotics.

Neuroleptic malignant syndrome (NMS) is a rare, toxic reaction to antipsychotics. The symptoms are severe muscle stiffness, rigidity, elevated body temperature, increased heart rate and blood pressure, irregular pulse, and profuse sweating. NMS may lead to delirium and coma. It can be fatal if medical intervention is not immediately provided. There are no tests to predict whether an individual is susceptible to developing NMS when exposed to an antipsychotic. Thus NMS must be recognized early because it is a medical emergency that requires immediate discontinuation of the antipsychotic, hospitalization, and intensive medical treatment.

Antipsychotics can lower the seizure threshold and induce **seizures** in susceptible individuals, especially those with a history of seizure disorder. Patients with a seizure disorder who are receiving anticonvulsants often receive antipsychotics without any increase in seizures.

The FDA found that the first-generation antipsychotic medicines may be associated with an increased risk of death when used in treating elderly patients with dementia-related psychosis. The FDA now deems that all antipsychotic medications, including trifluoperazine, are not indicated for treating elderly patients wit.dementia. Physicians who prescribe antipsychotic medications to elderly patients for dementia-related psychosis should discuss this fatal risk with the patient, the patient's family, or the patient's caretaker.

Use in Pregnancy and Breastfeeding: Pregnancy Category C

Trifluoperazine has not been tested in women to determine its safety in pregnancy. The effects of the medication on the developing fetus in pregnant women are unknown. In animal studies, there was no evidence of harm to the fetus when exposed to trifluoperazine. Animal studies, however, are not always predictive of effects in humans. Women who are pregnant or may become pregnant should discuss this with their physician. Some women may experience a recurrence of their psychosis when they stop trifluoperazine. In these circumstances, the physician may discuss the need to restart the medication or seek an alternative medication or treatment.

Nursing mothers should not take trifluoperazine, because small amounts will pass into breast milk and be ingested by the baby. If stopping the antipsychotic is not an alternative, breastfeeding should not be started or should be discontinued.

Possible Drug Interactions

Some medications when taken with trifluoperazine may result in drug interactions that alter their levels, which may produce undesired reactions. Use of medications for lowering blood pressure (antihypertensive medications) should be monitored closely because trifluoperazine may lower blood pressure and produce an additive effect. Medications that act on the central nervous system (CNS), including benzodiazepines (e.g., Valium), antihistamines, and narcotic pain medications, may possibly increase the risk and severity of CNS-related side effects of antipsychotics, including somnolence, drowsiness, dizziness, and fatigue.

Patients taking trifluoperazine should not consume alcohol because the combination may worsen drowsiness and sedation and impair thinking, judgment, and coordination.

Overdose

Depression of the CNS with deep somnolence, low blood pressure, and EPS are common signs of trifluoperazine overdose. More serious complications may include agitation, restlessness, convulsions, fever, arrhythmias, and coma. The risk of death from the overdose depends on the amount of trifluoperazine ingested and whether it was combined with other medications, especially CNS depressants.

Any suspected overdose should be treated as an emergency. The person should be taken to the emergency room for observation and treatment. The prescription bottle of medication (and any other medication suspected in the overdose) should be brought as well, because the information on the prescription label can be helpful to the treating physician in determining the number of pills ingested.

Special Considerations

- Do not discontinue trifluoperazine without consulting your physician.
- If you miss a dose, take it as soon as possible. If it is close to the next scheduled dose, skip the missed dose and continue on your regular dosing schedule. Do not take double doses.
- Trifluoperazine may be taken with or without food.
- Trifluoperazine may cause sedation and drowsiness, especially during initiation of therapy, and may impair your alertness. Use caution when driving or performing tasks that require alertness.
- Trifluoperazine may enhance ultraviolet light absorption and increase the risk of sunburn. Use a sunscreen, and avoid excessive exposure to sunlight.
- Store the medication in its originally labeled, light-resistant container, away from heat and moisture. Heat and moisture may precipitate breakdown of your medication, and the medication may lose its therapeutic effects.
- Keep your medication out of reach of children.

If you have any questions about your medication, consult your physician or pharmacist.

Notes

Second-Generation Antipsychotics

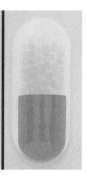

Abilify (aripiprazole)
Clozaril (clozapine)
Geodon (ziprasidone)
Invega (paliperidone)
Risperdal, Risperdal M-Tab, and Risperdal Consta (risperidone)
Seroquel (quetiapine)
Symbyax (Zyprexa [olanzapine] and Prozac [fluoxetine] combination)
Zyprexa and Zyprexa Zydis (olanzapine)

The **second-generation antipsychotics,** also commonly known as *atypical* antipsychotics, are among the most significant medicines developed in the past decade for the treatment of severe mental disorders such as schizophrenia, schizoaffective disorder, and mania. These agents are *atypical* because they are significantly different, both in structure and in overall activity, from the older, *typical* antipsychotic medications such as chlorpromazine, thioridazine, and Haldol (haloperidol). Having multiple mechanisms of action in the brain, the second-generation antipsychotics have wider applications than just for treating the **positive symptoms** of psychosis (e.g., hallucinations, delusions, bizarre behavior, disorganized speech). These medicines have proved to be highly effective for treating **negative symptoms** of schizophrenia, which are characterized by emotional and social withdrawal, flat affect, lack of spontaneity, inability to feel pleasure, attention impairment, and other restrictions in thought, speech, and behavior. Almost all the atypical antipsychotics (Geodon, Risperdal, Seroquel, Zyprexa, and Abilify) have received indications for treating acute mania in bipolar disorder. Zyprexa (olanzapine) has also been indicated for long-term treatment (maintenance treatment) of bipolar disorder. Thus most clinicians view second-generation antipsychotics not merely as antipsychotic medications but also as **psychotropic agents,** which are effective in treating a wide spectrum of mental disorders.

Clozaril (clozapine), the oldest of the second-generation antipsychotics, has been in use in Europe for more than 30 years. At one time, Clozaril held great promise for treatment of schizophrenia, but that hope was dashed when the drug was reported in the mid-1970s to cause **agranulocytosis,** a life-threatening condition in which white blood cells are fatally diminished. When deaths were reported from Clozaril-induced agranulocytosis, the drug was withdrawn from general use. Clozaril was not made available in the United States until the late 1980s, but the U.S. Food and Drug Administration (FDA) restricted its use, requiring close monitoring conditions and reserving the drug for treatment-resistant schizophrenia unresponsive to conventional antipsychotics. Clozaril was the prototype of the second-generation antipsychotics, and the renewed interest in such agents spurred the development of new antipsychotic agents with similar properties but without the risk of agranulocytosis. In a little more than a decade after the introduction of Clozaril in this country, Risperdal, Zyprexa, Seroquel, Geodon, and Abilify were developed.

How Antipsychotics Work

How antipsychotic drugs work may be explained by the *dopamine receptor antagonist hypothesis*. **Dopamine** is a neurotransmitter, a chemical produced by brain cells called **neurons** that enables neurons to communicate with each other. Dopamine is released by one neuron into the space between that neuron and the next neuron and then binds to specific sites on the other neuron called **receptors.** The interaction of the neurotransmitter with the receptors results in very specialized activities coded in the neuron, and it ultimately generates an electrical impulse that is transmitted down the nerve cell. At the end of the nerve terminal, the electrical impulse causes further release of dopamine. This form of communication between neurons is called **neurotransmission.** In specific areas of the brain, excessive dopamine neurotransmission may produce the psychotic symptoms (e.g., hallucinations, delusions, bizarre behavior) characteristic of schizophrenia and more severe cases of bipolar disorder. Drugs such as amphetamine and cocaine, for example, are known to increase dopamine release. In excessive amounts, these drugs induce psychotic symptoms not unlike schizophrenia.

Psychotic symptoms commonly seen in schizophrenia and other mental disorders, such as bipolar disorder, dementia, and drug-induced psychosis, include delusions, hallucinations, disorganized speech, and bizarre, agitated, or catatonic behavior. These symptoms are also called the positive symptoms of psychosis because of the excessive and overt nature of their clinical presentation.

Antipsychotics work principally by blocking, or antagonizing, the action of dopamine at its receptors, decreasing the chemical signals that drive psychotic behavior. That is, antipsychotics decrease neurotransmission by blocking dopamine from binding to the receptors. Excessive dopamine activity in selected areas of the brain may be the underlying cause of psychosis. Both conventional and second-generation antipsychotics are dopamine antagonists and are therefore effective in treating the positive symptoms of psychosis. In areas of the brain where antipsychotics have no therapeutic benefits, they may produce side effects.

There is a significant difference between the second-generation antipsychotics and the conventional antipsychotics in that the former also block the receptors of another neurotransmitter, **serotonin.** The action of serotonin is closely coupled with dopamine, and it has important influences on dopamine release in different areas of the brain. Serotonin antagonism is the defining feature of the second-generation antipsychotics and is the most important property that distinguishes these agents from conventional antipsychotics. In addition, the second-generation antipsychotics have low propensity to induce **extrapyramidal symptoms** (EPS) and have efficacy for negative symptoms. The second-generation antipsychotics are sometimes called **serotonin-dopamine antagonists.**

Advantages of the Second-Generation Antipsychotics

Second-generation antipsychotics have essentially replaced the older, conventional antipsychotics. The primary reason for this is that the second-generation antipsychotics are much better tolerated than their older counterparts. The second-generation agents are associated with a substantially lower risk of EPS and **tardive dyskinesia** (TD). EPS are acute-onset movement disorders characterized by muscular rigidity, tremors, shuffling movement, restlessness, and muscle spasms resulting in abnormal posture. TD is a delayed-onset condition that consists of abnormal involuntary movements usually involving the tongue and mouth and sometimes the arms and trunk. EPS and TD are substantial risks with conventional antipsychotics. Patients frequently cannot, and will not, tolerate the side effects of antipsychotics, and this becomes problematic if long-term treatment is needed. With their more favorable side-effect profile, the newer antipsychotics are better tolerated, and patients are more likely to take them consistently.

The other distinguishing advantage of the second-generation antipsychotics is that they are superior in treating negative symptoms. In areas of the brain where emotion and cognition are affected by the balance of serotonin and dopamine, the dual action of the second-generation agents resets this important balance when it has been altered. In patients with mental disorders such as schizophrenia, the balance of these neurotransmitters is disturbed, and patients may manifest negative symptoms.

For more information about a particular second-generation antipsychotic medication, refer to the handout for that medication.

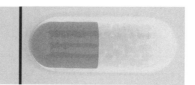

Abilify (aripiprazole)

Generic name: Aripiprazole
Available strengths: 2 mg, 5 mg, 10 mg, 20 mg, 30 mg tablets;
    10 mg, 15 mg oral disintegrating tablets (Abilify Discmelt);
    1 mg/mL oral solution; 7.5 mg/mL injection
Available in generic: No
Drug class: Second-generation antipsychotic

General Information

Abilify (aripiprazole) is one of the second-generation antipsychotic medications, which are also called *atypical* antipsychotics. (Refer to the handout "Second-Generation Antipsychotics" for an explanation of how these antipsychotics work.) Abilify is atypical in that it is significantly different, both in structure and in overall activity, from the earlier, *typical* antipsychotic medications such as chlorpromazine, thioridazine, and Haldol (haloperidol). The second-generation antipsychotics have a wider spectrum of activity, with fewer side effects associated with movement disorders, than the typical antipsychotics. The second-generation antipsychotics block both serotonin and dopamine receptors, whereas the typical antipsychotics are mainly dopamine-receptor antagonists. The use of Abilify is not limited to its antipsychotic action; it may also be useful as an antimanic or antidepressant agent.

When first marketed in the United States, Abilify was approved only for treatment of schizophrenia in adults. In following years, clinical studies showed that Abilify, like many of the other atypical antipsychotics, is effective for acute mania in bipolar disorder, and Abilify received approval for this use from the U.S. Food and Drug Administration (FDA), followed by approval for maintenance treatment of bipolar disorder. Most recently, in 2007 and 2008, the FDA made some major changes and approved Abilify for the treatment of schizophrenia in adults and in adolescents ages 13–17 years; the treatment of acute mania or mixed episodes in bipolar disorder in adults and in pediatric patients ages 10–17 years; and as an adjunctive (supplemental) treatment in major depression only in adults. Abilify, like many of the other atypical antipsychotics, has a spectrum of mood-stabilizing and antipsychotic activity.

The use of a medication for its approved indications is called its *labeled use*. In clinical practice, however, physicians often prescribe medications for *unlabeled* ("off-label") uses when published clinical studies, case reports, or their own clinical experiences support the efficacy and safety of those treatments. Like other second-generation antipsychotics, Abilify may be used to treat other psychiatric disorders, including psychotic depression and dementias such as Alzheimer's disease.

Dosing Information

The new dosage guidelines for Abilify, reflecting the changes by the FDA in 2007 and 2008, are as follows:

Indication—age group	Initial dosage (mg/day)	Recommended maintenance dosage (mg/day)	Maximum dosage (mg/day)
Schizophrenia—adults	10–15	10–15	30
Schizophrenia—adolescents	2	10	30
Bipolar mania—adults	15–30	15–30	30
Bipolar mania—pediatric	2	5–10	30
Adjunct to antidepressant for treatment of major depression—adults	2–5	5–10	15

Source. Abilify [package insert]. Bristol-Myers Squibb Company, Princeton, NJ, February 2008.

Common Side Effects

Abilify is generally well tolerated, with few bothersome side effects. Common side effects are headache, nausea, vomiting, insomnia, and tremor. In most cases these side effects are transient and are usually gone after the first week or two of therapy. Abilify is not associated with any significant weight gain and is notable among the second-generation antipsychotic agents (similar to Geodon) for its low propensity to affect weight.

Extrapyramidal symptoms (EPS) are infrequent with Abilify. EPS are neurological disturbances produced by antipsychotics (or other causes) in the area of the brain that controls motor coordination. These side effects include muscle rigidity, tremors, drooling, restlessness, a "mask-like" facial expression, shuffling gait, and muscle spasms that result in abnormal posture (**dystonia**). EPS mimic Parkinson's disease, and many of the signs and symptoms are common in both conditions. Some patients experience **akathisia,** which is a subjective sense of restlessness accompanied by fidgeting and inability to sit or stand still. EPS may be managed by decreasing the antipsychotic dosage or adding another medication (anticholinergic medication) to counteract the side effect.

Abilify may block a compensatory response—the narrowing of blood vessels—that counterbalances postural change, resulting in a momentary drop in blood pressure when the person rises too rapidly, which may cause dizziness and lightheadedness. This reaction is known as **orthostatic hypotension.** Patients, especially seniors and those taking antihypertensive medications, need to be cautious and rise slowly to allow the body to adjust to the change in position, avoiding a sudden drop in blood pressure.

Adverse Reactions and Precautions

Abilify may cause drowsiness and sedation and impair physical coordination and mental alertness. Patients should avoid potentially dangerous activities, such as driving a car or operating machinery, until they are sure that these side effects will not affect their ability to perform these tasks.

Tardive dyskinesia (TD) is a potential adverse reaction from antipsychotic medications. It is characterized by late-onset abnormal involuntary movements. TD is a potentially irreversible condition that commonly includes "pill-rolling" movements of the fingers, darting and writhing movements of the tongue, lip puckering, facial grimacing, and other irregular movements. The risk of TD associated with second-generation antipsychotics is significantly lower than with conventional antipsychotics. Because Abilify was introduced recently, there are few data available, but the risk of TD is expected to be very low.

Neuroleptic malignant syndrome (NMS) is a rare, toxic reaction to antipsychotics. The symptoms are severe muscle stiffness, rigidity, elevated body temperature, increased heart rate and blood pressure, irregular pulse, and profuse sweating. NMS may lead to delirium and coma. It can be fatal if medical intervention is not immediately provided. There are no tests to predict whether an individual is susceptible to developing NMS when exposed to an antipsychotic. Thus NMS must be recognized early because it is a medical emergency that requires immediate discontinuation of the antipsychotic, hospitalization, and intensive medical treatment.

Abilify and other second-generation antipsychotics are associated with abnormalities in glucose regulation. Abilify may elevate blood glucose (**hyperglycemia**) and in some cases cause **diabetes mellitus.** While glucose abnormalities and diabetes are sometimes related to weight gain, these conditions may occur in patients without significant weight gain. Patients who have excessive weight gain are more susceptible to the medication's negative impact on blood sugar and cholesterol. The FDA has required a warning of hyperglycemia and diabetes mellitus with use of Abilify and other second-generation antipsychotics in their labeling. Patients receiving Abilify, especially those who have a family history or an established diagnosis of diabetes, should be aware of this adverse reaction and should routinely monitor glucose levels while taking Abilify.

In elderly patients with dementia who are treated with a second-generation antipsychotic, including Abilify, there is an increased risk of death. The data from clinical studies show a higher risk in elderly patients with dementia treated with second-generation antipsychotics than with placebo-treated patients (i.e., patients taking a sugar pill). It is unclear why these medications have a higher risk in this group. Even though the risk is very low, the FDA requires Abilify to have in its package insert a warning about the associated risk in this population of taking an atypical antipsychotic medication.

With an indication for treatment of depression, Abilify must have in its labeling a warning of suicide risk associated with antidepressant medications. In short-term studies, antidepressants were found to increase the risk of suicidal thinking and behavior in children and adolescents with major depression and other psychiatric disorders. On the basis of these findings, the FDA requires a warning in the package insert that the prescriber be aware of the suicide risks in their patients who are starting antidepressant therapy, especially in the pediatric population. According to the FDA findings, the risk of suicidal thoughts and behaviors associated with antidepressants is age-related. This phenomenon tends to occur in the younger population and is most likely to occur early in the course of treatment. In adults over 24 years of age, there did not appear to be an increased risk of suicidality with antidepressants compared with placebo. In patients over age 65, the findings showed that antidepressants had a "protective effect" against suicidal thoughts and behavior.

After starting or changing antidepressant therapy, the patient, especially a child or adolescent, should be closely observed for worsening signs of depression.

Use in Pregnancy and Breastfeeding: Pregnancy Category C

Abilify has not been tested in women to determine its safety in pregnancy. The effects of the medication on the developing fetus in pregnant women are unknown. In animal studies, there may be effects on the development of the fetus, but there are not adequate and well-controlled studies in humans. Animal studies are not always predictive of effects in humans. Therefore, the use of Abilify in pregnant woman must always be weighed against the potential risks. Women who are pregnant or may become pregnant should discuss this with their physician. Some women may experience a recurrence of their psychosis when they stop Abilify. In these circumstances, the physician may discuss the need to restart the medication or seek an alternative medication or treatment.

Nursing mothers should not take Abilify, because small amounts will pass into breast milk and be ingested by the baby. If stopping the antipsychotic is not an alternative, breastfeeding should not be started or should be discontinued.

Possible Drug Interactions

Some medications when taken with Abilify may result in drug interactions that alter their levels, which may produce undesired reactions. The possible drug interactions with Abilify are summarized in the table below.

Prozac (fluoxetine) or Paxil (paroxetine)	Prozac and Paxil may decrease the metabolism of Abilify, thus increasing Abilify blood levels and the likelihood of unwanted side effects.
Nizoral (ketoconazole)	Nizoral, an antifungal agent, may decrease the metabolism of Abilify, thus increasing Abilify blood levels and the likelihood of unwanted side effects.
Tegretol (carbamazepine)	Tegretol may decrease the blood levels of Abilify, making it less effective in treating the symptoms of the illness.

Patients taking Abilify should not consume alcohol because the combination may impair thinking, judgment, and coordination.

Overdose

There are few data of acute overdose with Abilify. No fatalities have been reported in cases of Abilify overdose; in these cases, the largest identified amount taken was 180 mg, with which the only symptoms were somnolence and vomiting. The outcome may depend on the amount ingested and whether Abilify was combined with other medications.

Any suspected overdose should be treated as an emergency. The person should be taken to the emergency room for observation and treatment. The prescription bottle of medication (and any other medication suspected in the overdose) should be brought as well, because the information on the prescription label can be helpful to the treating physician in determining the number of pills ingested.

Special Considerations

- Do not discontinue Abilify without consulting your physician.
- If you miss a dose, take it as soon as possible that day. If into the next day, skip the missed dose and continue on your regular dosing schedule. Do not take double doses.
- Abilify may be taken with or without food.
- Abilify may cause sedation and drowsiness, especially during initiation of therapy, and may impair your alertness. Use caution when driving or performing tasks that require alertness.
- Store the medication in its originally labeled, light-resistant container, away from heat and moisture. Heat and moisture may precipitate breakdown of your medication, and the medication may lose its therapeutic effects.
- Keep your medication out of reach of children.

If you have any questions about your medication, consult your physician or pharmacist.

Notes

_____

_____

_____

_____

_____

_____

_____

_____

_____

_____

From Chew RH, Hales RE, Yudofsky SC: _What Your Patients Need to Know About Psychiatric Medications,_ Second Edition. Washington, DC, American Psychiatric Publishing, 2009

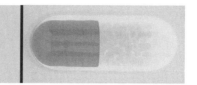

Clozaril (clozapine)

Generic name: Clozapine
Available strengths: 12.5 mg, 25 mg, 100 mg, 200 mg tablets;
    12.5 mg, 25 mg, 50 mg, 100 mg orally disintegrating tablets
    (FazaClo)
Available in generic: Yes, except FazaClo
Drug class: Second-generation antipsychotic

General Information

Clozaril (clozapine) is one of the second-generation antipsychotic medications, which are also called *atypical* antipsychotics. Clozaril was the first of the new class of second-generation antipsychotics developed for the treatment of schizophrenia. (Refer to the handout "Second-Generation Antipsychotics" for an explanation of how these antipsychotics work.) Clozaril is atypical in that it is significantly different, both in struture and in overall activity, from the earlier, *typical* antipsychotic medications such as chlorpromazine, thioridazine, and Haldol (haloperidol). The second-generation antipsychotics have a wider spectrum of activity, with fewer side effects associated with movement disorders, than the typical antipsychotics. The second-generation antipsychotics block both serotonin and dopamine receptors, whereas the typical antipsychotics are mainly dopamine-receptor antagonists.

Clozaril has been in use in Europe for more than 30 years. In the mid-1970s, the medication was reported to cause **agranulocytosis,** a life-threatening condition in which white blood cells are fatally diminished. When deaths were reported from Clozaril-induced agranulocytosis, the medication was withdrawn from general use. Clozaril was not made available in the United States until the late 1980s, but the U.S. Food and Drug Administration (FDA) restricted its use, requiring close monitoring conditions and reserving the medication for treatment-resistant schizophrenia (schizophrenia that does not respond adequately to standard, safer treatments). Recently, Clozaril was given an FDA approval for use in reducing the risk of suicidal behavior in patients with schizophrenia or schizoaffective disorder who display recurring suicidal behavior and are judged to be at chronic risk for suicide. The use of a medication for its approved indications is called its *labeled use.* In clinical practice, however, physicians often prescribe medications for *unlabeled* ("off-label") uses when published clinical studies, case reports, or their own clinical experiences support the efficacy and safety of those treatments. Unlabeled uses of Clozaril include treatment of other psychiatric disorders, such as bipolar disorder, schizoaffective disorder, and psychotic depression, when these disorders are refractory to other treatments.

Dosing Information

Use of Clozaril requires strict monitoring of the patient's white blood cell count (WBC) to ensure that therapy is quickly interrupted when agranulocytosis is suspected. There are four companies in the United States that market clozapine, and the brand Clozaril is also available. Every manufacturer must have a clozapine registry in place, which must track patients' blood tests while they are taking clozapine. The patient's pharmacy is responsible for registering the patient and the patient's physician with the manufacturer's registry. The pharmacy is also responsible for weekly reporting of the patient's WBC. A national databank maintains the history of patients whose clozapine treatment was discontinued because of a low WBC or agranulocytosis. These patients are then precluded from taking clozapine again, regardless of the company or system.

The recommended starting dosage of Clozaril is 25 mg at bedtime. The dosage is slowly increased over the first 2–3 weeks in increments of 25–50 mg every 4–5 days until a dosage of 200 mg/day is reached. If necessary, the dosage may be further increased to achieve a target dosage of 300–600 mg/day. At higher dosages, taking Clozaril on a twice-daily schedule may minimize some of the side effects. The median Clozaril dosage is approximately 600 mg/day, but some patients may require higher dosages. However, a maximum dosage of 900 mg/day should not be exceeded. The dosing for recurrent suicidal behavior follows similar dosing guidelines for treatment of schizophrenia and schizoaffective disorder.

Common Side Effects

The more common and bothersome side effects of Clozaril are sedation; gastrointestinal distress such as nausea, cramping, heartburn, and diarrhea; flulike symptoms; and excessive drooling, especially at night. Because Clozaril can inhibit **cholinergic neurons** in the nervous system, it frequently produces a cluster of side effects called **anticholinergic** side effects, which include blurred vision, dry mouth, constipation, and difficulty urinating. Seniors are particularly sensitive to anticholinergic side effects. Generally, as the patient develops greater tolerance to the medication, these side effects subside.

The advantage of Clozaril is that it rarely causes **extrapyramidal symptoms** (EPS), which are common with conventional antipsychotics. EPS are neurological disturbances produced by antipsychotics (or other causes) in the area of the brain that controls motor coordination.

Most people taking Clozaril will gain weight. For some, it may be significant and problematic. It appears that stimulation of appetite and overeating are the major causes of Clozaril-related weight gain. Weight should be monitored closely during therapy, and if weight gain occurs, an intervention program of diet and exercise should be started.

Clozaril may block a compensatory response—the narrowing of blood vessels—that counterbalances postural change, resulting in a momentary drop in blood pressure when the person rises too rapidly, which may cause dizziness and lightheadedness. This reaction is known as **orthostatic hypotension.** Patients, especially seniors and those taking antihypertensive medications, need to be cautious and rise slowly to allow the body to adjust to the change in position, avoiding a sudden drop in blood pressure.

Adverse Reactions and Precautions

Clozaril may cause drowsiness and sedation and impair physical coordination and mental alertness. Patients should avoid potentially dangerous activities, such as driving a car or operating machinery, until they are sure that these side effects will not affect their ability to perform these tasks.

The major concern with Clozaril is the danger of developing agranulocytosis. This adverse reaction affects about 1.2% of all treated patients in the United States. It starts with a drop in the level of white blood cells, which then may fall precipitously such that the WBC is almost undetectable. When all white blood cells are diminished, a particular type of white blood cells called **granulocytes** is also decreased. Granulocytes play an important role in the body's defense against infections. When granulocytes are drastically decreased (agranulocytosis), the body's immunity is compromised, and the person becomes susceptible to life-threatening infections.

There is no test to determine whether a person is susceptible to agranulocytosis from Clozaril. Therefore, Clozaril therapy requires weekly monitoring of the white blood cells. Therapy is quickly interrupted at the earliest sign of an adverse reaction. The monitoring system requires the patient to have weekly blood draws for a WBC, and the pharmacy may dispense only 1 week's supply at a time. If the patient has been treated for 6 months without interruption in therapy, blood tests are then only required every 2 weeks, and the patient can receive a 2-week supply of medication each time. Following 12 months of uninterrupted therapy, the interval can be increased to 4 weeks and the patient can receive up to a month of Clozaril.

Clozaril may induce seizures. The risk of seizures is associated with use of Clozaril at higher doses and when the medication is given to people with a history of seizures or other predisposing factors. The risk of Clozaril-induced seizures appears to be dose-related, and at dosages greater than 600 mg/day the incidence of seizures increases. A person with a history of epilepsy may not be a good candidate for Clozaril unless the seizures can be adequately controlled with anticonvulsant medications.

Tardive dyskinesia (TD) is a potential adverse reaction from antipsychotic medications. It is characterized by late-onset abnormal involuntary movements. TD is a potentially irreversible condition that commonly includes "pill-rolling" movements of the fingers, darting and writhing movements of the tongue, lip puckering, facial grimacing, and other irregular movements. Clozaril, however, is unlikely to cause TD. Moreover, patients with TD may benefit from Clozaril, which may reverse the dyskinetic symptoms caused by conventional antipsychotics.

Neuroleptic malignant syndrome (NMS) is a rare, toxic reaction to antipsychotics. The symptoms of NMS associated with Clozaril are generally milder than those associated with conventional antipsychotics. The symptoms may include increased heart rate and blood pressure, irregular pulse, and sweating. NMS may lead to delirium and coma. It can be fatal if medical intervention is not immediately provided. There are no tests to predict whether an individual is susceptible to developing NMS when exposed to an antipsychotic. Thus NMS must be recognized early because it is a medical emergency that requires immediate discontinuation of the antipsychotic, hospitalization, and intensive medical treatment.

Clozaril and other second-generation antipsychotics are associated with abnormalities in glucose regulation. Clozaril may elevate blood glucose levels (**hyperglycemia**) and in some cases cause **diabetes mellitus.** While glucose abnormalities and diabetes are sometimes related to weight gain, these conditions may occur in patients without significant weight gain. Patients who have excessive weight gain are more susceptible to the medication's negative impact on blood sugar and cholesterol. The FDA has required a warning of hyperglycemia and diabetes mellitus with use of Clozaril and other second-generation antipsychotics in their labeling. Patients receiving Clozaril, especially those with a family history or an established diagnosis of diabetes, should be aware of this adverse reaction and should routinely monitor glucose levels while taking Clozaril.

In elderly patients with dementia who are treated with a second-generation antipsychotic, including Clozaril, there is an increased risk of death. The data from clinical studies show a higher risk in elderly patients with dementia treated with second-generation antipsychotics than with placebo-treated patients (i.e., patients taking a sugar pill). It is unclear why these medications have a higher risk in this group. Even though the risk is very low, the FDA requires Clozaril to have in its package insert a warning about the associated risk in this population of taking an atypical antipsychotic medication.

From the pool of people reported taking Clozaril, the data show that Clozaril may be associated with an increased risk of inducing heart problems that can be fatal. The condition, known as **myocarditis,** is due to inflammation of the heart tissues, resulting in weakness of heart muscles. The symptoms associated with myocarditis are chest pain, shortness of breath (especially upon exertion), and palpitations, with awareness of a rapid or irregular heartbeat. This generally occurs during the first month of starting Clozaril therapy, but not in all cases. The required labeling warns physicians to alert patients taking Clozaril, especially those new to therapy, to report signs and symptoms of myocarditis and promptly discontinue Clozaril treatment if suspected.

Use in Pregnancy and Breastfeeding: Pregnancy Category B

Clozaril has not been tested in women to determine its safety in pregnancy. The effects of the medication on the developing fetus in pregnant women are unknown. In animal studies, there may be effects on the development of the fetus, but there are not adequate and well-controlled studies in humans. Animal studies are not always predictive of effects in humans. Therefore, the use of Clozaril in pregnant woman must always be weighed against the potential risks. Women who are pregnant or may become pregnant should discuss this with their physician. Some women may experience a recurrence of their psychosis when they stop Clozaril. In these circumstances, the physician may discuss the need to restart the medication or seek an alternative medication or treatment.

Nursing mothers should not take Clozaril, because small amounts will pass into breast milk and be ingested by the baby. If stopping the antipsychotic is not an alternative, breastfeeding should not be started or should be discontinued.

Possible Drug Interactions

Some medications when taken with Clozaril may result in drug interactions that alter their levels, which may produce undesired reactions. The possible drug interactions with Clozaril are summarized in the table below.

Tegretol (carbamazepine)	Tegretol, as well as other medications that may reduce white blood cells, should not be combined with Clozaril, because the combination may increase the risk of agranulocytosis. Moreover, Tegretol may significantly decrease the levels of Clozaril, decreasing its therapeutic effectiveness.
Antihypertensive medications	The combination of Clozaril and antihypertensive medications, such as Catapres (clonidine) and Inderal (propranolol), may increase the risk for orthostatic hypotension and exaggerate its effects.
Antihistamines, sedatives, and narcotic pain medication	When central nervous system depressants are combined with Clozaril, the sedative effects are additive and the sedation may be made worse, impairing the patient's ability to function.
Caffeine	Caffeine in coffee and cola beverages and in over-the-counter products may increase the blood levels of Clozaril, possibly increasing its adverse effects. Avoid caffeine if the interaction is suspected.
Selective serotonin reuptake inhibitors (SSRIs)	SSRIs such as Prozac, Celexa, Luvox, Zoloft, and Paxil may increase the blood levels of Clozaril, which may increase effects as well as toxicity. When an SSRI is started or discontinued, the Clozaril dosage may need to be adjusted accordingly.

Patients taking Clozaril should not consume alcohol because the combination may increase sedation and impair thinking, judgment, and coordination.

Overdose

Toxic symptoms from Clozaril overdose include confusion, excessive drooling, low blood pressure, irregular heartbeat (arrhythmias), and seizures. The outcome of an overdose depends on the amount ingested and whether Clozaril was combined with any other medications. Clozaril has significant anticholinergic properties. Anticholinergic toxicity may include diarrhea, elevated temperature, dilated pupils, rapid heart rate, delirium, hallucinations, and respiratory failure.

Any suspected overdose should be treated as an emergency. The person should be taken to the emergency room for observation and treatment. The prescription bottle of medication (and any other medication suspected in the overdose) should be brought as well, because the information on the prescription label can be helpful to the treating physician in determining the number of pills ingested.

Special Considerations

- Do not discontinue Clozaril without consulting your physician. Stopping Clozaril abruptly may result in rapid return of symptoms.
- If you miss a dose, take it as soon as possible. If it is close to the next scheduled dose, skip the missed dose and continue on your regular dosing schedule. Do not take double doses.
- Clozaril may be taken with or without food.
- Clozaril may cause sedation and drowsiness, especially during initiation of therapy, and may impair your alertness. Use caution when driving or performing tasks that require alertness.
- If you have signs of infection, including chills and fever that persist for more than 3–4 days, consult your physician. It is important to rule out Clozaril-induced decreases in white blood cells as a cause of the infection.
- Store the medication in its originally labeled, light-resistant container, away from heat and moisture. Heat and moisture may precipitate breakdown of your medication, and the medication may lose its therapeutic effects.
- Keep your medication out of reach of children.

If you have any questions about your medication, consult your physician or pharmacist.

Notes

From Chew RH, Hales RE, Yudofsky SC: *What Your Patients Need to Know About Psychiatric Medications*, Second Edition. Washington, DC, American Psychiatric Publishing, 2009

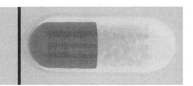

Geodon (ziprasidone)

Generic name: Ziprasidone
Available strengths: 20 mg, 40 mg, 60 mg, 80 mg capsules;
  20 mg/vial injection
Available in generic: No
Drug class: Second-generation antipsychotic

General Information

Geodon (ziprasidone) is one of the second-generation antipsychotic medications, which are also called atypical antipsychotics. (Refer to the handout "Second-Generation Antipsychotics" for an explanation of how these antipsychotics work.) Geodon is atypical in that it is significantly different, both in structure and in overall activity, from the earlier, *typical* antipsychotic medications such as chlorpromazine, thioridazine, and Haldol (haloperidol). The second-generation antipsychotics have a wider spectrum of activity, with fewer side effects associated with movement disorders, than the typical antipsychotics. The second-generation antipsychotics block both serotonin and dopamine receptors, whereas the typical antipsychotics are mainly dopamine-receptor antagonists. The use of Geodon is not limited to its antipsychotic action; it may also be useful as an antimanic agent.

The U.S. Food and Drug Administration (FDA) approved Geodon for the treatment of schizophrenia and acute mania or mixed episodes in bipolar disorder. The use of a medication for its approved indications is called its *labeled use*. In clinical practice, however, physicians often prescribe medications for *unlabeled* ("off-label") uses when published clinical studies, case reports, or their own clinical experiences support the efficacy and safety of those treatments. Like other second-generation antipsychotics, Geodon is used to treat a variety of psychiatric disorders, including schizoaffective disorder, psychotic depression, severe obsessive-compulsive disorder, and psychosis in Alzheimer's disease and other neuropsychiatric disorders.

Dosing Information

The recommended starting dosage of Geodon is 20–40 mg twice a day. The target dosage is between 120 mg/day and 160 mg/day, taken in divided doses twice a day. The usual maximum dosage is 160 mg/day. Geodon should be taken with meals to enhance absorption of the medication from the stomach into the bloodstream.

Geodon is also available in an injectable preparation, given intramuscularly, for the treatment of acute agitation.

Common Side Effects

Common side effects of Geodon are drowsiness, dizziness, indigestion, and constipation. Geodon is not associated with any significant weight gain and is notable among the second-generation antipsychotic agents (similar to Abilify) for its low propensity to affect weight.

There is a very low incidence of **extrapyramidal symptoms** (EPS) from Geodon. EPS are neurological disturbances produced by antipsychotics (or other causes) in the area of the brain that controls motor coordination. These side effects include muscle rigidity, tremors, drooling, restlessness, a "mask-like" facial expression, shuffling gait, and muscle spasms that result in abnormal posture (**dystonia**). EPS mimic Parkinson's disease, and many of the signs and symptoms are common in both conditions. Some patients experience **akathisia,** which is a subjective sense of restlessness accompanied by fidgeting and inability to sit or stand still. EPS may be managed by decreasing the antipsychotic dosage or adding another medication (anticholinergic medication) to counteract the side effect.

Geodon may block a compensatory response—the narrowing of blood vessels—that counterbalances postural change, resulting in a momentary drop in blood pressure when the person rises too rapidly, which may cause dizziness and lightheadedness. This reaction is known as **orthostatic hypotension.** Patients, especially seniors and those taking antihypertensive medications, need to be cautious and rise slowly to allow the body to adjust to the change in position, avoiding a sudden drop in blood pressure.

Adverse Reactions and Precautions

Geodon may cause sedation and drowsiness and impair physical coordination and mental alertness. Patients should avoid potentially dangerous activities, such as driving a car or operating machinery, until they are sure that these side effects will not affect their ability to perform these tasks.

Tardive dyskinesia (TD) is a potential adverse reaction from antipsychotic medications. It is characterized by late-onset abnormal involuntary movements. TD is a potentially irreversible condition that commonly includes "pill-rolling" movements of the fingers, darting and writhing movements of the tongue, lip puckering, facial grimacing, and other irregular movements. The risk of TD is believed to increase as the duration of treatment and the total cumulative amount of antipsychotic medications prescribed to the patient increase. The risk of TD associated with second-generation antipsychotics is significantly lower than with conventional antipsychotics.

Neuroleptic malignant syndrome (NMS) is a rare, toxic reaction to antipsychotics. The symptoms are severe muscle stiffness, rigidity, elevated body temperature, increased heart rate and blood pressure, irregular pulse, and profuse sweating. NMS may lead to delirium and coma. It can be fatal if medical intervention is not immediately provided. There are no tests to predict whether an individual is susceptible to developing NMS when exposed to an antipsychotic. Thus NMS must be recognized early because it is a medical emergency that requires immediate discontinuation of the antipsychotic, hospitalization, and intensive medical treatment.

Geodon may **slow electrical conduction in heart tissues** (myocardium). In earlier clinical studies, some patients showed on electrocardiogram (ECG) a prolongation of the electrical impulse as it traveled in the myocardium. This abnormal ECG finding, called *QTc prolongation*, may signal a potential for irregular heartbeat (**arrhythmia**). However, since the launch of Geodon in 2001 in the United States and from wider experience, physicians are more comfortable prescribing Geodon. The abnormal ECG finding associated with Geodon may not be clinically significant after all. However, patients who have a history of arrhythmia should have ECGs before starting Geodon and periodically during treatment to monitor any potential cardiac effect.

Geodon and other second-generation antipsychotics are associated with abnormalities in glucose regulation. Geodon may elevate blood glucose levels (**hyperglycemia**) and in some cases cause **diabetes mellitus.** While glucose abnormalities and diabetes are sometimes related to weight gain, these conditions may occur in patients without significant weight gain. Patients who have excessive weight gain are more susceptible to the medication's negative impact on blood sugar and cholesterol. The FDA has required a warning of hyperglycemia and diabetes mellitus with use of Geodon and other second-generation antipsychotics in their labeling. Patients receiving Geodon, especially those with a family history or an established diagnosis of diabetes, should be aware of this adverse reaction and should routinely monitor glucose levels while taking Geodon.

In elderly patients with dementia who are treated with a second-generation antipsychotic, including Geodon, there is an increased risk of death. The data from clinical studies show a higher risk in elderly patients with dementia treated with second-generation antipsychotics than with placebo-treated patients (i.e., patients taking a sugar pill). It is unclear why these medications have a higher risk in this group. Even though the risk is very low, the FDA requires Geodon to have in its package insert a warning about the associated risk in this population of taking an atypical antipsychotic medication.

Use in Pregnancy and Breastfeeding: Pregnancy Category C

Geodon has not been tested in women to determine its safety in pregnancy. The effects of the medication on the developing fetus in pregnant women are unknown. In animal studies, there may be effects on the development of the fetus, but there are not adequate and well-controlled studies in humans. Animal studies are not always predictive of effects in humans. Therefore, the use of Geodon in pregnant woman must always be weighed against the potential risks. Women who are pregnant or may become pregnant should discuss this with their physician. Some women may experience a recurrence of their psychosis when they stop Geodon. In these circumstances, the physician may discuss the need to restart the medication or seek an alternative medication or treatment.

Nursing mothers should not take Geodon, because small amounts will pass into breast milk and be ingested by the baby. If stopping the antipsychotic is not an alternative, breastfeeding should not be started or should be discontinued.

Possible Drug Interactions

Some medications when taken with Geodon may result in drug interactions that alter their levels, which may produce undesired reactions. The possible drug interactions with Geodon are summarized in the table below.

Antihypertensive medications	The combination of Geodon and antihypertensive medications, such as Catapres (clonidine) and Inderal (propranolol), may increase the risk for orthostatic hypotension and exaggerate its effects.
Nizoral (ketoconazole), Diflucan (fluconazole), and Sporanox (itraconazole)	These antifungal agents may decrease the metabolism of Geodon and cause increased Geodon blood levels, thus increasing the likelihood of unwanted side effects.
Tegretol (carbamazepine) and Dilantin (phenytoin)	Tegretol and Dilantin may decrease the blood levels of Geodon, making it less effective in treating the symptoms of the illness.
Central nervous system depressants	Sedating medications, such as barbiturates, benzodiazepines (e.g., Valium), narcotic analgesics, and antihistamines may exaggerate the sedative effect when combined with Geodon.
Some antiarrhythmic medications for controlling heart rate	The combination of certain antiarrhythmic medications and Geodon is contraindicated because it may increase the risk of life-threatening, irregular heartbeats (arrhythmias). Tell your doctor if you are taking heart medications or Geodon.

Patients taking Geodon should not consume alcohol because the combination may impair thinking, judgment, and coordination.

Overdose

The most common signs of Geodon overdose are extreme sedation, orthostatic hypotension, confusion, rapid and irregular heart rate, muscle rigidity, and seizures. The outcome depends on the amount ingested and whether Geodon was combined with other medications.

Any suspected overdose should be treated as an emergency. The person should be taken to the emergency room for observation and treatment. The prescription bottle of medication (and any other medication suspected in the overdose) should be brought as well, because the information on the prescription label can be helpful to the treating physician in determining the number of pills ingested.

Special Considerations

- Do not discontinue Geodon without consulting your physician.
- If you miss a dose, take it as soon as possible. If it is close to the next scheduled dose, skip the missed dose and continue on your regular dosing schedule. Do not take double doses.
- Geodon may be taken with or without food.
- Geodon may cause sedation and drowsiness, especially during initiation of therapy, and may impair your alertness. Use caution when driving or performing tasks that require alertness.
- Store the medication in its originally labeled, light-resistant container, away from heat and moisture. Heat and moisture may precipitate breakdown of your medication, and the medication may lose its therapeutic effects.
- Keep your medication out of reach of children.

If you have any questions about your medication, consult your physician or pharmacist.

Notes

_____

_____

_____

From Chew RH, Hales RE, Yudofsky SC: *What Your Patients Need to Know About Psychiatric Medications*, Second Edition. Washington, DC, American Psychiatric Publishing, 2009

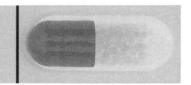

Invega (paliperidone)

Generic name: Paliperidone
Available strengths: 3 mg, 6 mg, 9 mg extended-release tablets
Available in generic: No
Drug class: Second-generation antipsychotic

General Information

Invega (paliperidone) was introduced in the United States in 2006. Invega is very similar to Risperdal (risperidone): it is the major, active metabolite of Risperdal. In the liver, Risperdal is converted to paliperidone. The manufacturer of Risperdal now markets this active metabolite as Invega. It comes in extended-release tablets, which deliver the drug at a controlled rate. The advantages of Invega, according to the manufacturer, are fewer side effects (possibly because Invega does not require the metabolite conversion as with Risperdal) and once-a-day dosing.

Invega is a **serotonin and dopamine antagonist** (SDA), belonging to the class of second-generation antipsychotics that are also called *atypical* antipsychotics. (Refer to the handout "Second-Generation Antipsychotics" for an explanation of how these antipsychotics work.) The second-generation antipsychotics are atypical in that they are significantly different, both in structure and in pharmacology, from the older, standard antipsychotics such as chlorpromazine, thioridazine, and Haldol (haloperidol). The second-generation antipsychotics have a wider spectrum of activity, with fewer side effects associated with movement disorders, than the typical antipsychotics. The second-generation antipsychotics block both serotonin and dopamine receptors, whereas the typical antipsychotics are mainly dopamine-receptor antagonists.

The U.S. Food and Drug Administration (FDA) approved Invega for the treatment of schizophrenia. It has not received an official approval for the treatment of acute mania in bipolar disorder, although it is believed that such approval is forthcoming. The use of a medication for its approved indications is called *labeled use*. In clinical practice, however, physicians often prescribe medications for *unlabeled* ("off-label") uses when published clinical studies, case reports, or their own clinical experiences support the efficacy and safety of those treatments. Like other second-generation antipsychotics, Invega may be used to treat other psychiatric disorders, including acute mania in bipolar disorder, schizoaffective disorder, psychotic depression, severe obsessive-compulsive disorder, and other neuropsychiatric disorders.

Dosing Information

The recommended starting dose of Invega extended-release tablets is 6 mg, taken once a day in the morning. However, some patients may benefit from higher doses, up to the maximum recommended dosage of 12 mg/

day, and for some patients, a lower dosage of 3 mg/day may be sufficient. For patients with severely impaired kidney function, for example, the recommended maximum dosage is 3 mg/day. With Invega, doctors can generally start with an optimal initial dose without having to increase the initial dose slowly.

Common Side Effects

Common side effects of Invega include drowsiness, dizziness, headache, nausea, and increased salivation. Invega can induce weight gain, although it does not usually cause as significant weight gain as some other antipsychotics. Weight gain can usually be managed by diet and exercise without stopping Invega.

There is a higher incidence of **extrapyramidal symptoms** (EPS) when the dosage of Invega exceeds 6 mg/day. EPS are neurological disturbances produced by antipsychotics (or other causes) in the area of the brain that controls motor coordination. These side effects include muscle rigidity, tremors, drooling, restlessness, a "mask-like" facial expression, shuffling gait, and muscle spasms that result in abnormal posture (**dystonia**). EPS mimic Parkinson's disease, and many of the signs and symptoms are common in both conditions. Some patients experience **akathisia,** which is a subjective sense of restlessness accompanied by fidgeting and inability to sit or stand still. EPS may be managed by decreasing the antipsychotic dosage or adding another medication (anticholinergic medication) to counteract the side effect. EPS may be managed by decreasing the antipsychotic dosage or adding another medication (anticholinergic medication) to counteract the side effect.

Invega may block a compensatory response—the narrowing of blood vessels—that counterbalances postural change, resulting in a momentary drop in blood pressure when the person rises too rapidly, which may cause dizziness and lightheadedness. This reaction is known as **orthostatic hypotension.** Patients, especially seniors and those taking antihypertensive medications, need to be cautious and rise slowly to allow the body to adjust to the change in position, avoiding a sudden drop in blood pressure.

Adverse Reactions and Precautions

Patients, especially seniors, need to be cautious of **orthostatic hypotension,** a momentary drop in blood pressure when a person goes from a sitting to a standing position. When rising too rapidly, the individual may experience dizziness and lightheadedness. If the drop in blood pressure is significant, the individual may faint. Patients should rise slowly from a supine or sitting position to avoid a possible sudden drop in blood pressure.

Tardive dyskinesia (TD) is a potential adverse reaction from antipsychotic medications. It is characterized by late-onset abnormal involuntary movements. TD is a potentially irreversible condition that commonly includes "pill-rolling" movements of the fingers, darting and writhing movements of the tongue, lip puckering, facial grimacing, and other irregular movements. The risk of TD is believed to increase as the duration of treatment and the total cumulative amount of antipsychotic medications prescribed to the patient increase. The risk of TD associated with second-generation antipsychotics is significantly lower than with conventional antipsychotics.

Neuroleptic malignant syndrome (NMS) is a rare, toxic reaction to antipsychotics. The symptoms are severe muscle stiffness, rigidity, elevated body temperature, increased heart rate and blood pressure, irregular pulse, and profuse sweating. NMS may lead to delirium and coma. It can be fatal if medical intervention is not immediately provided. There are no tests to predict whether an individual is susceptible to developing NMS when exposed to an antipsychotic. Thus, NMS must be recognized early because it is a medical emergency that requires immediate discontinuation of the antipsychotic, hospitalization, and intensive medical treatment.

Invega and other second-generation antipsychotics are associated with abnormalities in glucose regulation. Invega may elevate blood glucose levels (**hyperglycemia**) and in some cases cause **diabetes mellitus.**

While glucose abnormalities and diabetes are sometimes related to weight gain, these conditions may occur in patients without significant weight gain. Patients who have excessive weight gain are more susceptible to the medication's negative impact on blood sugar and cholesterol. The FDA has required a warning of hyperglycemia and diabetes mellitus with use of Invega and other second-generation antipsychotics in their labeling. Patients receiving Invega, especially those with a family history or an established diagnosis of diabetes, should be aware of this adverse reaction and should routinely monitor glucose levels while taking Invega.

In elderly patients with dementia who are treated with a second-generation antipsychotic, including Invega, there is an increased risk of death. The data from clinical studies show a higher risk in elderly patients with dementia treated with second-generation antipsychotics than with placebo-treated patients (i.e., patients taking a sugar pill). It is unclear why these medications have a higher risk in this group. Even though the risk is very low, the FDA requires Invega to have in its package insert a warning about the associated risk in this population of taking an atypical antipsychotic medication.

Use in Pregnancy and Breastfeeding: Pregnancy Category C

Invega has not been tested in women to determine its safety in pregnancy. The effects of the medication on the developing fetus in pregnant women are unknown. In animal studies, there may be effects on the development of the fetus, but there are not adequate and well-controlled studies in humans. Animal studies are not always predictive of effects in humans. Therefore, the use of Invega in pregnant woman must always be weighed against the potential risks. Women who are pregnant or may become pregnant should discuss this with their physician. Some women may experience a recurrence of their psychosis when they stop Invega. In these circumstances, the physician may discuss the need to restart the medication or seek an alternative medication or treatment.

Nursing mothers should not take Invega, because small amounts will pass into breast milk and be ingested by the baby. If stopping the antipsychotic is not an alternative, breastfeeding should not be started or should be discontinued.

Possible Drug Interactions

Invega is not expected to have any significant drug interactions with other medications. Given that Invega is a relatively new medication, there have been few reported drug interactions.

Patients taking Invega should not consume alcohol because the combination may impair thinking, judgment, and coordination.

Overdose

The experience of overdose with Invega is limited. The symptoms from overdose of Invega may include extreme sedation, hypotension, confusion, rapid heart rate, muscle rigidity, and seizures. The outcome also depends on the amount ingested and whether Invega was combined with other medications. Any suspected overdose should be treated as an emergency. The person should be taken to the emergency room for observation and treatment. The prescription bottle of medication (and any other medication suspected in the overdose) should be brought as well, because the information on the prescription label can be helpful to the treating physician in determining the number of pills ingested.

Special Considerations

- Invega may cause drowsiness and sedation and impair physical coordination and mental alertness. Until you are sure that these side effects will not impair your ability to perform daily tasks, it is important to avoid potentially dangerous activities, such as driving a car or operating machinery.
- Invega should only be taken once daily in the morning. Taking it at the beginning of the day allows for the controlled release of the medication throughout the day.
- Invega should be swallowed whole, not crushed or chewed, and should be taken with liquid to aid swallowing. It is normal to see the tablet shell along with other undissolved parts excreted in the stool.
- If you miss a dose, take it as soon as possible that day. However, if it is close to the next scheduled dose, skip the missed dose and continue on your regular dosing schedule the next morning. Do not take double doses.
- Do not discontinue Invega without consulting your physician.
- Invega may be taken with or without food.
- Store the medication in its originally labeled, light-resistant container, away from heat and moisture. Heat and moisture may precipitate breakdown of your medication, and the medication may lose its therapeutic effects.
- Keep your medication out of reach of children.

If you have any questions about your medication, consult your physician or pharmacist.

Notes

_____

_____

_____

_____

_____

_____

From Chew RH, Hales RE, Yudofsky SC: *What Your Patients Need to Know About Psychiatric Medications*, Second Edition. Washington, DC, American Psychiatric Publishing, 2009

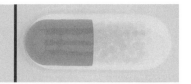

Risperdal, Risperdal M-Tab, and Risperdal Consta (risperidone)

Generic name: Risperidone
Available strengths: 0.25 mg, 0.5 mg, 1 mg, 2 mg, 3 mg, 4 mg tablets;
   0.5 mg, 1 mg, 2 mg, 3 mg, 4 mg rapid-disintegrating tablets
   (Risperdal M-Tab); 1 mg/mL oral solution;
   25 mg, 37.5 mg, 50 mg long-acting injection (Risperdal Consta)
Available in generic: Yes, but only the tablets
Drug class: Second-generation antipsychotic

General Information

Risperdal (risperidone) is one of the second-generation antipsychotic medications, which are also called *atypical* antipsychotics. (Refer to the handout "Second-Generation Antipsychotics" for an explanation of how these antipsychotics work.) Risperdal is atypical in that it is significantly different, both in structure and in overall activity, from the earlier, *typical* antipsychotic medications such as chlorpromazine, thioridazine, and Haldol (haloperidol). The second-generation antipsychotics have a wider spectrum of activity, with fewer side effects associated with movement disorders, than the typical antipsychotics. The second-generation antipsychotics block both serotonin and dopamine receptors, whereas the typical antipsychotics are mainly dopamine-receptor antagonists.

When first marketed in the United States in 1993, Risperdal was approved only for treatment of schizophrenia in adults. Subsequently, clinical studies showed that Risperdal, like many of the other atypical antipsychotics, is effective for treating acute mania in bipolar disorder, and the U.S. Food and Drug Administration (FDA) approved Risperdal for this use. In 2007, the FDA expanded the use of Risperdal to include treatment of schizophrenia in adults and in adolescents 13–17 years of age; short-term treatment of acute mania or mixed episodes in bipolar disorder in adults and in pediatric patients 10–17 years of age; and treatment of irritability associated with autistic disorder, including symptoms of aggression, self-injurious behavior, and uncontrollable temper tantrums.

The use of a medication for its approved indications is called its *labeled use*. In clinical practice, however, physicians often prescribe medications for *unlabeled* ("off-label") use when published clinical studies, case reports, or their own clinical experiences support the efficacy and safety of those treatments. Like other second-generation antipsychotics, Risperdal may be used to treat other psychiatric disorders, including psychotic depression, Tourette's syndrome (a chronic tic disorder), and obsessive-compulsive disorder.

Dosing Information

The new dosage guidelines for Risperdal, reflecting recent changes by the FDA, are as follows:

Indication—age group	Initial dosage (mg/day)	Increasing by	Target dosage (mg/day)	Effective dosage range (mg/day)
Schizophrenia—adults	2	1–2 mg daily	4–8	4–16
Schizophrenia—adolescents ages 13–17 years	0.5	0.5–1 mg daily	3	1–6
Bipolar mania—adults	2–3	1 mg daily	1–6	1–6
Bipolar mania—children and adolescents ages 10–17 years	0.5	0.5–1 mg daily	2.5	0.5–6
Irritability associated with autistic disorder	0.25 (<20 kg) 0.5 (≥20 kg)	0.25–0.5 mg daily after 2 weeks	0.5 (<20 kg) 1 (≥20 kg)	0.5–3

Source.   Risperdal [package insert]. Janssen Pharmaceutica Products, L.P., August 2007.

Risperdal comes in a rapid-disintegrating tablet form (Risperdal M-Tab), which dissolves in the mouth. It also comes in a solution that can be mixed in water or other liquids, but it is not compatible with tea or cola.

Risperdal Consta is a long-acting injectable form of Risperdal. The recommended starting dosage is 25 mg every 2 weeks. It takes about 3 weeks for Risperdal Consta to build up adequate blood levels, thus oral Risperdal or another antipsychotic medication must be continued for 3 weeks after the first dose of Risperdal Consta is given in order to prevent worsening of symptoms. Most patients' symptoms respond to 25 mg given every 2 weeks. If symptoms do not respond to 25 mg, a higher dosage of 37.5 or 50 mg every 2 weeks may be needed. The dosage should not exceed the maximum of 50 mg every 2 weeks.

Common Side Effects

At lower doses, Risperdal is generally well tolerated. Common side effects include sedation, dizziness, headache, nausea, vomiting, constipation, insomnia, and agitation. There is a higher incidence of **extrapyramidal symptoms** (EPS) when the dosage of Risperdal exceeds 6 mg/day. EPS are neurological disturbances produced by antipsychotics (or other causes) in the area of the brain that controls motor coordination. These side effects include muscle rigidity, tremors, drooling, restlessness, a "mask-like" facial expression, shuffling gait, and muscle spasms that result in abnormal posture (**dystonia**). EPS mimic Parkinson's disease, and many of the signs and symptoms are common in both conditions. Some patients experience **akathisia,** which is a subjective sense of restlessness accompanied by fidgeting and inability to sit or stand still. EPS may be managed by decreasing the antipsychotic dosage or adding another medication (anticholinergic medication) to counteract the side effect.

Generally, Risperdal does not induce significant weight gain as compared with some other antipsychotics. Control of weight can usually be managed by diet and exercise without stopping Risperdal.

Risperdal may block a compensatory response—the narrowing of blood vessels—that counterbalances postural change, resulting in a momentary drop in blood pressure when the person rises too rapidly, which may cause dizziness and lightheadedness. This reaction is known as **orthostatic hypotension.** Patients, especially seniors and those taking antihypertensive medications, need to be cautious and rise slowly to allow the body to adjust to the change in position, avoiding a sudden drop in blood pressure.

Adverse Reactions and Precautions

Risperdal may cause drowsiness and sedation and impair physical coordination and mental alertness. Patients should avoid potentially dangerous activities, such as driving a car or operating machinery, until they are sure that these side effects will not affect their ability to perform these tasks.

Tardive dyskinesia (TD) is a potential adverse reaction from antipsychotic medications. It is characterized by late-onset abnormal involuntary movements. TD is a potentially irreversible condition that commonly includes "pill-rolling" movements of the fingers, darting and writhing movements of the tongue, lip puckering, facial grimacing, and other irregular movements. The risk of TD is believed to increase as the duration of treatment and the total cumulative amount of antipsychotic medications prescribed to the patient increase. The risk of TD associated with second-generation antipsychotics is significantly lower than with conventional antipsychotics.

Neuroleptic malignant syndrome (NMS) is a rare, toxic reaction to antipsychotics. The symptoms are severe muscle stiffness, rigidity, elevated body temperature, increased heart rate and blood pressure, irregular pulse, and profuse sweating. NMS may lead to delirium and coma. It can be fatal if medical intervention is not immediately provided. There are no tests to predict whether an individual is susceptible to developing NMS when exposed to an antipsychotic. Thus NMS must be recognized early because it is a medical emergency that requires immediate discontinuation of the antipsychotic, hospitalization, and intensive medical treatment.

Risperdal and other second-generation antipsychotics are associated with abnormalities in glucose regulation. Risperdal may elevate blood glucose levels (**hyperglycemia**) and in some cases cause **diabetes mellitus.** While glucose abnormalities and diabetes are sometimes related to weight gain, these conditions may occur in patients without significant weight gain. Patients who have excessive weight gain are more susceptible to the medication's negative impact on blood sugar and cholesterol. The FDA has required a warning of hyperglycemia and diabetes mellitus with use of Risperdal and other second-generation antipsychotics in their labeling. Patients receiving Risperdal, especially those with a family history or an established diagnosis of diabetes, should be aware of this adverse reaction and should routinely monitor glucose levels while taking Risperdal.

In elderly patients with dementia who are treated with a second-generation antipsychotic, including Risperdal, there is an increased risk of death. The data from clinical studies show a higher risk in elderly patients with dementia treated with second-generation antipsychotics than with placebo-treated patients (i.e., patients taking a sugar pill). It is unclear why these medications have a higher risk in this group. Even though the risk is very low, the FDA requires Risperdal to have in its package insert a warning about the associated risk in this population of taking an atypical antipsychotic medication.

With an indication for treatment of acute mania in bipolar disorder, Risperdal must have in its labeling a warning of suicide risk associated with antidepressant medications. In short-term studies, antidepressants were found to increase the risk of suicidal thinking and behavior in children and adolescents with major depression and other psychiatric disorders. On the basis of these findings, the FDA requires a warning in the package insert that the prescriber be aware of the suicide risks in their patients who are starting antidepressant therapy, especially in the pediatric population. According to the FDA findings, the risk of suicidal thoughts and behaviors associated with antidepressants is age-related. This phenomenon tends to occur in the younger population and is most likely to occur early in the course of treatment. In adults over 24 years of age, there did not appear to be an increased risk of suicidality with antidepressants compared with placebo. In patients over age 65, the findings showed that antidepressants had a "protective effect" against suicidal thoughts and behavior.

After starting or changing antidepressant therapy, the patient, especially a child or adolescent, should be closely observed for worsening signs of depression.

Use in Pregnancy and Breastfeeding: Pregnancy Category C

Risperdal has not been tested in women to determine its safety in pregnancy. The effects of the medication on the developing fetus in pregnant women are unknown. In animal studies, there may be effects on the development of the fetus, but there are not adequate and well-controlled studies in humans. Animal studies are not always predictive of effects in humans. Therefore, the use of Risperdal in pregnant woman must always be weighed against the potential risks. Women who are pregnant or may become pregnant should discuss this with their physician. Some women may experience a recurrence of their psychosis when they stop Risperdal. In these circumstances, the physician may discuss the need to restart the medication or seek an alternative medication or treatment.

Nursing mothers should not take Risperdal, because small amounts will pass into breast milk and be ingested by the baby. If stopping the antipsychotic is not an alternative, breastfeeding should not be started or should be discontinued.

Possible Drug Interactions

Some medications when taken with Risperdal may result in drug interactions that alter their levels, which may produce undesired reactions. The possible drug interactions with Risperdal are summarized in the table below.

Selective serotonin reuptake inhibitors (SSRIs)	Prozac, Paxil, and other SSRI antidepressants may decrease the metabolism of Risperdal, thus increasing Risperdal blood levels and the likelihood of unwanted side effects.
Nizoral (ketoconazole), Diflucan (fluconazole), and Sporanox (itraconazole)	These antifungal agents may decrease the metabolism of Risperdal, thus increasing Risperdal blood levels and the likelihood of unwanted side effects.
Tegretol (carbamazepine)	Tegretol may decrease the blood levels of Risperdal, making it less effective in treating the symptoms of the illness.

Patients taking Risperdal should not consume alcohol because the combination may impair thinking, judgment, and coordination.

Overdose

The most common signs of Risperdal overdose include extreme sedation, orthostatic hypotension, confusion, rapid heart rate, muscle rigidity, and seizures. The outcome depends on the amount ingested and whether Risperdal was combined with other medications.

Any suspected overdose should be treated as an emergency. The person should be taken to the emergency room for observation and treatment. The prescription bottle of medication (and any other medication suspected in the overdose) should be brought as well, because the information on the prescription label can be helpful to the treating physician in determining the number of pills ingested.

Special Considerations

- Do not discontinue Risperdal without consulting your physician.
- If you miss a dose, take it as soon as possible that day. If it is close to the next schedule dose, skip the missed dose and continue on your regular dosing schedule. Do not take double doses.
- Risperdal may be taken with or without food.
- Risperdal may cause sedation and drowsiness, especially during initiation of therapy, and may impair your alertness. Use caution when driving or performing tasks that require alertness.
- Store the medication in its originally labeled, light-resistant container, away from heat and moisture. Heat and moisture may precipitate breakdown of your medication, and the medication may lose its therapeutic effects.
- Keep your medication out of reach of children.

If you have any questions about your medication, consult your physician or pharmacist.

Notes

_____

_____

_____

_____

_____

_____

_____

From Chew RH, Hales RE, Yudofsky SC: *What Your Patients Need to Know About Psychiatric Medications*, Second Edition. Washington, DC, American Psychiatric Publishing, 2009

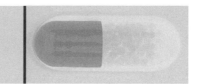

Seroquel (quetiapine)

Generic name: Quetiapine
Available strengths: 25 mg, 50 mg, 100 mg, 200 mg,
    300 mg, 400 mg tablets; 200 mg, 300 mg, 400 mg
    extended-release tablets (Seroquel XR)
Available in generic: No
Drug class: Second-generation antipsychotic

General Information

Seroquel (quetiapine) is one of the second-generation antipsychotic medications, which are also called *atypical* antipsychotics. (Refer to the handout "Second-Generation Antipsychotics" for an explanation of how these antipsychotics work.) Seroquel is atypical in that it is significantly different, both in structure and in pharmacology, from the older, *typical* antipsychotic medications such as chlorpromazine, thioridazine, and Haldol (haloperidol). The second-generation antipsychotics have a wider spectrum of activity, with fewer side effects associated with movement disorders, than the typical antipsychotics. The second-generation antipsychotics block both serotonin and dopamine receptors, whereas the typical antipsychotics are mainly dopamine-receptor antagonists.

When first marketed in the United States in 1997, Seroquel was approved only for the treatment of schizophrenia in adults. In the following years, clinical studies showed that Seroquel, like many of the other atypical antipsychotics, is effective for treating acute mania in bipolar disorder. In 2006, the U.S. Food and Drug Administration (FDA) approved Seroquel (but not the XR form) for the treatment of depressive episodes and acute mania associated with bipolar disorder. It is also approved for the maintenance treatment of bipolar disorder in conjunction with lithium or divalproex (Depakote), However, Seroquel has not been approved by the FDA for use in children or adolescents.

The use of a medication for its approved indications is called its *labeled* use. In clinical practice, however, physicians often prescribe medications for *unlabeled* uses when published clinical studies, case reports, or their own clinical experiences support the efficacy and safety of those treatments. Like other second-generation antipsychotics, Seroquel may be used to treat other psychiatric disorders, including off-label in pediatric patients.

Dosing Information

For schizophrenia, the recommended starting dosage of Seroquel is 25–50 mg twice a day. The dosage is increased by 25–50 mg every day or two until a target dosage of 300–400 mg/day, taken twice a day, is reached. After several weeks, if needed, the dosage may be increased to a maximum of 800 mg/day. Seroquel has a wide dosing range. Effective dosages for schizophrenia may range from 150 mg/day to 800 mg/day.

In treatment of depressive episodes associated with bipolar disorder, the recommended dosing is 50 mg at bedtime on day 1, 100 mg on day 2, 200 mg on day 3, and 300 mg on day 4 and thereafter.

In treatment of acute mania in bipolar disorder, the usual starting dosage is 100 mg/day, given in two divided doses, and the dosage is rapidly increased to 400 mg/day by the fourth day. If needed, the dosage is increased by 200 mg/day to a maximum of 800 mg/day by day 7. As acute mania abates, Seroquel may be continued as a single agent or in combination with another mood stabilizer, such as Depakote. Dosage adjustments may be needed to find the lowest dosage required to maintain remission.

A more cautious dosing approach is recommended for seniors or for patients with a medical condition, such as liver disease. The dosage should be increased slowly, with a lower starting and ending dosage.

Common Side Effects

The common side effects of Seroquel are drowsiness and dizziness. Drowsiness may be problematic during the daytime. Taking a larger portion of the divided dosage at bedtime and a smaller one in the morning may minimize daytime sleepiness. For example, if the total dosage were 300 mg/day, the patient would take 200 mg at bedtime and 100 mg in the morning.

There is a very low incidence of **extrapyramidal symptoms** (EPS) from Seroquel. EPS are neurological disturbances produced by antipsychotics (or other causes) in the area of the brain that controls motor coordination. These side effects include muscle rigidity, tremors, drooling, restlessness, a "mask-like" facial expression, shuffling gait, and muscle spasms that result in abnormal posture (**dystonia**). EPS mimic Parkinson's disease, and many of the signs and symptoms are common in both conditions. Some patients experience **akathisia,** which is a subjective sense of restlessness accompanied by fidgeting and inability to sit or stand still. EPS may be managed by decreasing the antipsychotic dosage or adding another medication (anticholinergic medication) to counteract the side effect.

Patients frequently will gain weight when treated with Seroquel. It appears that Seroquel increases appetite and may produce some underlying metabolic changes. The major concern of this weight gain is the health consequences to the patient, including the potential for developing diabetes and increasing cholesterol and other lipids, which may increase the risk for cardiovascular disease. Furthermore, patients may want to stop taking their medication if they become self-conscious about putting on excessive weight. If this side effect becomes problematic, patients should not stop their medication but should consult their physician. Weight can usually be managed by diet and exercise without stopping Seroquel.

Seroquel may block a compensatory response—the narrowing of blood vessels—that counterbalances postural change, resulting in a momentary drop in blood pressure when the person rises too rapidly, which may cause dizziness and lightheadedness. This reaction is known as **orthostatic hypotension.** Patients, especially seniors and those taking antihypertensive medications, need to be cautious and rise slowly to allow the body to adjust to the change in position, avoiding a sudden drop in blood pressure.

Adverse Reactions and Precautions

Seroquel may cause drowsiness and sedation and impair physical coordination and mental alertness. Patients should avoid potentially dangerous activities, such as driving a car or operating machinery, until they are sure that these side effects will not affect their ability to perform these tasks.

Tardive dyskinesia (TD) is a potential adverse reaction from antipsychotic medications. It is characterized by late-onset abnormal involuntary movements. TD is a potentially irreversible condition that commonly includes "pill-rolling" movements of the fingers, darting and writhing movements of the tongue, lip puckering, facial grimacing, and other irregular movements. The risk of TD is believed to increase as the duration of treatment and the total cumulative amount of antipsychotic medications prescribed to the patient increase. The risk of TD associated with second-generation antipsychotics is significantly lower than with conventional antipsychotics.

Neuroleptic malignant syndrome (NMS) is a rare, toxic reaction to antipsychotics. The symptoms are severe muscle stiffness, rigidity, elevated body temperature, increased heart rate and blood pressure, irregular pulse, and profuse sweating. NMS may lead to delirium and coma. It can be fatal if medical intervention is not immediately provided. There are no tests to predict whether an individual is susceptible to developing NMS when exposed to an antipsychotic. Thus NMS must be recognized early because it is a medical emergency that requires immediate discontinuation of the antipsychotic, hospitalization, and intensive medical treatment.

There have been reports of patients who showed transient and asymptomatic increases in liver enzymes, but it was concluded that the elevated enzymes were temporary and not serious. Nevertheless, patients' liver function should be monitored by laboratory tests before beginning treatment with Seroquel and then periodically during treatment.

Seroquel and other second-generation antipsychotics are associated with abnormalities in glucose regulation. Seroquel may elevate blood glucose levels (**hyperglycemia**) and in some cases cause **diabetes mellitus.** While glucose abnormalities and diabetes are sometimes related to weight gain, these conditions may occur in patients without significant weight gain. Patients who have excessive weight gain are more susceptible to the medication's negative impact on blood sugar and cholesterol. The FDA has required a warning of hyperglycemia and diabetes mellitus with use of Seroquel and other second-generation antipsychotics in their labeling. Patients receiving Seroquel, especially those with a family history or an established diagnosis of diabetes, should be aware of this adverse reaction and should routinely monitor glucose levels while taking Seroquel.

In elderly patients with dementia who are treated with a second-generation antipsychotic, including Seroquel, there is an increased risk of death. The data from clinical studies show a higher risk in elderly patients with dementia treated with second-generation antipsychotics than with placebo-treated patients (i.e., patients taking a sugar pill). It is unclear why these medications have a higher risk in this group. Even though the risk is very low, the FDA requires Seroquel to have in its package insert a warning about the associated risk in this population of taking an atypical antipsychotic medication.

With an indication for treatment of depression, Seroquel must have in its labeling a warning of suicide risk associated with antidepressant medications. In short-term studies, antidepressants were found to increase the risk of suicidal thinking and behavior in children and adolescents with major depression and other psychiatric disorders. On the basis of these findings, the FDA requires a warning in the package insert that the prescriber be aware of the suicide risks in their patients who are starting antidepressant therapy, especially in the pediatric population. According to the FDA findings, the risk of suicidal thoughts and behaviors associated with antidepressants is age-related. This phenomenon tends to occur in the younger population and is most likely to occur early in the course of treatment. In adults over 24 years of age, there did not appear to be an increased risk of suicidality with antidepressants compared with placebo. In patients over age 65, the findings showed that antidepressants had a "protective effect" against suicidal thoughts and behavior.

After starting or changing antidepressant therapy, the patient, especially a child or adolescent, should be closely observed for worsening signs of depression.

Use in Pregnancy and Breastfeeding: Pregnancy Category C

Seroquel has not been tested in women to determine its safety in pregnancy. The effects of the medication on the developing fetus in pregnant women are unknown. In animal studies, there may be effects on the development of the fetus, but there are not adequate and well-controlled studies in humans. Animal studies are not always predictive of effects in humans. Therefore, the use of Seroquel in pregnant woman must always be weighed against the potential risks. Women who are pregnant or may become pregnant should discuss this with their physician. Some women may experience a recurrence of their psychosis when they stop Seroquel. In these circumstances, the physician may discuss the need to restart the medication or seek an alternative medication or treatment.

Nursing mothers should not take Seroquel, because small amounts will pass into breast milk and be ingested by the baby. If stopping the antipsychotic is not an alternative, breastfeeding should not be started or should be discontinued.

Possible Drug Interactions

Some medications when taken with Seroquel may result in drug interactions that alter their levels, which may produce undesired reactions. The possible drug interactions with Seroquel are summarized in the table below.

Antihypertensive medications	The combination of Seroquel and antihypertensive medications, such as Catapres (clonidine) and Inderal (propranolol), may increase the risk for orthostatic hypotension and exaggerate its effects.
Nizoral (ketoconazole), Diflucan (fluconazole), and Sporanox (itraconazole)	Antifungal agents may decrease the metabolism of Seroquel, thus increasing blood levels and the likelihood of unwanted side effects.
Tegretol (carbamazepine) and Dilantin (phenytoin)	Tegretol and Dilantin may decrease the blood levels of Seroquel, making it less effective in treating the symptoms of the illness.
Central nervous system depressants	Sedating medications, such as barbiturates, benzodiazepines (e.g., Valium), narcotic analgesics, and antihistamines, may increase sedation when combined with Seroquel.

Patients taking Seroquel should not consume alcohol because the combination may impair thinking, judgment, and coordination.

Overdose

The most common signs of Seroquel overdose include extreme sedation, orthostatic hypotension, confusion, rapid and irregular heart rate, muscle rigidity, and seizures. The outcome depends on the amount ingested and whether Seroquel was combined with other medications.

Any suspected overdose should be treated as an emergency. The person should be taken to the emergency room for observation and treatment. The prescription bottle of medication (and any other medication suspected in the overdose) should be brought as well, because the information on the prescription label can be helpful to the treating physician in determining the number of pills ingested.

Special Considerations

- Do not discontinue Seroquel without consulting your physician.
- If you miss a dose, take it as soon as possible that day. If it is close to the next schedule dose, skip the missed dose and continue on your regular dosing schedule. Do not take double doses.
- Seroquel may be taken with or without food.
- Seroquel may cause sedation and drowsiness, especially during initiation of therapy, and may impair your alertness. Use caution when driving or performing tasks that require alertness.
- Store the medication in its originally labeled, light-resistant container, away from heat and moisture. Heat and moisture may precipitate breakdown of your medication, and the medication may lose its therapeutic effects.
- Keep your medication out of reach of children.

If you have any questions about your medication, consult your physician or pharmacist.

Notes

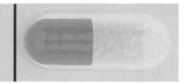

Symbyax (Zyprexa [olanzapine] and Prozac [fluoxetine] combination)

Generic name: Olanzapine and fluoxetine combination
Available strengths: 3 mg/25 mg, 6 mg/25 mg, 6 mg/50 mg,
   12 mg/25 mg, 12 mg/50 mg capsules (Zyprexa/Prozac)
Available in generic: No
Drug class: Second-generation antipsychotic and
   selective serotonin reuptake inhibitor antidepressant

General Information

Symbyax is a combination medication containing the antipsychotic **Zyprexa (olanzapine)** and the antidepressant **Prozac (fluoxetine).** Zyprexa is one of the second-generation antipsychotics, which are also called *atypical* antipsychotics. (Refer to the handout "Second-Generation Antipsychotics" for an explanation of how these antipsychotics work.) Zyprexa possesses mood-stabilizing (i.e., controlling mood swings) and antipsychotic properties that are effective in treating a wide spectrum of mental disorders. The second-generation antipsychotics have a wider spectrum of activity, with fewer side effects associated with movement disorders, than the typical antipsychotics. The second-generation antipsychotics block both serotonin and dopamine receptors, whereas the typical antipsychotics are mainly dopamine-receptor antagonists.

The antidepressant Prozac contained in Symbyax is a **selective serotonin reuptake inhibitor** (SSRI). Prozac and other SSRI antidepressants work by blocking the reuptake of the neurotransmitter serotonin back into brain cells, thereby increasing the levels of serotonin in the brain. Depression and other mental disorders may be due to abnormally low levels of serotonin. The presumed action of Prozac and other SSRIs is to increase serotonin levels, which may help to restore those areas of the brain to normal function.

Symbyax was approved by the U.S. Food and Drug Administration (FDA) for the treatment of depressive episodes associated with bipolar disorder. The use of a medication for its approved indications is called its *labeled* use. In clinical practice, however, physicians often prescribe medications for *unlabeled* uses, when published clinical studies, case reports, or their own clinical experiences support the efficacy and safety of those treatments. Symbyax is used off-label to treat other psychiatric disorders.

Dosing Information

Symbyax comes in fixed combinations of Zyprexa and Prozac in different strengths. It is available in the combinations of 3 mg/25 mg, 6 mg/25 mg, 6 mg/50 mg, 12 mg/25 mg, and 12 mg/50 mg of Zyprexa/Prozac, respectively. The recommended starting dosage for Symbyax is 6 mg/25 mg taken once a day. Dosage adjustments are made according to response and tolerability to the medication. The dosage may range from 6 mg to 12 mg of Zyprexa and 25 mg to 50 mg of Prozac, all taken in a single daily dose.

Common Side Effects

The common side effects reported with Symbyax are sleepiness, tiredness, tremor, peripheral edema (accumulation of fluid in the legs and ankles), dry mouth, increased appetite, and weight gain. As tolerance to the medication develops, these side effects should subside. Taking Symbyax in a single bedtime dose may minimize daytime sedation and drowsiness. For dry mouth, chewing sugarless gum or sucking on sugarless candy may promote salivation.

Zyprexa in Symbyax may induce **extrapyramidal symptoms** (EPS), although these effects are very uncommon with the second-generation antipsychotics. EPS are neurological disturbances produced by antipsychotics (or other causes) in the area of the brain that controls motor coordination. These side effects include muscle rigidity, tremors, drooling, restlessness, a "mask-like" facial expression, shuffling gait, and muscle spasms that result in abnormal posture (**dystonia**). At dosages greater than 10 mg/day, some patients may experience **akathisia,** which is a subjective sense of restlessness accompanied by fidgeting and inability to sit or stand still. EPS may be managed by decreasing the antipsychotic dosage or adding another medication (anticholinergic medication) to counteract the side effect.

Symbyax may increase appetite and caloric intake, causing significant weight gain. In clinical studies, the mean weight increase in patients who took Symbyax was approximately 8 pounds, compared with placebo-treated groups. The major concern of weight gain is the health consequences to the patient, including the potential for developing diabetes and increasing cholesterol and other lipids, which may increase the risk for cardiovascular disease. Furthermore, patients may want to stop taking their medication if they become self-conscious about putting on excessive weight. If this side effect becomes problematic, patients should not stop their medication but should consult their physician. Weight can usually be managed by diet and exercise without stopping Symbyax.

Symbyax may block a compensatory response—the narrowing of blood vessels—that counterbalances postural change, resulting in a momentary drop in blood pressure when the person rises too rapidly, which may cause dizziness and lightheadedness. This reaction is known as **orthostatic hypotension.** Patients, especially seniors and those taking antihypertensive medications, need to be cautious and rise slowly to allow the body to adjust to the change in position, avoiding a sudden drop in blood pressure.

Adverse Reactions and Precautions

Symbyax may cause drowsiness and sedation and impair physical coordination and mental alertness. Patients should avoid potentially dangerous activities, such as driving a car or operating machinery, until they are sure that these side effects will not affect their ability to perform these tasks.

Tardive dyskinesia (TD) is a potential adverse reaction from antipsychotic medications. It is characterized by late-onset abnormal involuntary movements. TD is a potentially irreversible condition that commonly includes "pill-rolling" movements of the fingers, darting and writhing movements of the tongue, lip puckering, facial grimacing, and other irregular movements. The risk of TD is believed to increase as the duration of treatment and the total cumulative amount of antipsychotic medications prescribed to the patient increase. The risk of TD associated with second-generation antipsychotics, such as Zyprexa in Symbyax, is significantly lower than with conventional antipsychotics. In rare cases, however, Prozac has been associated with TD. It is too early to determine whether the combination of Zyprexa and Prozac may increase the incidence of TD, because the condition usually requires years of exposure to the medication.

Neuroleptic malignant syndrome (NMS) is a rare, toxic reaction to antipsychotics, including Zyprexa in Symbyax. The symptoms are severe muscle stiffness, rigidity, elevated body temperature, increased heart rate and blood pressure, irregular pulse, and profuse sweating. NMS may lead to delirium and coma. It can be fatal if medical intervention is not immediately provided. There are no tests to predict whether an individual is susceptible to developing NMS when exposed to an antipsychotic. Thus NMS must be recognized early because it is a medical emergency that requires immediate discontinuation of the antipsychotic, hospitalization, and intensive medical treatment.

Antipsychotic medications, including Zyprexa in Symbyax, may disrupt the body's ability to dissipate heat. Fatal cases from disruption of the body's ability to lower core temperature have been reported with antipsychotics, particularly the older, first-generation antipsychotics. Therefore, individuals taking Symbyax need to be cautious of conditions that may contribute to elevation in temperature, including exposure to extreme heat, dehydration, strenuous exercise, and concomitant medications, such as anticholinergic agents, which may reduce the body's ability to dissipate heat.

Zyprexa and other second-generation antipsychotics are associated with abnormalities in glucose regulation. Zyprexa may elevate blood glucose levels (**hyperglycemia**) and in some cases cause **diabetes mellitus.** While glucose abnormalities and diabetes are sometimes related to weight gain, these conditions may occur in patients without significant weight gain. Patients who have excessive weight gain are more susceptible to the medication's negative impact on blood sugar and cholesterol. The FDA has required a warning of hyperglycemia and diabetes mellitus with use of Zyprexa and other second-generation antipsychotics in their labeling. Patients receiving Symbyax, especially those with a family history or an established diagnosis of diabetes, should be aware of this adverse reaction and should routinely monitor glucose levels while taking Symbyax.

In elderly patients with dementia who are treated with a second-generation antipsychotic, including Zyprexa in Symbyax, there is an increased risk of death. The data from clinical studies show a higher risk in elderly patients with dementia treated with second-generation antipsychotics than with placebo-treated patients (i.e., patients taking a sugar pill). It is unclear why these medications have a higher risk in this group. Even though the risk is very low, the FDA requires Symbyax to have in its package insert a warning about the associated risk in this population of taking an atypical antipsychotic medication.

With an indication for treatment of depression, Symbyax must have in its labeling a warning of suicide risk associated with antidepressant medications. In short-term studies, antidepressants were found to increase the risk of suicidal thinking and behavior in children and adolescents with major depression and other psychiatric disorders. On the basis of these findings, the FDA requires a warning in the package insert that the prescriber be aware of the suicide risks in their patients who are starting antidepressant therapy, especially in the pediatric population. According to FDA findings, the risk of suicidal thoughts and behaviors associated with antidepressants is age-related. This phenomenon tends to occur in the younger population and, most likely, to occur early in the course of treatment. In adults over 24 years of age, there did not appear to be an increased risk of suicidality with antidepressants compared with placebo. In patients over age 65, the findings showed that antidepressants had a "protective effect" against suicidal thoughts and behavior.

After starting or changing antidepressant therapy, the patient, especially a child or adolescent, should be closely observed for worsening signs of depression.

Use in Pregnancy and Breastfeeding: Pregnancy Category C

Symbyax has not been tested in women to determine its safety in pregnancy. The effects of the medication on the developing fetus in pregnant women are unknown. In animal studies, there may be effects on the development of the fetus, but there are not adequate and well-controlled studies in humans. Animal studies are not always predictive of effects in humans. Therefore, the use of Symbyax in pregnant woman must always be weighed against the potential risks. Women who are pregnant or may become pregnant should discuss this with their physician. Some women may experience a recurrence of their symptoms when they stop Symbyax. In these circumstances, the physician may discuss the need to restart the medication or seek an alternative medication or treatment.

Nursing mothers should not take Symbyax, because small amounts will pass into breast milk and be ingested by the baby. If stopping the antipsychotic/antidepressant is not an alternative, breastfeeding should not be started or should be discontinued.

Possible Drug Interactions

Some medications when taken with Symbyax may result in drug interactions that alter their levels, which may produce undesired reactions. The antidepressants known as **monoamine oxidase inhibitors** (MAOIs), such as Nardil (phenelzine), should not be taken with Symbyax. Furthermore, an MAOI should not be started for at least 2 weeks and preferably 4–5 weeks after the discontinuation of Symbyax, because of the long duration of action of Prozac and its metabolites. The combination of an MAOI and Prozac may precipitate a dangerous elevation of blood pressure.

Other possible drug interactions with Symbyax are summarized in the table below.

Luvox (fluvoxamine)	Luvox may decrease the metabolism of Symbyax, thus increasing blood levels of Symbyax and the likelihood of unwanted side effects.
Tegretol (carbamazepine)	Tegretol may increase the metabolism of Zyprexa and thus decrease the blood levels and effectiveness of Symbyax in treating the symptoms of the illness.
Clozaril (clozapine)	Clozaril blood levels may be elevated by the Prozac in Symbyax, increasing the potential for toxicity.
Dilantin (phenytoin)	Prozac may elevate the blood levels of the anticonvulsant Dilantin, increasing the potential for toxicity from Dilantin.
Coumadin (warfarin)	Prozac may increase the anticoagulant effect of Coumadin and increase the risk of bleeding; the Coumadin dosage may need to be adjusted.

Patients taking Symbyax should not consume alcohol because the combination may impair thinking, judgment, and coordination.

Overdose

There are few data on acute overdose with Symbyax. Fatal cases have been reported with patients who overdosed on Prozac alone. The most common symptoms associated with Prozac overdose include somnolence, confusion, nausea, vomiting, rapid heart rate, and seizures. In cases of Zyprexa overdose, common signs include agitation, rapid heart rate, EPS, and reduced level of consciousness ranging from sedation to coma. Among the serious and sometimes fatal cases from acute overdose with Zyprexa, seizures, cardiac arrhythmias, respiratory depression, and cardiopulmonary arrest were reported. Acute overdose with Symbyax, which contains two active ingredients, may be potentially more hazardous than overdose with Zyprexa or Prozac alone.

Any suspected overdose should be treated as an emergency. The person should be taken to the emergency room for observation and treatment. The prescription bottle of medication (and any other medication suspected in the overdose) should be brought as well, because the information on the prescription label can be helpful to the treating physician in determining the number of pills ingested.

Special Considerations

- **Warning:** Always let your physician or a family member know if you have suicidal thoughts. Notify your psychiatrist or your family physician whenever your depressive symptoms worsen or whenever you feel unable to control suicidal urges or thoughts.
- Do not discontinue Symbyax without consulting your physician.
- If you miss a dose, take it as soon as possible. If it is close to the next scheduled dose, skip the missed dose and continue on your regular dosing schedule. Do not take double doses.
- Symbyax may be taken with or without food.
- Symbyax may cause sedation and drowsiness, especially during initiation of therapy, and may impair your alertness. Use caution when driving or performing tasks that require alertness.
- Store the medication in its originally labeled, light-resistant container, away from heat and moisture. Heat and moisture may precipitate breakdown of the medication, and the medication may lose its therapeutic effects.
- Keep your medication out of reach of children.

If you have any questions about your medication, consult your physician or pharmacist.

Notes

_____

_____

_____

_____

_____

From Chew RH, Hales RE, Yudofsky SC: *What Your Patients Need to Know About Psychiatric Medications*, Second Edition. Washington, DC, American Psychiatric Publishing, 2009

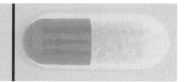

Zyprexa and Zyprexa Zydis (olanzapine)

Generic name: Olanzapine
Available strengths: 2.5 mg, 5 mg, 7.5 mg, 10 mg,
    15 mg, 20 mg tablets; 5 mg, 10 mg, 15 mg, 20 mg
    orally disintegrating tablets (Zyprexa Zydis);
    10 mg/vial injection
Available in generic: No
Drug class: Second-generation antipsychotic

General Information

Zyprexa (olanzapine) is one of the second-generation antipsychotics, which are also called *atypical* antipsychotics. (Refer to the handout "Second-Generation Antipsychotics" for an explanation of how these antipsychotics work.) Zyprexa is atypical in that it is significantly different, both in structure and in pharmacology, from the older, *typical* antipsychotic medications such as chlorpromazine, thioridazine, and Haldol (haloperidol). The second-generation antipsychotics have a wider spectrum of activity, with fewer side effects associated with movement disorders, than the typical antipsychotics. The second-generation antipsychotics block both serotonin and dopamine receptors, whereas the typical antipsychotics are mainly dopamine-receptor antagonists. Zyprexa possesses mood-stabilizing (i.e., controlling mood swings) and antipsychotic properties that are effective in treating a wide spectrum of mental disorders.

Zyprexa was approved by the U.S. Food and Drug Administration (FDA) for treatment of schizophrenia and acute mania or mixed episodes associated with bipolar disorder—used alone or in combination with lithium or valproate (e.g., Depakote). In addition, Zyprexa was given an indication that allows it to be used alone (monotherapy) in maintenance treatment of bipolar disorder. The use of a medication for its approved indications is called its *labeled* use. In clinical practice, however, physicians often prescribe medications for *unlabeled* uses when published clinical studies, case reports, or their own clinical experiences support the efficacy and safety of those treatments. Like other second-generation antipsychotics, Zyprexa may be used to treat other psychiatric disorders, including off-label in pediatric patients.

Dosing Information

The recommended starting dosage for Zyprexa for treatment of schizophrenia is 5–10 mg/day, taken once daily, preferably in the evening or at bedtime. It may be taken without regard to meals. The dosage may be increased, usually in weekly increments of 5 mg/day. The dosage range is usually between 10 mg/day and 20 mg/day. However, dosages greater than 20 mg/day may be required for some patients.

In treatment of acute mania in bipolar disorder, the initial dosage is 10–15 mg/day, taken in a single daily dose. The dosage may be increased in increments of 5 mg/day, but not in less than 24 hours. When the acute episode is stabilized, the patient may continue maintenance therapy with Zyprexa alone (monotherapy) to prevent relapse, using a maintenance dosage of 15–20 mg/day. If Zyprexa is used in combination with another mood stabilizer, such as lithium or Depakote, the dosage is generally lowered to 10 mg/day.

Zyprexa also comes in an orally disintegrating tablet under the brand Zyprexa Zydis. The preparation rapidly melts in the mouth.

Common Side Effects

Frequent and bothersome side effects from Zyprexa are sedation, constipation, and dry mouth. As tolerance to the medication develops, these side effects usually subside. Taking Zyprexa in a single bedtime dose may minimize daytime sedation. For dry mouth, chewing sugarless gum or sucking on sugarless candy may promote salivation. To prevent constipation, patients should increase fluid intake and dietary fiber and should exercise regularly. Bulk laxatives or a stool softener such as Colace may be needed at times to relieve constipation.

Extrapyramidal symptoms (EPS), which are commonly associated with conventional antipsychotics, are infrequent with Zyprexa. EPS are neurological disturbances produced by antipsychotics (or other causes) in the area of the brain that controls motor coordination. These side effects include muscle rigidity, tremors, drooling, restlessness, a "mask-like" facial expression, shuffling gait, and muscle spasms that result in abnormal posture (**dystonia**). At dosages greater than 10 mg/day, some patients may experience **akathisia,** which is a subjective sense of restlessness accompanied by fidgeting and inability to sit or stand still. EPS may be managed by decreasing the antipsychotic dosage or adding another medication (anticholinergic medication) to counteract the side effect.

Zyprexa may induce significant weight gain. This may be due to increased appetite or to some underlying metabolic changes. The major concern of weight gain is the health consequences to the patient, including the potential for developing diabetes and increasing cholesterol and other lipids, which may increase the risk for cardiovascular disease. Furthermore, patients may want to stop taking their medication if they become self-conscious about putting on excessive weight. If this side effect becomes problematic, patients should not stop their medication but should consult their physician.

Zyprexa may block a compensatory response—the narrowing of blood vessels—that counterbalances postural change, resulting in a momentary drop in blood pressure when the person rises too rapidly, which may cause dizziness and lightheadedness. This reaction is known as **orthostatic hypotension.** Patients, especially seniors and those taking antihypertensive medications, need to be cautious and rise slowly to allow the body to adjust to the change in position, avoiding a sudden drop in blood pressure.

Adverse Reactions and Precautions

Zyprexa may cause drowsiness and sedation and impair physical coordination and mental alertness. Patients should avoid potentially dangerous activities, such as driving a car or operating machinery, until they are sure that these side effects will not affect their ability to perform these tasks.

Tardive dyskinesia (TD) is a potential adverse reaction from antipsychotic medications. It is characterized by late-onset abnormal involuntary movements. TD is a potentially irreversible condition that commonly includes "pill-rolling" movements of the fingers, darting and writhing movements of the tongue, lip puckering, facial grimacing, and other irregular movements. The risk of TD is believed to increase as the duration of treatment and the total cumulative amount of antipsychotic medications prescribed to the patient increase. The risk of TD associated with second-generation antipsychotics is significantly lower than with conventional antipsychotics.

Neuroleptic malignant syndrome (NMS) is a rare, toxic reaction to antipsychotics. The symptoms are severe muscle stiffness, rigidity, elevated body temperature, increased heart rate and blood pressure, irregular pulse, and profuse sweating. NMS may lead to delirium and coma. It can be fatal if medical intervention is not immediately provided. There are no tests to predict whether an individual is susceptible to developing NMS when exposed to an antipsychotic. Thus NMS must be recognized early because it is a medical emergency that requires immediate discontinuation of the antipsychotic, hospitalization, and intensive medical treatment.

Zyprexa and other second-generation antipsychotics are associated with abnormalities in glucose regulation. Zyprexa may elevate blood glucose levels (**hyperglycemia**) and in some cases cause **diabetes mellitus.** While glucose abnormalities and diabetes are sometimes related to weight gain, these conditions may occur in patients without significant weight gain. Patients who have excessive weight gain are more susceptible to the medication's negative impact on blood sugar and cholesterol. The FDA has required a warning of hyperglycemia and diabetes mellitus with use of Zyprexa and other second-generation antipsychotics in their labeling. Patients receiving Zyprexa, especially those with a family history or an established diagnosis of diabetes, should be aware of this adverse reaction and should routinely monitor glucose levels while taking Zyprexa.

In elderly patients with dementia who are treated with a second-generation antipsychotic, including Zyprexa, there is an increased risk of death. The data from clinical studies show a higher risk in elderly patients with dementia treated with second-generation antipsychotics than with placebo-treated patients (i.e., patients taking a sugar pill). It is unclear why these medications have a higher risk in this group. Even though the risk is very low, the FDA requires Zyprexa to have in its package insert a warning about the associated risk in this population of taking an atypical antipsychotic medication.

Use in Pregnancy and Breastfeeding: Pregnancy Category C

Zyprexa has not been tested in women to determine its safety in pregnancy. The effects of the medication on the developing fetus in pregnant women are unknown. In animal studies, there may be effects on the development of the fetus, but there are not adequate and well-controlled studies in humans. Animal studies are not always predictive of effects in humans. Therefore, the use of Zyprexa in pregnant woman must always be weighed against the potential risks. Women who are pregnant or may become pregnant should discuss this with their physician. Some women may experience a recurrence of their psychosis when they stop Zyprexa. In these circumstances, the physician may discuss the need to restart the medication or seek an alternative medication or treatment.

Nursing mothers should not take Zyprexa, because small amounts will pass into breast milk and be ingested by the baby. If stopping the antipsychotic is not an alternative, breastfeeding should not be started or should be discontinued.

Possible Drug Interactions

Some medications when taken with Zyprexa may result in drug interactions that alter their levels, which may produce undesired reactions. The possible drug interactions with Zyprexa are summarized in the table on the next page.

Patients taking Zyprexa should not consume alcohol because the combination may impair thinking, judgment, and coordination.

Luvox (fluvoxamine)	Luvox may decrease the metabolism of Zyprexa, thus increasing blood levels of Zyprexa and the likelihood of unwanted side effects.
Tegretol (carbamazepine)	Tegretol may decrease the blood levels of Zyprexa, reducing its effectiveness in treating the symptoms of the illness.

Overdose

There are few data on acute overdose with Zyprexa, but fatalities in association with overdose of Zyprexa alone have been reported. Common signs of Zyprexa overdose are agitation, rapid heart rate, EPS, and reduced level of consciousness ranging from sedation to coma. Among the serious and sometimes fatal cases from acute overdose with Zyprexa, seizures, cardiac arrhythmias, respiratory depression, and cardiopulmonary arrest were reported.

Any suspected overdose should be treated as an emergency. The person should be taken to the emergency room for observation and treatment. The prescription bottle of medication (and any other medication suspected in the overdose) should be brought as well, because the information on the prescription label can be helpful to the treating physician in determining the number of pills ingested.

Special Considerations

- Do not discontinue Zyprexa without consulting your physician.
- If you miss a dose, take it as soon as possible. If it is close to the next scheduled dose, skip the missed dose and continue on your regular dosing schedule. Do not take double doses.
- Zyprexa may be taken with or without food.
- Zyprexa may cause sedation and drowsiness, especially during initiation of therapy, and may impair your alertness. Use caution when driving or performing tasks that require alertness.
- Store the medication in its originally labeled, light-resistant container, away from heat and moisture. Heat and moisture may precipitate breakdown of your medication, and the medication may lose its therapeutic effects.
- Keep your medication out of reach of children.

If you have any questions about your medication, consult your physician or pharmacist.

Notes

From Chew RH, Hales RE, Yudofsky SC: *What Your Patients Need to Know About Psychiatric Medications*, Second Edition. Washington, DC, American Psychiatric Publishing, 2009

Treatment of Attention-Deficit/Hyperactivity Disorder in Adults

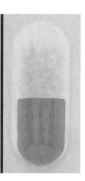

Stimulants

Adderall and Adderall XR (amphetamine mixture)

Concerta (methylphenidate, extended release)

Daytrana (methylphenidate topical patch)

DextroStat and Dexedrine Spansules (dextroamphetamine)

Focalin and Focalin XR (dexmethylphenidate, immediate and extended release)

Metadate ER and Metadate CD (methylphenidate, extended release)

Ritalin, Ritalin-SR, and Ritalin LA (methylphenidate, immediate and extended release)

Vyvanse (lisdexamfetamine)

Nonstimulants

Catapres (clonidine)

Strattera (atomoxetine)

Tenex (guanfacine)

Attention-deficit/hyperactivity disorder (ADHD) is a common childhood or adolescent psychiatric diagnosis. Although most children outgrow symptoms of hyperactivity, many continue to have residual attention problems in their teenage years, and a significant percentage (about 25%) of childhood ADHD persists into adulthood. It is estimated that 1%–2% of men and women in United States, some 5 million adults, have ADHD. These individuals have problems sustaining attention, sitting still, and controlling their impulses. The prevalence of adulthood ADHD is almost equal among men and women, whereas in childhood ADHD the diagnosis is higher in boys than girls.

Adults with ADHD generally do not have the extent of hyperactivity seen in the childhood disorder, and the disorder in adults is diagnosed as **attention-deficit disorder** (ADD). Their principal difficulty is distractibility; they have a hard time sustaining attention and maintaining their focus. Impulse control is also lacking, and often these individuals act or speak without thinking. They may rush into misguided ventures or business deals without much forethought. Others may view their behavior and judgment as immature and impulsive. Untreated, adults with ADD are prone to abuse alcohol and drugs, get into accidents or trouble with the law, or develop other mental health disorders; sadly, they are also prone to commit suicide.

Studies show that ADHD runs in families, particularly in male relatives of ADHD children, but it is unclear exactly how the disorder is transmitted. There is no evidence that ADHD is caused by a single, identifiable genetic defect. Genetic transmission of ADHD will probably be explained by a group of genes that controls or modifies the inheritance of the disorder.

There are nongenetic explanations of ADHD as well. Recognized causes of ADHD also include brain damage, low birth weight, and prenatal factors such as inadequate maternal nutrition and alcohol and substance abuse. Brain damage may result from obstetrical complications, viral infections, and exposure to toxins. Low birth weight is correlated with ADHD, with or without birth complications. In some cases, low birth weight may be attributed to lack of prenatal care (e.g., malnutrition) and substance abuse. Fetal exposure to toxic substances, including alcohol and lead, may predispose the child to ADHD and cognitive deficits. For example, **fetal alcohol syndrome** includes hyperactivity, attention deficit, and impulsivity as well as other physical problems.

The symptoms of ADHD may be explained by aberrations of neurotransmitter systems in areas of the brain that mediate attention. ADHD is associated with the brain cells (neurons) that require **dopamine** and **norepinephrine** as their neurotransmitters (i.e., brain chemicals that facilitate transmission of impulses between neurons). Low levels of these neurotransmitters in specific and interrelated areas of the brain that regulate attention, regardless of the cause, may result in the symptoms of attention-deficit and hyperactivity. A depletion of dopamine may result in difficulties in sustaining attention, and depletion of norepinephrine may be responsible for hyperactivity. The most compelling evidence to support this hypothesis is that treatments prescribed for ADHD—medications such as dextroamphetamine and methylphenidate (e.g., Ritalin)—work by enhancing the levels of dopamine and norepinephrine in the brain.

The principal medications used in treatment of ADHD are stimulants. It may seem paradoxical that stimulants, which excite the central nervous system, are effective in blunting the symptoms of hyperactivity, inattention, and impulsivity in ADHD. The explanation may be that ADHD is a disorder of deficit caused by deficient levels of two important neurotransmitters, dopamine and norepinephrine, in the brain. Increasing the levels of these neurotransmitters with stimulants may help reduce and control the symptoms of the disorder.

Because an array of stimulants is available to treat ADHD, physicians should explain the available treatment options to their patients. Essentially there are two primary stimulants used in treating ADHD: amphetamine and methylphenidate. There are several ways to change these stimulants to enhance or alter their effects. One way is to add another chemical group to the parent molecule to enhance its effect. For example, adding another chemical group to amphetamine—the parent molecule—will change it to methamphetamine (Desoxyn) and increase its potency. Another way is to isolate the more active **isomer** of the molecule. Isomers are mirror images of the drug that are not superimposable on top of each other. Our right and left hands, for example, are mirror images that are not superimposable. Dextroamphetamine is an isomer of amphetamine, and dexmethylphenidate (Focalin) is an isomer of methylphenidate. A third way is by changing the formulation of the stimulant to alter its duration of action. For example, methylphenidate comes in several formulations, including an immediate-release tablet (Ritalin), an extended-release tablet (Ritalin-SR), and a long-acting capsule (Ritalin-LA).

Amphetamine and methylphenidate stimulants have a high potential for abuse. Chronic abuse can lead to dependence. However, if they are properly prescribed by a physician and closely monitored, the risk of dependence is minimized. For this reason, prescribing of these stimulants is tightly controlled by state and federal regulations. They are classified as Schedule II controlled substances—the most closely regulated group of controlled medications.

Other medications used in the treatment of ADHD are the so-called nonstimulants. This mixed group of medications is unlike the stimulants, and there is not the concern of abuse and dependence with these medications that there is with amphetamines and methylphenidate. The only nonstimulant approved by the U.S. Food and Drug Administration (FDA) for the treatment of ADHD is Strattera (atomoxetine). The other nonstimulants used by physicians for treatment of ADHD include Tenex (guanfacine), Catapres (clonidine), and antidepressants such as Wellbutrin (bupropion) and Effexor (venlafaxine). These medications are not approved by the FDA for treatment of ADHD, and they are prescribed "off-label." The use of a medication for its approved indications is called its *labeled use*. In clinical practice, however, physicians often prescribe medications for *unlabeled* ("off-label") uses when published clinical studies, case reports, or their own clinical experiences support the efficacy and safety of those treatments. The nonstimulants are not as commonly used as the amphetamines and methylphenidate for ADHD. Except for Strattera, the nonstimulants have not been widely studied for treatment of ADHD, and evidence of their effectiveness is, at best, based on limited clinical trials but mostly clinical experience.

For more information on a particular medication, refer to the handout on that medication.

Stimulants and Nonstimulants for ADHD

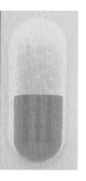

Stimulants
Adderall and Adderall XR (amphetamine mixtures)
Concerta (methylphenidate, extended release)
Daytrana (methylphenidate topical patch)
Dexedrine and Dexedrine Spansules (dextroamphetamine)
Focalin and Focalin XR (dexmethylphenidate,
immediate and extended release)
Metadate ER and and Metadate CD
(methylphenidate, extended release)
Ritalin, Ritalin-SR, and Ritalin LA (methylphenidate,
immediate and extended release)
Vyvanse (lisdexamfetamine)

Nonstimulants
Catapres (clonidine)
Strattera (atomoxetine)
Tenex (guanfacine)

The psychostimulants, more simply known as stimulants, are used primarily in treating attention-deficit/hyperactivity disorder (ADHD) and narcolepsy, a condition characterized by daytime somnolence in which the patient periodically falls into a deep sleep during the day. Narcolepsy is a disorder of the sleep–wake control mechanisms within the brain that interferes with both daytime wakefulness and nighttime sleep.

Other medications used in the treatment of ADHD are the so-called nonstimulants. This mixed group of medications is unlike the stimulants, and there is not the concern of abuse and dependence with these medications as with amphetamines and methylphenidate. The only nonstimulant approved by the U.S. Food and Drug Administration (FDA) for treatment of ADHD is Strattera (atomoxetine). The other nonstimulants, including Tenex (guanfacine), Catapres (clonidine), and Wellbutrin (bupropion), are not approved by the FDA for treatment of ADHD, and they are prescribed "off-label." The use of a medication for its approved indications is called its *labeled use*. In clinical practice, however, physicians often prescribe medications for *unlabeled* (off-label) uses when published clinical studies, case reports, or their own clinical experiences support the efficacy and safety of those treatments.

For those who do not like to take pills, methylphenidate can be introduced into circulation through the skin by a topical patch. The methylphenidate topical patch, called Daytrana, can be worn for up to 9 hours to deliver a controlled rate of methylphenidate through the skin. After absorption of the medication into circulation, there is no difference in the action of the medication than had it been taken orally. For more information on Daytrana, refer to the handout for this medication.

Vyvanse (lisdexamfetamine) is a unique extended-release formulation of dextroamphetamine, or *d*-amphetamine. The extended release is accomplished through modification of the active molecule dextroamphetamine to form lisdexamfetamine, which is inactive. After Vyvanse is taken, it is rapidly absorbed and distributed to the liver, where it is converted back to the active stimulant, *d*-amphetamine. The time to absorb and convert lisdexamfetamine to dextroamphetamine essentially makes Vyvanse an extended-release formulation of *d*-amphetamine. For more information on Vyvanse, refer to the handout for this medication.

In numerous clinical studies and decades of clinical experience, the stimulants have clearly demonstrated improvement of outcome for children with ADHD. They increase children's ability to concentrate, extend their attention span, and decrease hyperactivity. Adults with ADHD also benefit from therapy with stimulants. Stimulants help adults concentrate and remain focused on their tasks, increase their attention span, and decrease impulsivity and hyperactivity.

The nonstimulants are not as commonly used as the amphetamines and methylphenidate for ADHD. Except for Strattera, the nonstimulants have not been widely studied for treatment of ADHD, and evidence of their effectiveness is, at best, based on limited clinical trials but mostly clinical experience.

Dosing Information

Dosing of stimulants in adults is based on clinical presentation and individualized to the patient's response and reported side effects. In children, dosing is also based on age and weight. The other consideration in dosing is selection of a formulation with the duration of action tailored to the needs of the patient. For example, Ritalin-SR, a long-acting methylphenidate, produces sustained release of medication for about 8 hours, whereas Concerta, another methylphenidate, provides immediate and delayed-release action for about 12 hours of action.

Ritalin is the most widely prescribed stimulant for ADHD, but Dexedrine (dextroamphetamine) is equally effective. Immediate-release Ritalin is short acting and begins to work in 30–60 minutes after administration, with duration of 2–5 hours. The advantage is that it works quickly, but the duration of action is short and requires dosing two or three times a day. Similarly, Dexedrine is a short-acting stimulant with peak effects 1–2 hours after administration, and the effects last 2–5 hours.

Because multiple dosing may be difficult for patients, especially school-age children, Ritalin and Dexedrine come in long-acting preparations that provide 6–8 hours of benefit from a single morning dose. The long-acting preparations of Ritalin and Dexedrine provide flexible dosing options, but the formulations of stimulants are made confusing by their different designations: for Ritalin, "SR" denotes *sustained-release* and "LA" denotes *long-acting*; for Metadate, "ER" denotes *extended-release* and "CD" denotes *controlled-delivery*; for Adderall, "XR" denotes *extended-release*; and for Dexedrine, the "Spansule" is a trademark for a *long-acting* capsule form.

Adderall is mixture of dextroamphetamine and amphetamine, and Adderall XR is the extended-release preparation of the mixture. Adderall provides about 5 hours of effect, whereas Adderall XR extends the duration to 8–10 hours.

With recent advances in drug delivery systems, manufacturers have incorporated new technology in the formulation of stimulants to provide a bimodal action from a single tablet or capsule. This bimodal delivery system can release 20%–50% of the medication immediately and the remainder in the 10–12 hours following. For example, Concerta (methylphenidate) uses a system that provides immediate and extended delivery of medication. It releases about 22% of the medication within 1–2 hours and the remainder of the drug over 10–12 hours. Similarly, Adderall XR, Metadate CD, and Ritalin LA use this bimodal delivery system. The advantage of this preparation is that it provides immediate effect from a single morning dose and extended action into the evening, but by bedtime the effects of the medication wear off without affecting sleep. The different preparations of amphetamine and methylphenidate are summarized in the table on the next two pages.

Brand name	Generic name	Available strengths	Dosing frequency (approximate duration of action)
		STIMULANTS	
Amphetamines			
Short-acting			
DextroStat	Dextroamphetamine (immediate release)	5, 10 mg tablets	Two to three times a day (4–6 hours)
Liquadd	Dextroamphetamine oral solution	5 mg/5 mL	
Adderall	Amphetamine mixture (immediate release)	5, 7.5, 10, 12.5, 15, 20, 30 mg tablets	Two times a day (4–6 hours)
Long-acting			
Dexedrine Spansules	Dextroamphetamine (sustained release)	5, 10, 15 mg capsules	Once a day in the morning (6–8 hours)
Adderall XR	Amphetamine mixture (extended release)	5, 10, 15, 20, 25, 30 mg capsules	Once a day in the morning (8–10 hours)
Vyvanse	Lisdexamfetamine	20, 30, 40, 50, 60, 70 mg capsules	Once a day in the morning (up to 12 hours)
Methylphenidates			
Short-acting			
Ritalin	Methylphenidate	5, 10, 20 mg tablets	Two to three times a day (2–5 hours)
Methylin	Methylphenidate	2.5, 5, 10 mg chewable tablets	Two to three times a day (3–5 hours)
Methylin Oral Solution	Methylphenidate	5 mg/5 mL, 10 mg/5 mL	Two to three times a day (3–5 hours)
Intermediate-acting			
Ritalin-SR	Methylphenidate (sustained release)	20 mg tablet	Once a day (6–8 hours)
Methylin ER	Methylphenidate (extended release)	10, 20 mg tablets	One to two times a day (6–8 hours)
Metadate ER	Methylphenidate (extended release)	10, 20 mg tablets	One to two times a day (6–8 hours)
Long-acting			
Ritalin LA	Methylphenidate (extended release)	10, 20, 30, 40 mg capsules	Once a day in the morning (8–10 hours)
Metadate CD	Methylphenidate (extended release)	10, 20, 30, 40, 50, 60 mg capsules	Once a day in the morning (8–10 hours)

321

Brand name	Generic name	Available strengths	Dosing frequency (approximate duration of action)
STIMULANTS *(continued)*			
Methylphenidates *(continued)*			
Long-acting (continued)			
Concerta	Methylphenidate (extended release)	18, 27, 36, 54 mg tablets	Once a day in the morning (8–12 hours)
Daytrana	Methylphenidate (topical patch)	10, 15, 20, 30 mg patch	Once a day in the morning (9 hours/day, off 15 hours)
Dexmethylphenidate			
Focalin	Dexmethylphenidate (immediate action)	2.5, 5, 10 mg tablets	Two times a day (2–5 hours)
Focalin XR	Dexmethylphenidate (delayed action)	5, 10, 15, 20 mg capsules	Once a day (5–8 hours)
NONSTIMULANTS			
Catapres	Clonidine*	0.1, 0.2, 0.3 mg tablets	Once a day
Tenex	Guanfacine*	1, 2 mg tablets	Once a day
Strattera	Atomoxetine	10, 18, 25, 40, 60, 80, 100 mg capsules	Once a day in the morning (24 hours)

*Off-label use for attention-deficit/hyperactivity disorder (ADHD).

Common Side Effects

The common side effects associated with stimulants are rapid heart rate, palpitations, restlessness, insomnia, dry mouth, constipation, nausea, diarrhea, loss of appetite, weight loss, and elevation of blood pressure. (See individual handouts for common side effects of nonstimulants.)

Adverse Reactions and Precautions

Stimulants, particularly the amphetamines, have a high potential for abuse. Individuals with a history of alcohol and substance abuse may be at risk for abusing stimulants. Individuals who abuse stimulants develop tolerance and psychological dependence that may result in addiction. With long-term abuse of stimulants and the resulting sleepless nights, the individual may develop psychotic symptoms.

Stimulants may increase blood pressure. Individuals with a history of high blood pressure or heart disease should be cautious about taking stimulants because these agents can exacerbate these conditions. Uncontrolled high blood pressure can have serious consequences, including stroke and heart attacks. Patients taking stimulants should routinely check their blood pressure.

Individuals with a history of seizure disorder should be cautious while taking stimulants because these agents can lower the seizure threshold.

In children and adolescents who are still in their growth period, stimulants can suppress linear growth. Physicians commonly interrupt treatment, if possible, on weekends and holidays, when children are not in school, for growth catch-up. Children and adolescents taking stimulants require close monitoring for growth suppression and periodic measuring of their height. This effect is not a concern in the adult population.

Stimulants may make tics worse in individuals with a tic disorder (i.e., twitching of a muscle group, especially in the face).

Stimulants should be avoided, or used with caution, by patients with a diagnosis of schizophrenia or bipolar disorder. Stimulants are frequently abused in this population, and high doses of stimulants may trigger psychosis and mania.

Use in Pregnancy and Breastfeeding: Pregnancy Category C

The stimulants have not been tested in women to determine their safety in pregnancy. The effects of these medications on the developing fetus in pregnant women are unknown. Women who are pregnant or may become pregnant should discuss this with their physician.

Nursing mothers should not take any stimulant, because small amounts will pass into breast milk and be ingested by the baby. If stopping the stimulant is not an alternative, breastfeeding should not be started or should be discontinued.

Possible Drug Interactions

Stimulants should not be taken in combination with a group of antidepressants known as **monoamine oxidase inhibitors** (MAOIs). The combination may precipitate increases in blood pressure. This and other significant drug interactions reported with stimulants are summarized in the table below.

Monoamine oxidase inhibitors (MAOIs) (e.g., Parnate, Emsam, Nardil, Marplan)	MAOIs should not be taken with methylphenidates (e.g., Concerta, Ritalin, Focalin), dextroamphetamines (e.g., DextroStat, Adderall, Adderall XR), and Strattera. The combination may precipitate dangerous elevation of blood pressure.
Weight-loss medications (e.g., Meridia)	Weight-loss medications, prescription and nonprescription, should not be taken with dextroamphetamines/amphetamines or methylphenidates. The combination may increase blood pressure or cause irritability, insomnia, and other adverse reactions from excessive stimulation.
Coumadin (warfarin)	Methylphenidate may increase the anticoagulant action of Coumadin.
Prozac (fluoxetine), Paxil (paroxetine), Tagamet (cimetidine), Wellbutrin (bupropion), and Norvir (ritonavir)	These medications may inhibit the metabolism of Strattera and should be monitored closely when used together.

Overdose

The severity of acute amphetamine and methylphenidate overdose depends on the amount ingested. The individual may experience a progression of the following symptoms from an acute overdose: restlessness, agitation, irritability, insomnia, hyperactivity, confusion, elevated blood pressure, rapid heart rate, delirium, hallucinations, irregular heartbeat, convulsions, coma, circulatory collapse, and death.

Any suspected overdose should be treated as an emergency. The person should be taken to the emergency room for observation and treatment. The prescription bottle of medication (and any other medication suspected in the overdose) should be brought as well, because the information on the prescription label can be helpful to the treating physician in determining the number of pills ingested.

Special Considerations

- Dexedrine and Ritalin should be taken early in the morning, especially the sustained-release preparations, so the action of the medication does not extend into bedtime hours and interfere with sleep.
- Do not chew or crush the sustained-release or long-acting preparations; swallow the tablet or capsule whole.
- Do not take more than instructed by your physician.
- If the stimulant causes pronounced nervousness, restlessness, insomnia, loss of appetite, or weight loss, notify your physician.
- If you miss a dose, take it as soon as possible. If it is close to the next scheduled dose, skip the missed dose and continue on your regular dosing schedule. Do not take double doses.
- Store the medication in its originally labeled, light-resistant container, away from heat and moisture. Heat and moisture may precipitate breakdown of your medication, and the medication may lose its therapeutic effects.
- Keep your medications out of reach of children.

If you have any questions about your medication, consult your physician or pharmacist.

Notes

_____

_____

_____

_____

Adderall and Adderall XR (amphetamine mixture)

Generic name: Amphetamine mixture
Available strengths: 5 mg, 7.5 mg, 10 mg, 12.5 mg, 15 mg, 20 mg,
   30 mg immediate-release tablets; 5 mg, 10 mg, 15 mg, 20 mg,
   25 mg, 30 mg extended-release capsules (Adderall XR)
Available in generic: Yes, but only Adderall immediate-release
Drug class: Stimulant

General Information

Adderall (dextroamphetamine and amphetamine mixture) and **Adderall XR (extended release)** are psychostimulants, better known as stimulants. Adderall is used primarily in treating attention-deficit/hyperactivity disorder (ADHD) and narcolepsy, a condition characterized by daytime somnolence in which the patient periodically falls into a deep sleep during the day. Narcolepsy is a disorder of the sleep–wake control mechanisms within the brain that interferes with both daytime wakefulness and nighttime sleep.

The use of a medication for its approved indications is called its *labeled use*. In clinical practice, however, physicians often prescribe medications for *unlabeled* ("off-label") uses when published clinical studies, case reports, or their own clinical experiences support the efficacy and safety of those treatments. Adderall is often used to augment antidepressants in treating refractory depression. For patients with chronic treatment-resistant depression, for example, Adderall in combination with antidepressants can provide symptomatic relief and improvement beyond that experienced with antidepressants alone.

In numerous clinical studies and substantial clinical experience, Adderall has clearly demonstrated improvement in outcome for children with ADHD. Adderall increases the child's ability to concentrate, extends attention span, and decreases hyperactivity. Adults with ADHD also benefit from therapy with Adderall. Adderall helps them concentrate and remain focused on their tasks, increases their attention span, and decreases impulsivity and hyperactivity.

Adderall and Adderall XR are mixtures of amphetamine and dextroamphetamine salts in different combinations. For example, a 20 mg tablet of Adderall contains 5 mg of dextroamphetamine sulfate, 5 mg of dextroamphetamine saccharate, 5 mg of amphetamine sulfate, and 5 mg of amphetamine aspartate. The given strength of an Adderall tablet or capsule is the sum of all the stimulants in the mixture. Adderall has a duration of action of approximately 5 hours, whereas Adderall XR lasts 8–10 hours.

Because Adderall and Adderall XR are stimulants, they are closely regulated controlled substances. The physician must write a new prescription each time they are dispensed, and a prescription cannot be refilled.

325

Dosing Information

For adults, the recommended starting dosage of Adderall is 5 mg twice a day. The dosage is adjusted based on the individual's response. The usual therapeutic dosage may range from 10 mg/day to 40 mg/day, administered two times a day. The maximum dosage should not exceed 60 mg/day.

Adderall may be converted to once-daily dosing with Adderall XR using an equivalent dosage of the extended-release form. However, the maximum recommended dosage is 30 mg/day with Adderall XR. The capsules should be swallowed whole and not chewed or crushed. The capsules may be opened and sprinkled in applesauce and swallowed without chewing.

Common Side Effects

The common side effects associated with taking Adderall are rapid heart rate, palpitations, nervousness, restlessness, insomnia, dry mouth, constipation, nausea, diarrhea, loss of appetite, weight loss, and elevation of blood pressure.

Adverse Reactions and Precautions

Adderall has a high potential for abuse. Individuals with a history of alcohol and substance abuse may be at risk for abusing stimulants. Individuals who abuse Adderall develop tolerance and psychological dependence that may result in addiction. With long-term abuse of Adderall and the resulting sleepless nights, the individual may develop psychotic symptoms.

Adderall may increase blood pressure. Individuals with a history of high blood pressure or heart disease should be cautious about taking Adderall because it can exacerbate these conditions. Uncontrolled high blood pressure can have serious consequences, including stroke and heart attack. Patients taking Adderall should routinely check their blood pressure.

Individuals with a history of seizure disorder should be cautious while taking Adderall, because it can lower the seizure threshold and increase susceptibility for seizures.

In children and adolescents who are still in their growth period, Adderall can suppress linear growth. Physicians commonly interrupt treatment on weekends and holidays when children are not in school, for growth catch-up. Children and adolescents taking Adderall require close monitoring for growth suppression and periodic measuring of their height. This effect is not a concern in the adult population.

Adderall may make tics worse in individuals with a tic disorder (i.e., twitching of a muscle group, especially in the face).

Adderall should be avoided, or used with caution, by patients with a diagnosis of schizophrenia or bipolar disorder. Stimulants are frequently abused in this population, and high doses of Adderall may trigger psychosis and mania.

Use in Pregnancy and Breastfeeding: Pregnancy Category C

Adderall has not been tested in women to determine its safety in pregnancy. The effects of the medication on the developing fetus in pregnant women are unknown. Women who are pregnant or may become pregnant should discuss this with their physician.

Nursing mothers should not take any stimulant, because small amounts will pass into breast milk and be ingested by the baby. If stopping the stimulant is not an alternative, breastfeeding should not be started or should be discontinued.

Possible Drug Interactions

Adderall should not be taken in combination with a group of antidepressants known as **monoamine oxidase inhibitors** (MAOIs). The combination may precipitate increases in blood pressure. This and other significant drug interactions reported with Adderall are summarized in the table below.

Monoamine oxidase inhibitors (MAOIs) (e.g., Parnate, Emsam, Nardil, Marplan)	MAOIs should not be taken with methylphenidates (e.g., Concerta, Ritalin, Focalin), dextroamphetamines (e.g., DextroStat, Adderall, Adderall XR), or Strattera. The combination may precipitate dangerous elevation of blood pressure.
Weight-loss medications (e.g., Meridia)	Weight-loss medications, prescription and nonprescription, should not be taken with dextroamphetamines/amphetamines or methylphenidates. The combination may increase blood pressure or cause irritability, insomnia, and other adverse reactions from excessive stimulation.

Overdose

The severity of Adderall overdose depends on the amount ingested. The individual may experience a progression of the following symptoms from an acute overdose: restlessness, agitation, irritability, insomnia, hyperactivity, confusion, elevated blood pressure, rapid heart rate, delirium, hallucinations, irregular heartbeat, convulsions, coma, circulatory collapse, and death.

Any suspected overdose should be treated as an emergency. The person should be taken to the emergency room for observation and treatment. The prescription bottle of medication (and any other medication suspected in the overdose) should be brought as well, because the information on the prescription label can be helpful to the treating physician in determining the number of pills ingested.

Special Considerations

- To avoid insomnia, the last daily dose of Adderall should not be taken late in the evening. Adderall XR should be taken only once a day in the morning.
- Adderall may be taken with or without food.
- Do not take more than instructed by your physician.
- If Adderall causes pronounced nervousness, restlessness, insomnia, loss of appetite, or weight loss, notify your physician.
- If you miss a dose, take it as soon as possible. If it is close to the next scheduled dose, skip the missed dose and continue on your regular dosing schedule. Do not take double doses. If you missed your dose of Adderall XR in the morning and it is late in the evening, skip the dose and continue on your regular dosing schedule the next morning.
- Do not chew or crush Adderall tablets or Adderall XR capsules; swallow them whole. Take with a full glass of water to help swallow the medication.

- Store the medication in its originally labeled, light-resistant container, away from heat and moisture. Heat and moisture may precipitate breakdown of your medication, and the medication may lose its therapeutic effects.
- Keep your medication out of reach of children.

If you have any questions about your medication, consult your physician or pharmacist.

Notes

_____

_____

_____

_____

_____

_____

_____

_____

_____

_____

From Chew RH, Hales RE, Yudofsky SC: *What Your Patients Need to Know About Psychiatric Medications*, Second Edition. Washington, DC, American Psychiatric Publishing, 2009

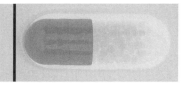

Concerta (methylphenidate, extended release)

Generic name: Methylphenidate, extended release
Available strengths: 18 mg, 27 mg, 36 mg, 54 mg tablets
Available in generic: No
Drug class: Stimulant

General Information

Concerta (methylphenidate, controlled release) is a psychostimulant, better known as a stimulant. Concerta is used primarily in treating attention-deficit/hyperactivity disorder (ADHD) and narcolepsy, a condition characterized by daytime somnolence in which the patient periodically falls into a deep sleep during the day. Narcolepsy is a disorder of the sleep–wake control mechanisms within the brain that interferes with both daytime wakefulness and nighttime sleep.

The use of a medication for its approved indications is called its *labeled use*. In clinical practice, however, physicians often prescribe medications for *unlabeled* ("off-label") uses when published clinical studies, case reports, or their own clinical experiences support the efficacy and safety of those treatments. Concerta is often used to augment antidepressants in treating refractory depression. For patients with chronic treatment-resistant depression, for example, Concerta in combination with antidepressants can provide symptomatic relief and improvement beyond that experienced with antidepressants alone.

In numerous clinical studies and substantial clinical experience, Concerta has clearly demonstrated improvement in outcome for children with ADHD. Concerta increases the child's ability to concentrate, extends attention span, and decreases hyperactivity. Adults with ADHD also benefit from therapy with Concerta. Concerta helps them concentrate and remain focused on their tasks, increases their attention span, and decreases impulsivity and hyperactivity.

Concerta tablets deliver methylphenidate in two phases using advanced technology. In the first phase, the stimulant is released within 1–2 hours from the outer coat of the tablet to provide rapid onset of action; in the second phase, the remainder is released at a controlled rate over 10–12 hours. The tablet is composed of a core, containing the stimulant, which is surrounded by a membrane that controls the time-released system. The core is enveloped by an outer coat containing a layer of methylphenidate. When the Concerta tablet is ingested, the outer coat dissolves within 1–2 hours, providing the initial dose of methylphenidate. During gastrointestinal passage of the tablet, the remainder of the stimulant is gradually released from the core of the tablet. The empty tablet shell is expelled in the stool.

Because Concerta is a stimulant, it is a closely regulated controlled substance. The physician must write a new prescription each time it is dispensed, and a prescription cannot be refilled.

Dosing Information

For adults, the usual starting dosage of immediate-release methylphenidate is 5 mg twice a day, and the dosage is adjusted based on the individual's response. The average dosage is 20–30 mg/day, administered two or three times daily. The maximum dosage should not exceed 60 mg/day. Concerta may be used in place of immediate-release methylphenidate, Ritalin-SR, or Metadate ER by replacing the total daily dosage with the nearest equivalent dose of Concerta. For example, 5 mg of methylphenidate twice daily (10 mg/day) or three times a day (15 mg/day) could be replaced with 18 mg of Concerta once a day. In addition, 20 mg/day of Ritalin-SR or Metadate ER could be converted to 18 mg of Concerta once a day.

Individuals new to methylphenidate may initially take 18 mg of Concerta once a day in the morning. The dosage may be adjusted at weekly intervals to the next higher strength, depending on response, up to a maximum dosage of 54 mg/day.

Concerta tablets should be swallowed whole and never chewed or crushed. Chewing or crushing the tablets destroys the controlled-release system. Concerta should be taken early in the morning with or without food. If taken late in the day, the stimulant effect can be prolonged into the night and interfere with sleep.

Common Side Effects

The common side effects associated with taking Concerta are rapid heart rate, palpitations, nervousness, restlessness, insomnia, dry mouth, constipation, nausea, diarrhea, loss of appetite, weight loss, and elevation of blood pressure.

Adverse Reactions and Precautions

Concerta has a high potential for abuse. Individuals with a history of alcohol and substance abuse may be at risk for abusing stimulants. Individuals who abuse Concerta develop tolerance and psychological dependence that may result in addiction. With long-term abuse of Concerta and the resulting sleepless nights, the individual may develop psychotic symptoms.

Concerta may increase blood pressure. Individuals with a history of high blood pressure or heart disease should be cautious about taking Concerta because it can exacerbate these conditions. Uncontrolled high blood pressure can have serious consequences, including stroke and heart attack. Patients taking Concerta should routinely check their blood pressure.

Individuals with a history of seizure disorder should be cautious while taking Concerta, because it can lower the seizure threshold and increase susceptibility for seizures.

In children and adolescents who are still in their growth period, Concerta can suppress linear growth. Physicians commonly interrupt treatment on weekends and holidays when children are not in school, for growth catch-up. Children and adolescents taking Concerta require close monitoring for growth suppression and periodic measuring of their height. This effect is not a concern in the adult population.

Concerta may make tics worse in individuals with a tic disorder (i.e., twitching of a muscle group, especially in the face).

Concerta should be avoided, or used with caution, by patients with a diagnosis of schizophrenia or bipolar disorder. Stimulants are frequently abused in this population, and high doses of Concerta may trigger psychosis and mania.

Use in Pregnancy and Breastfeeding: Pregnancy Category C

Concerta has not been tested in women to determine its safety in pregnancy. The effects of the medication on the developing fetus in pregnant women are unknown. Women who are pregnant or may become pregnant should discuss this with their physician.

Nursing mothers should not take any stimulant, because small amounts will pass into breast milk and be ingested by the baby. If stopping the stimulant is not an alternative, breastfeeding should not be started or should be discontinued.

Possible Drug Interactions

Concerta should not be taken in combination with a group of antidepressants known as **monoamine oxidase inhibitors** (MAOIs). The combination may precipitate increases in blood pressure. This and other significant drug interactions reported with Concerta are summarized in the table below.

Monoamine oxidase inhibitors (MAOIs) (e.g., Parnate, Emsam, Nardil, Marplan)	MAOIs should not be taken with methylphenidates or dexmethylphenidate (e.g., Concerta, Ritalin, Focalin). The combination may precipitate dangerous elevation of blood pressure.
Weight-loss medications (e.g., Meridia)	Weight-loss medications, prescription and nonprescription, should not be taken with methylphenidates or dexmethylphenidate. The combination may increase blood pressure or cause irritability, insomnia, and other adverse reactions from excessive stimulation.
Coumadin (warfarin)	Methylphenidate and dexmethylphenidate may increase the anticoagulant action of Coumadin.

Overdose

The severity of Concerta overdose depends on the amount ingested. The individual may experience a progression of the following symptoms from an acute overdose: restlessness, agitation, irritability, insomnia, hyperactivity, confusion, elevated blood pressure, rapid heart rate, delirium, hallucinations, irregular heart beat, convulsions, coma, circulatory collapse, and death.

Any suspected overdose should be treated as an emergency. The person should be taken to the emergency room for observation and treatment. The prescription bottle of medication (and any other medication suspected in the overdose) should be brought as well, because the information on the prescription label can be helpful to the treating physician in determining the number of pills ingested.

Special Considerations

- To avoid insomnia, the daily dose of Concerta should be taken early in the morning and not late in the day.
- Concerta may be taken with food to avoid stomach upset.
- Do not take more than instructed by your physician.
- If Concerta causes pronounced nervousness, restlessness, insomnia, loss of appetite, or weight loss, notify your physician.
- If you miss a dose, take it as soon as possible. If it is late in the afternoon or evening, skip the missed dose and continue on your regular dosing schedule the next morning. Do not take double doses.
- Do not chew or crush Concerta tablets; swallow them whole. Take with a full glass of water to help swallow the medication.
- Do not be alarmed by the empty tablet shell in your stool.
- Store the medication in its originally labeled, light-resistant container, away from heat and moisture. Heat and moisture may precipitate breakdown of your medication, and the medication may lose its therapeutic effects.
- Keep your medication out of reach of children.

If you have any questions about your medication, consult your physician or pharmacist.

Notes

_____

_____

_____

_____

_____

_____

From Chew RH, Hales RE, Yudofsky SC: *What Your Patients Need to Know About Psychiatric Medications*, Second Edition. Washington, DC, American Psychiatric Publishing, 2009

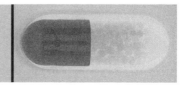

Daytrana (methylphenidate topical patch)

Generic name: methylphenidate topical patch
Available strengths: 10 mg, 15 mg, 20 mg, 30 mg
   per 9 hours
Available in generic: No
Drug class: Stimulant

General Information

Daytrana incorporates the stimulant **methylphenidate** in a transdermal system to deliver the medication at a constant rate for up to 9 hours, but the effects of the stimulant can continue for 3 hours more after the patch is removed. A 10 mg topical patch, for example, delivers approximately 10 mg of methylphenidate over 9 hours and provides duration of action for up to 12 hours. The stimulant is absorbed through the skin into general circulation and delivered to the brain where it exerts its action.

As with oral methylphenidate, Daytrana is approved for use in attention-deficit disorder (ADD), attention-deficit/hyperactivity disorder (ADHD), and narcolepsy, a condition characterized by daytime somnolence, in which the patient periodically falls into a deep sleep during the day.

Dosing Information

The dosing for Daytrana is managed by the patch size (milligrams) and the wear time (typically 9 hours on and 15 hours off the patch, but wear time can be individualized; see below). The recommended starting dosage is a 10 mg patch for the first week, and if response is not maximized, a 15 mg patch the second week, a 20 mg patch the third week, and up to a 30 mg patch by the fourth week. The final dosage and wear time are individualized to the patient's response and needs.

When the patient is being switched from oral methylphenidate to Daytrana, the manfacturer recommends following the titration schedule above because of differences in absorption and duration of action with the patch compared with oral products.

Individualization of the wear time for Daytrana can help manage side effects and optimize therapy. The patch may be removed before 9 hours have elapsed if a shorter duration of action is desired or late-day side effects (e.g., irritation) appear. The patient should consult his or her physician before altering the wear time.

Because Daytrana is a stimulant, it is a closely regulated controlled substance. The physician must write a new prescription each time it is dispensed, and a prescription cannot be refilled.

Common Side Effects

The common side effects associated with taking Daytrana include nausea, vomiting, decreased appetite, weight loss, insomnia, irritability, and tics. These side effects are generally mild to moderate.

Adverse Reactions and Precautions

Stimulants have a high potential for abuse. Individuals with a history of alcohol and substance abuse may be at risk for abusing stimulants, including Daytrana. Individuals who abuse stimulants develop tolerance and psychological dependence that may result in addiction. With long-term abuse of stimulants and the resulting sleepless nights, the individual may develop psychotic symptoms. Daytrana may have less potential for abuse compared with the oral methylphenidates, but it must be prescribed cautiously, as with all stimulants.

Daytrana may increase blood pressure. Individuals with a history of high blood pressure or heart disease should be cautious about taking Daytrana because it can exacerbate these conditions. Uncontrolled high blood pressure can have serious consequences, including stroke and heart attack. Patients taking Daytrana should routinely check their blood pressure.

Individuals with a history of seizure disorder should be cautious while using Daytrana, because it can lower seizure threshold and increase susceptibility for seizures.

In children and adolescents who are still in their growth period, Daytrana can suppress linear growth. Physicians commonly interrupt treatment on weekends and holidays when children are not in school, for growth catch-up. Children and adolescents taking Daytrana require close monitoring for growth suppression and periodic measuring of their height. This effect is not a concern in the adult population.

Daytrana may make tics worse in individuals with a tic disorder (i.e., twitching of a muscle group, especially in the face).

Daytrana should be avoided, or used with caution, by patients with a diagnosis of schizophrenia or bipolar disorder. Stimulants are frequently abused in these populations, and high doses of Daytrana may trigger psychosis and mania.

A skin reaction called **contact sensitization** has been reported in some patients using Daytrana patches. With contact sensitization, the area of the skin is red and inflamed, with some swelling, and there may be small, hard, round bumps (papules) or small vesicles. If the skin reaction does not improve in 1 or 2 days or if it spreads beyond the patch site, a physician should be consulted.

The application site should not be exposed to external heat sources, including heating pad, electric blanket, or heated waterbed, while the patient is wearing the patch. Increasing the temperature around the application site may enhance absorption of methylphenidate and cause adverse reactions.

Use in Pregnancy and Breastfeeding: Pregnancy Category C

Daytrana has not been tested in women to determine its safety in pregnancy. The effects of the medication on the developing fetus in pregnant women are unknown. Women who are pregnant or may become pregnant should discuss this with their physician.

Nursing mothers should not take any stimulant, because small amounts will pass into breast milk and be ingested by the baby. If stopping the stimulant is not an alternative, breastfeeding should not be started or should be discontinued.

Possible Drug Interactions

Daytrana should not be taken in combination with a group of antidepressants known as **monoamine oxidase inhibitors** (MAOIs). The combination may precipitate an increase in blood pressure. This and other significant drug interactions reported with Daytrana are summarized in the following table.

Monoamine oxidase inhibitors (MAOIs) (e.g., Parnate, Emsam, Nardil, Marplan)	MAOIs should not be taken with methylphenidates or dexmethylphenidate (e.g., Concerta, Ritalin, Focalin). The combination may precipitate dangerous elevation of blood pressure.
Weight-loss medications (e.g., Meridia)	Weight-loss medications, prescription and nonprescription, should not be taken with methylphenidates or dexmethylphenidate. The combination may increase blood pressure or cause irritability, insomnia, and other adverse reactions from excessive stimulation.
Coumadin (warfarin)	Methylphenidate and dexmethylphenidate may increase the anticoagulant action of Coumadin.

Overdose

The severity of Daytrana overdose depends on the amount of methylphenidate absorbed through the skin. The individual may experience a progression of the following symptoms from an acute overdose: restlessness, agitation, irritability, insomnia, hyperactivity, confusion, elevated blood pressure, rapid heart rate, delirium, hallucinations, irregular heartbeat, convulsions, coma, circulatory collapse, and death.

In suspected overdose, all patches should be removed immediately. Even after removal of the patches, methylphenidate may continue to be absorbed from the skin into circulation. The person should be brought to the emergency room for evaluation and treatment.

Special Considerations

In each box of Daytrana, instructions are provided for application, disposal, and storage of the topical patches (Daytrana package insert; Shire US, Inc., 01/08). These instructions are summarized below:

Application

- A Daytrana patch should be applied to the hip area 2 hours before the effect of the stimulant is needed.
- Use the patch immediately after opening the pouch and removing the protective liner. If it is not used immediately, do not put it back in the pouch for later use.
- Do not use a patch that has been cut or damaged in any way.
- Apply to clean, dry, non-oily skin. Do not apply to skin that is irritated (e.g., rash) or inflamed. Apply to the hip below the waistline to prevent clothing from rubbing the patch off.

- Press the patch firmly with the palm of the hand for about 30 seconds, ensuring a tight seal around the edges of the patch. Water should not affect adherence if the patch is correctly applied.
- If a patch falls off, a new patch may be applied to a different area of the hip. The combined wear time of both patches, however, should not exceed 9 hours. If a patch falls off, do not use tape or adhesives to hold it on the skin.
- Do not use electric blankets, heating pads or other heat sources, including a heated waterbed, while wearing Daytrana. Heat promotes circulation, which can increase the absorption of methylphenidate and, therefore, the amount getting into the body, and cause serious side effects.

Disposal

- On removal, fold the patch in half with the sticky sides together. Flush the used patch down a toilet or dispose of it in a lidded container right away.
- Dispose of unused Daytrana patches when they are no longer needed in the same manner.
- Wash your hands after handling the patch.

Storage

- Daytrana patches should be stored at room temperature (77°F) for optimal stability. For outings, patches may be kept at temperature range of 59°to 86°F for short periods.
- Do not store patches in the refrigerator or freezer.
- Do not store patches out of their pouches.
- Once the tray is opened, the contents should be used within 2 months.
- Store the medication in its originally labeled, light-resistant container, away from heat and moisture. Heat and moisture may cause breakdown of the medication, and the medication may lose its therapeutic effects.
- Keep your medication out of reach of children.

If you have any questions about your medication, consult your physician or pharmacist.

Notes

_____

_____

_____

_____

_____

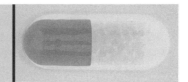

DextroStat and Dexedrine Spansules (dextroamphetamine)

Generic name: Dextroamphetamine
Available strengths: 5 mg, 10 mg immediate-release tablets (DextroStat);
   5 mg, 10 mg, 15 mg sustained-release capsules
   (Dexedrine Spansules)
Available in generic: Yes
Drug class: Stimulant

General Information

DextroStat (immediate-release dextroamphetamine) and **Dexedrine Spansules (dextroamphetamine sustained-release capsules)** are psychostimulants, better known as stimulants. Dextroamphetamine is used primarily in treating attention-deficit/hyperactivity disorder (ADHD) and narcolepsy, a condition characterized by daytime somnolence in which the patient periodically falls into a deep sleep during the day. Narcolepsy is a disorder of the sleep–wake control mechanisms within the brain that interferes with both daytime wakefulness and nighttime sleep.

The use of a medication for its approved indications is called its *labeled use.* In clinical practice, however, physicians often prescribe medications for *unlabeled* ("off-label") uses when published clinical studies, case reports, or their own clinical experiences support the efficacy and safety of those treatments. Dextroamphetamine is often used to augment antidepressants in treating refractory depression. For patients with chronic treatment-resistant depression, for example, dextroamphetamine in combination with antidepressants can provide symptomatic relief and improvement beyond that experienced with antidepressants alone.

In numerous clinical studies and decades of clinical experience, dextroamphetamine has clearly demonstrated improvement in outcome for children with ADHD. Dextroamphetamine increases the child's ability to concentrate, extends attention span, and decreases hyperactivity. Adults with ADHD also benefit from therapy with dextroamphetamine. Dextroamphetamine helps them concentrate and remain focused on their tasks, increases their attention span, and decreases impulsivity and hyperactivity.

Because DextroStat and Dexedrine Spansules are stimulants, they are closely regulated controlled substances. The physician must write a new prescription each time they are dispensed, and a prescription cannot be refilled.

Dosing Information

Dextroamphetamine is available in immediate-release tablets (DextroStat) and sustained-release capsules (Dexedrine Spansules). For adults, the recommended starting dosage of dextroamphetamine is 5 mg twice a day. The dosage is adjusted based on the individual's response. The usual therapeutic dosage range is between 10 mg/day and 40 mg/day, administered two times daily. The dosing of dextroamphetamine in the immediate-release form may be converted to once-daily dosing with an equivalent dosage of sustained-release capsules.

Common Side Effects

The common side effects associated with taking dextroamphetamine are rapid heart rate, palpitations, nervousness, restlessness, insomnia, dry mouth, constipation, nausea, diarrhea, loss of appetite, weight loss, and elevation of blood pressure.

Adverse Reactions and Precautions

Dextroamphetamine has a high potential for abuse. Individuals with a history of alcohol and substance abuse may be at risk for abusing stimulants. Individuals who abuse dextroamphetamine develop tolerance and psychological dependence that may result in addiction. With long-term abuse of dextroamphetamine and the resulting sleepless nights, the individual may develop psychotic symptoms.

Dextroamphetamine may increase blood pressure. Individuals with a history of high blood pressure or heart disease should be cautious about taking dextroamphetamine because it can exacerbate these conditions. Uncontrolled high blood pressure can have serious consequences, including stroke and heart attack. Patients taking dextroamphetamine should routinely check their blood pressure.

Individuals with a history of seizure disorder should be cautious while taking dextroamphetamine, because it can lower the seizure threshold and increase susceptibility for seizures.

In children and adolescents who are still in their growth period, dextroamphetamine can suppress linear growth. Physicians commonly interrupt treatment on weekends and holidays when children are not in school, for growth catch-up. Children and adolescents taking dextroamphetamine require close monitoring for growth suppression and periodic measuring of their height. This effect is not a concern in the adult population.

Dextroamphetamine may make tics worse in individuals with a tic disorder (i.e., twitching of a muscle group, especially in the face).

Dextroamphetamine should be avoided, or used with caution, by patients with a diagnosis of schizophrenia or bipolar disorder. Stimulants are frequently abused in this population, and high doses of dextroamphetamine may trigger psychosis and mania.

Use in Pregnancy and Breastfeeding: Pregnancy Category C

Dextroamphetamine has not been tested in women to determine its safety in pregnancy. The effects of the medication on the developing fetus in pregnant women are unknown. Women who are pregnant or may become pregnant should discuss this with their physician.

Nursing mothers should not take any stimulant, because small amounts will pass into breast milk and be ingested by the baby. If stopping the stimulant is not an alternative, breastfeeding should not be started or should be discontinued.

338

Possible Drug Interactions

Dextroamphetamine should not be taken in combination with a group of antidepressants known as **monoamine oxidase inhibitors** (MAOIs). The combination may precipitate increases in blood pressure. This and other significant drug interactions reported with dextroamphetamine are summarized in the table below.

Monoamine oxidase inhibitors (MAOIs) (e.g., Parnate, Emsam, Nardil, Marplan)	MAOIs should not be taken with methylphenidates (e.g., Concerta, Ritalin, Focalin), dextroamphetamines (e.g., DextroStat, Adderall, Adderall XR), or Strattera. The combination may precipitate dangerous elevation of blood pressure.
Weight-loss medications (e.g., Meridia)	Weight-loss medications, prescription and nonprescription, should not be taken with dextroamphetamines/amphetamines or methylphenidates. The combination may increase blood pressure or cause irritability, insomnia, and other adverse reactions from excessive stimulation.

Overdose

The severity of dextroamphetamine overdose depends on the amount ingested. The individual may experience a progression of the following symptoms from an acute overdose: restlessness, agitation, irritability, insomnia, hyperactivity, confusion, elevated blood pressure, rapid heart rate, delirium, hallucinations, irregular heartbeat, convulsions, coma, circulatory collapse, and death.

Any suspected overdose should be treated as an emergency. The person should be taken to the emergency room for observation and treatment. The prescription bottle of medication (and any other medication suspected in the overdose) should be brought as well, because the information on the prescription label can be helpful to the treating physician in determining the number of pills ingested.

Special Considerations

- To avoid insomnia, the last daily dose of dextroamphetamine should not be taken late in the evening. Dexedrine Spansules should be taken once a day in the morning.
- Dextroamphetamine may be taken with or without food.
- Do not take more than instructed by your physician.
- If dextroamphetamine causes pronounced nervousness, restlessness, insomnia, loss of appetite, or weight loss, notify your physician.
- If you miss a dose, take it as soon as possible. If it is close to the next scheduled dose, skip the missed dose and continue on your regular dosing schedule. Do not take double doses. If you missed your dose of Dexedrine Spansules in the morning and it is late in the evening, skip the dose and continue on your regular dosing schedule the next morning.
- Do not chew or crush dextroamphetamine capsules; swallow them whole. Take with a full glass of water to help swallow the medication.

- Store the medication in its originally labeled, light-resistant container, away from heat and moisture. Heat and moisture may precipitate breakdown of your medication, and the medication may lose its therapeutic effects.
- Keep your medication out of reach of children.

If you have any questions about your medication, consult your physician or pharmacist.

Notes

From Chew RH, Hales RE, Yudofsky SC: *What Your Patients Need to Know About Psychiatric Medications*, Second Edition. Washington, DC, American Psychiatric Publishing, 2009

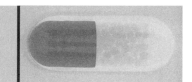

Focalin and Focalin XR (dexmethylphenidate)

Generic name: Dexmethylphenidate
Available strengths: 2.5 mg, 5 mg, 10 mg tablets;
   5 mg, 10 mg, 15 mg, 20 mg capsules (Focalin XR)
Available in generic: No
Drug class: Stimulant

General Information

Focalin (dexmethylphenidate) and **Focalin XR (extended release)** are psychostimulants, or better known as stimulants. Focalin is used primarily in treating attention-deficit/hyperactivity disorder (ADHD) and narcolepsy, a condition characterized by daytime somnolence in which the patient periodically falls into a deep sleep during the day. Narcolepsy is a disorder of the sleep–wake control mechanisms within the brain that interferes with both daytime wakefulness and nighttime sleep.

The use of a medication for its approved indications is called its *labeled use*. In clinical practice, however, physicians often prescribe medications for *unlabeled* ("off-label") uses when published clinical studies, case reports, or their own clinical experiences support the efficacy and safety of those treatments.

In numerous clinical studies and substantial clinical experience, Focalin has clearly demonstrated improvement in outcome for children with ADHD. Focalin increases the child's ability to concentrate, extends attention span, and decreases hyperactivity. Adults with ADHD also benefit from therapy with Focalin. Focalin helps them concentrate and remain focused on tasks, increases their attention span, and decreases impulsivity and hyperactivity.

Focalin (dexmethylphenidate) is chemically similar to Ritalin (methylphenidate). Methylphenidate has two mirror-image forms, which are called **isomers** (*d*-, *l*-isomers). Focalin is the active isomer (*d*-isomer) of methylphenidate, whereas the *l*-isomer has little or no activity. Isomers are mirror-image chemicals, similar to right and left hands, and are not superimposable (i.e., cannot be placed over each other). The advantage of Focalin is that the patient is taking the active isomer of methylphenidate, but at equivalent dosages, there is little difference between Focalin and Ritalin.

Because Focalin and Focalin XR are stimulants, they are closely regulated controlled substances. The physician must write a new prescription each time they are dispensed, and a prescription cannot be refilled.

Dosing Information

The recommended starting dosage of Focalin for individuals who are not currently taking methylphenidate (Ritalin, Metadate) is 2.5 mg two times a day (5 mg/day). The dosage is adjusted in 2.5- to 5-mg daily increments at weekly intervals to a maximum of 10 mg twice daily (20 mg/day). Focalin XR can be given once a day. Focalin may be switched to the XR formulation with an equivalent daily dose. Instead of taking Focalin 2.5 mg two times a day, for example, it may be more convenient to take Focalin XR 5 mg once a day in the morning. Focalin XR 5 mg, 10 mg, 15 mg, and 20 mg are equivalent to Focalin 2.5 mg, 5 mg, 7.5, and 10 mg twice a day. For individuals currently taking methylphenidate and switching to Focalin or Focalin XR, the starting dosage is half the dosage of methylphenidate.

The dosing of Focalin in adults is based on clinical presentation and individualized to the patient's response and report of side effects. In children, dosing is also based on age and weight. The other consideration in dosing is selection of a formulation with the duration of action tailored to the needs of the patient. Focalin is short acting and begins to work in 30–60 minutes after administration, with duration of 2–5 hours. The advantage is that it works quickly, but the duration of action is short and requires dosing two or three times a day.

Common Side Effects

The common side effects associated with taking Focalin are rapid heart rate, palpitations, nervousness, restlessness, insomnia, dry mouth, constipation, nausea, diarrhea, loss of appetite, weight loss, and elevation of blood pressure.

Adverse Reactions and Precautions

Focalin has a high potential for abuse. Individuals with a history of alcohol and substance abuse may be at risk for abusing stimulants. Individuals who abuse Focalin develop tolerance and psychological dependence that may result in addiction. With long-term abuse of Focalin and the resulting sleepless nights, the individual may develop psychotic symptoms.

Focalin may increase blood pressure. Individuals with a history of high blood pressure or heart disease should be cautious about taking Focalin because it can exacerbate these conditions. Uncontrolled high blood pressure can have serious consequences, including stroke and heart attack. Patients taking Focalin should routinely check their blood pressure.

Individuals with a history of seizure disorder should be cautious while taking Focalin, because it can lower the seizure threshold and increase susceptibility for seizures.

In children and adolescents who are still in their growth period, Focalin can suppress linear growth. Physicians commonly interrupt treatment on weekends and holidays when children are not in school, for growth catch-up. Children and adolescents taking Focalin require close monitoring for growth suppression and periodic measuring of their height. This effect is not a concern in the adult population.

Focalin may make tics worse in individuals with a tic disorder (i.e., twitching of a muscle group, especially in the face).

Focalin should be avoided, or used with caution, by patients with a diagnosis of schizophrenia or bipolar disorder. Stimulants are frequently abused in this population, and high doses of Focalin may trigger psychosis and mania.

Use in Pregnancy and Breastfeeding: Pregnancy Category C

Focalin has not been tested in women to determine its safety in pregnancy. The effects of the medication on the developing fetus in pregnant women are unknown. Women who are pregnant or may become pregnant should discuss this with their physician.

Nursing mothers should not take any stimulant, because small amounts will pass into breast milk and be ingested by the baby. If stopping the stimulant is not an alternative, breastfeeding should not be started or should be discontinued.

Possible Drug Interactions

Focalin should not be taken in combination with a group of antidepressants known as **monoamine oxidase inhibitors** (MAOIs). The combination may precipitate increases in blood pressure. This and other significant drug interactions reported with amphetamine and methylphenidate are summarized in the table below.

Monoamine oxidase inhibitors (MAOIs) (e.g., Parnate, Emsam, Nardil, Marplan)	MAOIs should not be taken with methylphenidates or dexmethylphenidate (e.g., Concerta, Ritalin, Focalin). The combination may precipitate dangerous elevation of blood pressure.
Weight-loss medications (e.g., Meridia)	Weight-loss medications, prescription and nonprescription, should not be taken with methylphenidates or dexmethylphenidate. The combination may increase blood pressure or cause irritability, insomnia, and other adverse reactions from excessive stimulation.
Coumadin (warfarin)	Methylphenidate and dexmethylphenidate may increase the anticoagulant action of Coumadin.

Overdose

The severity of Focalin overdose depends on the amount ingested. The individual may experience a progression of the following symptoms from an acute overdose: restlessness, agitation, irritability, insomnia, hyperactivity, confusion, elevated blood pressure, rapid heart rate, delirium, hallucinations, irregular heart beat, convulsions, coma, circulatory collapse, and death.

Any suspected overdose should be treated as an emergency. The person should be taken to the emergency room for observation and treatment. The prescription bottle of medication (and any other medication suspected in the overdose) should be brought as well, because the information on the prescription label can be helpful to the treating physician in determining the number of pills ingested.

Special Considerations

- To avoid insomnia, the last daily dose of Focalin should be taken early in the evening, and not close to bedtime.
- Focalin may be taken with food to avoid stomach upset.
- Do not take more than instructed by your physician.
- If Focalin causes pronounced nervousness, restlessness, insomnia, loss of appetite, or weight loss, notify your physician.
- If you miss a dose, take it as soon as possible. If it is close to the next scheduled dose, skip the missed dose and continue on your regular dosing schedule. Do not take double doses.

- Store the medication in its originally labeled, light-resistant container, away from heat and moisture. Heat and moisture may precipitate breakdown of your medication, and the medication may lose its therapeutic effects.
- Keep your medication out of reach of children.

If you have any questions about your medication, consult your physician or pharmacist.

Notes

_____

_____

_____

_____

_____

_____

_____

_____

_____

_____

From Chew RH, Hales RE, Yudofsky SC: *What Your Patients Need to Know About Psychiatric Medications*, Second Edition. Washington, DC, American Psychiatric Publishing, 2009

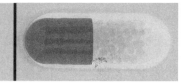

Metadate ER and Metadate CD (methylphenidate, extended release)

Generic name: Methylphenidate, extended release
Available strengths: 10 mg, 20 mg extended-release tablets (Metadate ER);
    10 mg, 20 mg, 30 mg, 40 mg, 50 mg, 60 mg extended-release capsules
    (Metadate CD)
Available in generic: No
Drug class: Stimulant

General Information

Metadate ER and **Metadate CD (methylphenidate, extended release)** are psychostimulants, or better known as stimulants. Metadate is used primarily in treating attention-deficit/hyperactivity disorder (ADHD) and narcolepsy, a condition characterized by daytime somnolence in which the patient periodically falls into a deep sleep during the day. Narcolepsy is a disorder of the sleep–wake control mechanisms within the brain that interferes with both daytime wakefulness and nighttime sleep.

The use of a medication for its approved indications is called its *labeled use*. In clinical practice, however, physicians often prescribe medications for *unlabeled* ("off-label") uses when published clinical studies, case reports, or their own clinical experiences support the efficacy and safety of those treatments. Metadate is often used to augment antidepressants in treating refractory depression. For patients with chronic treatment-resistant depression, for example, Metadate in combination with antidepressants can provide symptomatic relief and improvement beyond that experienced with antidepressants alone.

In numerous clinical studies and substantial clinical experience, Metadate has clearly demonstrated improvement in outcome for children with ADHD. Metadate increases the child's ability to concentrate, extends attention span, and decreases hyperactivity. Adults with ADHD also benefit from therapy with Metadate. Metadate helps them concentrate and remain focused on their tasks, increases their attention span, and decreases impulsivity and hyperactivity.

Metadate ER incorporates methylphenidate in an extended-release tablet composed of a wax matrix, allowing slow release of the stimulant as the tablet passes through the gastrointestinal tract. The ER tablet has duration of approximately 6–8 hours, and a single tablet provides a duration of effect corresponding to the total daily dosage of immediate-release methylphenidate. The disadvantage of the ER tablet is that it takes about 2–3 hours before peak clinical effects are seen, which may be problematic, especially for school-age children. Metadate CD, a dual-action preparation, overcomes this drawback. Metadate CD provides both immediate and extended release of the stimulant. The CD capsules contain methylphenidate incorporated into two types of beads: one type releases the medication immediately after ingestion, while a second type provides sustained release of methylphenidate lasting up to 8 hours. The immediate-release beads account for about 30% of the total methylphenidate in the capsule. From a single dose of Metadate CD taken early in morning, there is an initial release of methylphenidate followed by sustained release throughout the afternoon. By evening, the methylphenidate in the body decreases, so that by bedtime the medication should not interfere with sleep.

Because Metadate ER and Metadate CD are stimulants, they are closely regulated controlled substances. The physician must write a new prescription each time they are dispensed, and a prescription cannot be refilled.

Dosing Information

For adults, the usual starting dosage for immediate-release methylphenidate is 5 mg twice a day, and the dosage is adjusted based on the individual's response. The average dosage is 20–30 mg/day, administered two or three times daily. The maximum dosage should not exceed 60 mg/day. Metadate ER may be used in place of regular methylphenidate by replacing the total daily dosage of methylphenidate with an equivalent dosage of Metadate ER. For example, the dosage of an individual taking 10 mg of methylphenidate twice daily could be switched to 20 mg of Metadate ER once a day in the morning.

Individuals new to methylphenidate may initially take 10–20 mg of Metadate CD in the morning, and the dosage may be increased in weekly intervals by 10 mg, based on response, up to a maximum dosage of 60 mg/day. For individuals currently taking immediate-release methylphenidate or Metadate ER, the previous daily dosage may be converted to the nearest dosage of Metadate CD. For example, the dosage of an individual taking 5 mg three times a day (15 mg/day) of immediate-release methylphenidate could be converted to 20 mg of Metadate CD once a day. Metadate ER could be substituted with an equivalent dose of Metadate CD.

Metadate tablets and capsules should be swallowed whole and not chewed or crushed. The CD capsules may be opened and sprinkled over a spoonful of applesauce and swallowed without chewing.

Common Side Effects

The common side effects associated with taking Metadate are rapid heart rate, palpitations, nervousness, restlessness, insomnia, dry mouth, constipation, nausea, diarrhea, loss of appetite, weight loss, and elevation of blood pressure.

Adverse Reactions and Precautions

Metadate has a high potential for abuse. Individuals with a history of alcohol and substance abuse may be at risk for abusing stimulants. Individuals who abuse Metadate develop tolerance and psychological dependence that may result in addiction. With long-term abuse of Metadate and the resulting sleepless nights, the individual may develop psychotic symptoms.

Metadate may increase blood pressure. Individuals with a history of high blood pressure or heart disease should be cautious about taking Metadate because it can exacerbate these conditions. Uncontrolled high blood pressure can have serious consequences, including stroke and heart attack. Patients taking Metadate should routinely check their blood pressure.

Individuals with a history of seizure disorder should be cautious while taking Metadate, because it can lower the seizure threshold and increase susceptibility for seizures.

In children and adolescents who are still in their growth period, Metadate can suppress linear growth. Physicians commonly interrupt treatment on weekends and holidays when children are not in school, for growth catch-up. Children and adolescents taking Metadate require close monitoring for growth suppression and periodic measuring of their height. This effect is not a concern in the adult population.

Metadate may make tics worse in individuals with a tic disorder (i.e., twitching of a muscle group, especially in the face).

Metadate should be avoided, or used with caution, by patients with a diagnosis of schizophrenia or bipolar disorder. Stimulants are frequently abused in this population, and high doses of Metadate may trigger psychosis and mania.

Use in Pregnancy and Breastfeeding: Pregnancy Category C

Metadate has not been tested in women to determine its safety in pregnancy. The effects of the medication on the developing fetus in pregnant women are unknown. Women who are pregnant or may become pregnant should discuss this with their physician.

Nursing mothers should not take any stimulant, because small amounts will pass into breast milk and be ingested by the baby. If stopping the stimulant is not an alternative, breastfeeding should not be started or should be discontinued.

Possible Drug Interactions

Metadate should not be taken in combination with a group of antidepressants known as **monoamine oxidase inhibitors** (MAOIs). The combination may precipitate increases in blood pressure. This and other significant drug interactions reported with Metadate are summarized in the table below.

Monoamine oxidase inhibitors (MAOIs) (e.g., Parnate, Emsam, Nardil, Marplan)	MAOIs should not be taken with methylphenidates or dexmethylphenidate (e.g., Concerta, Ritalin, Focalin). The combination may precipitate dangerous elevation of blood pressure.
Weight-loss medications (e.g., Meridia)	Weight-loss medications, prescription and non-prescription, should not be taken with methylphenidates or dexmethylphenidate. The combination may increase blood pressure or cause irritability, insomnia, and other adverse reactions from excessive stimulation.
Coumadin (warfarin)	Methylphenidate and dexmethylphenidate may increase the anticoagulant action of Coumadin.

Overdose

The severity of Metadate overdose depends on the amount ingested. The individual may experience a progression of the following symptoms from an acute overdose: restlessness, agitation, irritability, insomnia, hyperactivity, confusion, elevated blood pressure, rapid heart rate, delirium, hallucinations, irregular heartbeat, convulsions, coma, circulatory collapse, and death.

Any suspected overdose should be treated as an emergency. The person should be taken to the emergency room for observation and treatment. The prescription bottle of medication (and any other medication suspected in the overdose) should be brought as well, because the information on the prescription label can be helpful to the treating physician in determining the number of pills ingested.

Special Considerations

- The last daily dose of Metadate should be taken early in the evening, and not close to bedtime, to avoid insomnia.
- Metadate may be taken with food to avoid stomach upset.
- Do not take more than instructed by your physician.
- If Metadate causes pronounced nervousness, restlessness, insomnia, loss of appetite, or weight loss, notify your physician.
- If you miss a dose, take it as soon as possible. If it is late in the afternoon or evening, skip the missed dose and continue on your regular dosing schedule the next morning. Do not take double doses.
- Do not chew or crush Metadate tablets or capsules; swallow them whole. Take with a full glass of water to help swallow the medication.
- Store the medication in its originally labeled, light-resistant container, away from heat and moisture. Heat and moisture may precipitate breakdown of your medication, and the medication may lose its therapeutic effects.
- Keep your medication out of reach of children.

If you have any questions about your medication, consult your physician or pharmacist.

Notes

_____

_____

_____

_____

_____

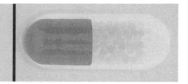

Ritalin, Ritalin-SR, and Ritalin LA (methylphenidate)

Generic name: Methylphenidate
Available strengths: 5 mg, 10 mg, 20 mg immediate-release tablets;
 20 mg sustained-release tablet (Ritalin-SR);
 10 mg, 20 mg, 30 mg, 40 mg extended-release capsules (Ritalin LA)
Available in generic: Yes, except Ritalin-SR
Drug class: Stimulant

General Information

Ritalin (methylphenidate), Ritalin-SR (methylphenidate sustained release), and **Ritalin LA (methylphenidate extended release)** are psychostimulants, better known as stimulants. Ritalin is used primarily in treating attention-deficit/hyperactivity disorder (ADHD) and narcolepsy, a condition characterized by daytime somnolence in which the patient periodically falls into a deep sleep during the day. Narcolepsy is a disorder of the sleep–wake control mechanisms within the brain that interferes with both daytime wakefulness and nighttime sleep.

The use of a medication for its approved indications is called its *labeled use*. In clinical practice, however, physicians often prescribe medications for *unlabeled* ("off-label") uses when published clinical studies, case reports, or their own clinical experiences support the efficacy and safety of those treatments. Ritalin is often used to augment antidepressants in treating refractory depression. For patients with chronic treatment-resistant depression, for example, Ritalin in combination with antidepressants can provide symptomatic relief and improvement beyond that experienced with antidepressants alone.

In numerous clinical studies and decades of clinical experience, Ritalin has clearly demonstrated improvement in outcome for children with ADHD. Ritalin increases the child's ability to concentrate, extends attention span, and decreases hyperactivity. Adults with ADHD also benefit from therapy with Ritalin. Ritalin helps them concentrate and remain focused on their tasks, increases their attention span, and decreases impulsivity and hyperactivity.

Ritalin comes in an immediate-release tablet that lasts 2–5 hours and should be administered two or three times a day for consistent daytime response. Ritalin-SR, a sustained-release tablet, has a duration of approximately 6–8 hours and can be taken once a day in the morning in place of regular Ritalin. A single tablet provides a duration of effect corresponding to the total daily dosage of regular Ritalin. The disadvantage of the SR tablet is that it takes about 2–3 hours before peak clinical effects are seen, which may be problematic, especially for school-age children. Ritalin LA, a dual action preparation, overcomes this drawback. Ritalin LA provides both immediate and extended release of the stimulant. The LA capsules contain methylphenidate incorporated into two types of beads: one type releases the medication immediately after ingestion, while a second type provides gradual release of methylphenidate lasting up to 8 hours. The stimulant in the body decreases by evening, so that by bedtime the medication should not interfere with sleep.

Because Ritalin, Ritalin-SR, and Ritalin LA are stimulants, they are closely regulated controlled substances. The physician must write a new prescription each time they are dispensed, and a prescription cannot be refilled.

Dosing Information

For adults, the recommended starting dosage of Ritalin is 5 mg twice a day, and the dosage is adjusted based on the individual's response. The average dosage is 20–30 mg/day, administered two or three times daily. The maximum dosage should not exceed 60 mg/day. Immediate-release Ritalin may be converted to once-a-day dosing with the Ritalin-SR tablet by replacing the total daily dosage of Ritalin with an equivalent dose of Ritalin-SR. The SR tablet should be swallowed whole and not chewed or crushed.

Individuals new to methylphenidate may initially take 20 mg of Ritalin LA once a day in the morning. The dosage may be increased in weekly intervals by 10 mg, based on response, up to a maximum dosage of 60 mg/day. The medication of individuals who are currently taking Ritalin or Ritalin-SR may be converted to Ritalin LA by substituting the daily dosage with the nearest equivalent dosage of the LA capsule. For example, the dosage of an individual taking 20 mg of Ritalin two times a day (40 mg/day) may be converted to a single dose of 40 mg of Ritalin LA once a day.

Ritalin-SR tablets and Ritalin LA capsules should be swallowed whole and not chewed or crushed. The LA capsules may be opened and sprinkled over a spoonful of applesauce and swallowed without chewing.

Common Side Effects

The common side effects associated with taking Ritalin are rapid heart rate, palpitations, nervousness, restlessness, insomnia, dry mouth, constipation, nausea, diarrhea, loss of appetite, weight loss, and elevation of blood pressure.

Adverse Reactions and Precautions

Ritalin has a high potential for abuse. Individuals with a history of alcohol and substance abuse may be at risk for abusing stimulants. Individuals who abuse Ritalin develop tolerance and psychological dependence that may result in addiction. With long-term abuse of Ritalin and the resulting sleepless nights, the individual may develop psychotic symptoms.

Ritalin may increase blood pressure. Individuals with a history of high blood pressure or heart disease should be cautious about taking Ritalin because it can exacerbate these conditions. Uncontrolled high blood pressure can have serious consequences, including stroke and heart attack. Patients taking Ritalin should routinely check their blood pressure.

Individuals with a history of seizure disorder should be cautious while taking Ritalin, because it can lower the seizure threshold and increase susceptibility for seizures.

In children and adolescents who are still in their growth period, Ritalin can suppress linear growth. Physicians commonly interrupt treatment on weekends and holidays when children are not in school, for growth catch-up. Children and adolescents taking Ritalin require close monitoring for growth suppression and periodic measuring of their height. This effect is not a concern in the adult population.

Ritalin may make tics worse in individuals with a tic disorder (i.e., twitching of a muscle group, especially in the face).

Ritalin should be avoided, or used with caution, by patients with a diagnosis of schizophrenia or bipolar disorder. Stimulants are frequently abused in this population, and high doses of Ritalin may trigger psychosis and mania.

Use in Pregnancy and Breastfeeding: Pregnancy Category C

Ritalin has not been tested in women to determine its safety in pregnancy. The effects of the medication on the developing fetus in pregnant women are unknown. Women who are pregnant or may become pregnant should discuss this with their physician.

Nursing mothers should not take any stimulant, because small amounts will pass into breast milk and be ingested by the baby. If stopping the stimulant is not an alternative, breastfeeding should not be started or should be discontinued.

Possible Drug Interactions

Ritalin should not be taken in combination with a group of antidepressants known as **monoamine oxidase inhibitors** (MAOIs). The combination may precipitate increases in blood pressure. This and other significant drug interactions reported with Ritalin are summarized in the table below.

Monoamine oxidase inhibitors (MAOIs) (e.g., Parnate, Emsam, Nardil, Marplan)	MAOIs should not be taken with methylphenidates or dexmethylphenidate (e.g., Concerta, Ritalin, Focalin). The combination may precipitate dangerous elevation of blood pressure.
Weight-loss medications (e.g., Meridia)	Weight-loss medications, prescription and non-prescription, should not be taken with methylphenidates or dexmethylphenidate. The combination may increase blood pressure or cause irritability, insomnia, and other adverse reactions from excessive stimulation.
Coumadin (warfarin)	Methylphenidate and dexmethylphenidate may increase the anticoagulant action of Coumadin.

Overdose

The severity of Ritalin overdose depends on the amount ingested. The individual may experience a progression of the following symptoms from an acute overdose: restlessness, agitation, irritability, insomnia, hyperactivity, confusion, elevated blood pressure, rapid heart rate, delirium, hallucinations, irregular heartbeat, convulsions, coma, circulatory collapse, and death.

Any suspected overdose should be treated as an emergency. The person should be taken to the emergency room for observation and treatment. The prescription bottle of medication (and any other medication suspected in the overdose) should be brought as well, because the information on the prescription label can be helpful to the treating physician in determining the number of pills ingested.

Special Considerations

- The last daily dose of Ritalin should be taken early in the evening, and not close to bedtime, to avoid insomnia. Ritalin-SR and Ritalin LA should be taken early in the morning.
- Ritalin may be taken with food to avoid stomach upset.
- Do not take more than instructed by your physician.
- If Ritalin causes pronounced nervousness, restlessness, insomnia, loss of appetite, or weight loss, notify your physician.
- If you miss a dose, take it as soon as possible. If it is late in the afternoon or evening, skip the missed dose of Ritalin-SR or Ritalin LA and continue on your regular dosing schedule the next morning. Do not take double doses.
- Do not chew or crush Ritalin-SR tablets or Ritalin-LA capsules; swallow them whole. Take with a full glass of water to help swallow the medication.
- Store the medication in its originally labeled, light-resistant container, away from heat and moisture. Heat and moisture may precipitate breakdown of your medication, and the medication may lose its therapeutic effects.
- Keep your medication out of reach of children.

If you have any questions about your medication, consult your physician or pharmacist.

Notes

_____

_____

_____

_____

_____

_____

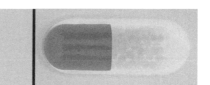

Vyvanse
(lisdexamfetamine)

Generic name: lisdexamfetamine
Available strengths: 20 mg, 30 mg, 40 mg, 50 mg,
    60 mg, 70 mg capsules
Available in generic: No
Drug class: Stimulant

General Information

Vyvanse (lisdexamfetamine) is a unique extended-release formulation of **dextroamphetamine** (*d*-amphetamine). The extended release is achieved through modification of the active molecule dextroamphetamine to form lisdexamfetamine, which is inactive. After Vyvanse is taken, it is rapidly absorbed and distributed to the liver, where it is converted back to the active stimulant, dextroamphetamine. The time to absorb and convert lisdexamfetamine to dextroamphetamine essentially makes Vyvanse an extended-release formulation of dextroamphetamine. Upon activation, Vyvanse is similar to Dexedrine Spansules (dextroamphetamine extended-release capsules) and has a duration of action of 8–12 hours.

The use of a medication for its approved indications is called its *labeled use*. In clinical practice, however, physicians often prescribe medications for *unlabeled* ("off-label") uses when published clinical studies, case reports, or their own clinical experiences support the efficacy and safety of those treatments. Vyvanse is approved by the U.S. Food and Drug Administration (FDA) for treatment of attention-deficit/hyperactivity disorder (ADHD). Physicians, however, may also use it to treat narcolepsy, a condition characterized by daytime somnolence, in which the person periodically falls into a deep sleep during the day.

Because Vyvanse is a stimulant, it is a closely regulated controlled substance. The physician must write a new prescription each time it is dispensed, and a prescription cannot be refilled.

Dosing Information

The dosage of Vyvanse varies according to age, weight, and response. Because Vyvanse was studied primarily in children with ADHD, dosing information for adults is limited.

The recommended starting dosage in children ages 6–12 years with ADHD who are either starting treatment for the first time or switching from another medication is 30 mg daily in the morning, taken with or without food. If needed, the dosage may be adjusted by 20 mg/day at weekly intervals. The maximum recommended dosage for children is 70 mg/day. The dosage for adults may vary.

Common Side Effects

The side effects reported with Vyvanse are mainly from early clinical studies of children ages 6–12 years. More frequently occurring side effects include headache, decreased appetite, weight loss, insomnia, irritability, and abdominal pain. Sometimes these side effects are caused by starting the medication at too high a dosage, and they should subside when the dosage is decreased. In general, side effects become less bothersome as patients get used to the medicine.

Adverse Reactions and Precautions

Like other amphetamine products, Vyvanse has a high potential for abuse. Individuals with a history of alcohol and substance abuse may be at risk for abusing stimulants. Individuals who abuse Vyvanse develop tolerance and psychological dependence that may result in addiction.

Vyvanse may increase blood pressure and heart rate. Patients with a history of high blood pressure or heart disease should be cautious about taking Vyvanse because it can exacerbate these conditions. Uncontrolled high blood pressure can have serious consequences, including stroke and heart attack. Patients taking Vyvanse should routinely check their blood pressure.

Individuals with a history of seizure disorder should be cautious while taking Vyvanse because it can lower the seizure threshold and increase susceptibility for seizures.

In children and adolescents who are still in their growth period, Vyvanse can suppress linear growth. Physicians commonly interrupt treatment on weekends and holidays when children are not in school, for growth catch-up. Children and adolescents taking Vyvanse require close monitoring for growth suppression and periodic measuring of their height. This effect is not a concern in the adult population.

Vyvanse may make tics worse in individuals with a tic disorder (i.e., twitching of a muscle group, especially in the face).

Vyvanse should be avoided, or used with caution, in patients with schizophrenia or bipolar disorder. Stimulants are frequently abused in this population, and high doses of Vyvanse may trigger psychosis and mania.

Use in Pregnancy and Breastfeeding: Pregnancy Category C

Vyvanse has not been tested in women to determine its safety in pregnancy. The effects of the medication on the developing fetus are unknown. Women who are pregnant or may become pregnant should discuss this with their physician.

Nursing mothers should not take any stimulant, because small amounts will pass into breast milk and be ingested by the baby. If stopping the stimulant is not an alternative, breastfeeding should not be started or should be discontinued.

Possible Drug Interactions

Vyvanse should not be taken in combination with antidepressants known as **monoamine oxidase inhibitors** (MAOIs). The combination may precipitate increases in blood pressure. This and other significant drug interactions reported with Vyvanse are summarized in the table on the next page.

Monoamine oxidase inhibitors (MAOIs) (e.g., Parnate, Emsam, Nardil, Marplan)	MAOIs should not be taken with methylphenidates (e.g., Concerta, Ritalin, Focalin), dextroamphetamines (e.g., DextroStat, Adderall, Adderall XR), or Strattera. The combination may precipitate dangerous elevation of blood pressure.
Weight-loss medications (e.g., Meridia)	Weight-loss medications, prescription and non-prescription, should not be taken with dextroamphetamines/amphetamines or methylphenidates. The combination may increase blood pressure or cause irritability, insomnia, and other adverse reactions from excessive stimulation.

Overdose

The severity of Vyvanse overdose depends on the amount ingested. An individual may experience the progression of the following symptoms from an acute overdose: restlessness, agitation, irritability, insomnia, hyperactivity, confusion, elevated blood pressure, rapid heart rate, delirium, hallucinations, irregular heartbeat, convulsions, coma, circulatory collapse, and death.

Any suspected overdose should be treated as an emergency. The person should be taken to the emergency room for observation and treatment. The prescription bottle of medication (and any other medication suspected in the overdose) should be brought as well, because the information on the prescription label can be helpful to the treating physician in determining the number of pills ingested.

Special Considerations

- Vyvanse is only taken once a day, generally in the morning. If you miss a dose, take it as soon as possible. Skip the dose if it is late afternoon, and return to your regular scheduled dose the next morning. Taking the medication too late in the afternoon may cause sleeping difficulty. To avoid insomnia, take Vyvanse in the morning.
- The capsule should be taken whole. It may also be opened and the contents emptied into a glass of water and consumed immediately.
- Vyvanse may be taken with or without food.
- Do not take more than instructed by your physician.
- If Vyvanse causes pronounced nervousness, restlessness, insomnia, loss of appetite, or weight loss, notify your physician.
- Store the medication in its originally labeled, light-resistant container, away from heat and moisture. Heat and moisture may precipitate breakdown of your medication, and the medication may lose its therapeutic effects, and the medication may lose its therapeutic effects.
- Keep your medications out of the reach of children.

If you have any questions about your medication, consult your physician or pharmacist.

Notes

_____

_____

_____

_____

_____

_____

_____

_____

_____

_____

_____

_____

From Chew RH, Hales RE, Yudofsky SC: _What Your Patients Need to Know About Psychiatric Medications_, Second Edition. Washington, DC, American Psychiatric Publishing, 2009

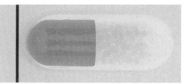

Catapres (clonidine)

Generic name: Clonidine
Available strengths: 0.1 mg, 0.2 mg, 0.3 mg tablets; 0.1 mg/24 hr,
   0.2 mg/24 hr, 0.3 mg/24 hr transdermal patches (Catapres-TTS)
Available in generic: Yes, but only the tablets
Drug class: Noradrenergic agonist

General Information

Catapres (clonidine) was originally developed for the treatment of high blood pressure (**antihypertensive**), but because of its unique action, it is effective in treating many other conditions as well. The U.S. Food and Drug Administration, however, approved Catapres only for use as an antihypertensive. The use of a medication for its approved indications is called its *labeled use*. In clinical practice, however, physicians often prescribe medications for *unlabeled* ("off-label") uses when published clinical studies, case reports, or their own clinical experiences support the efficacy and safety of those treatments.

There are many off-label uses of Catapres, including the treatment of attention-deficit/hyperactivity disorder (ADHD), tic disorders, Tourette's syndrome, sleep difficulties in children with ADHD being treated with stimulants during the daytime, treatment of aggressive youth with disruptive behavior disorders, alcohol withdrawal, opiate (narcotic) detoxification, and restless legs syndrome. Catapres may also be used off-label in treating posttraumatic stress disorder (PTSD). In patients with PTSD, stress triggers hyperactivity of their nervous system, which commonly results in nightmares, panic, startled reactions, and outbursts of rage. Catapres may help reduce these symptoms by its action in the central nervous system.

Catapres exerts its action in the brain stem by stimulating certain types of receptors known as α-**adrenergic receptors.** This decreases activity in that part of the nervous system that regulates heart rate and blood pressure, thereby lowering the heart rate and blood pressure.

How exactly Catapres works in ADHD is unknown. In areas of the brain that regulate attention, **neurotransmitters** such as **norepinephrine** (nerve cells that utilize norepinephrine are called **noradrenergic neurons**) and **dopamine** play a crucial role in maintaining attention and focus. Neurotransmitters are the chemicals in the brain that facilitate **neurotransmission,** the propagation of a signal to different neurons. ADHD may be due to the abnormal regulation of neurotransmission in the area of the brain that regulates attention and focus, and ADHD-associated impairments may be related to diminished levels of dopamine and norepinephrine. Medications that enhance levels of norepinephrine and dopamine, such as amphetamines and methylphenidate (stimulants), are effective in diminishing symptoms of ADHD. Catapres, a nonstimulant, may be effective in ADHD by its action on α-adrenergic receptors in areas of the brain that regulate attention and behavior.

Dosing Information

In the treatment of ADHD and Tourette's syndrome, Catapres is usually used in combination with a stimulant, such as Ritalin, but it may also be used alone. Depending on the use, the dosage of Catapres can range from 0.1 to 0.3 mg/day. In younger children, the dosage can vary depending on the weight of the child, with a range from 3 to 5 μg/kg weight of the child per day. For example, a child weighing 50 pounds (about 23 kilograms) requiring a 5 μg dose would receive 0.1 mg/day. The dose can be given in divided doses of 0.05 mg, two times a day.

Catapres is also available in a skin patch (Catapres-TTS), which has a transdermal delivery system that provides the medication at a dosage of 0.1, 0.2, or 0.3 mg/day, depending on the strength of the patch. Catapres-TTS-1, for example, will deliver 0.1 mg/day of clonidine through the skin into the body for 7 days. The skin patch is applied once every 7 days to a hairless area of the upper outer arm or chest.

Before Catapres is started, pulse and blood pressure should be obtained to establish a baseline level. Measurements should be obtained after the dosage is increased and repeated every 4–6 weeks when the patient is stable at a continuing dosage. The physician may order an electrocardiogram (ECG) to rule out any cardiac problems before starting Catapres. After the patient stabilizes while taking Catapres, the physician may repeat the ECG to monitor for any cardiac changes that may be due to the medication. Patients with preexisting heart disease, including problems with cardiac rhythm, are not good candidates for Catapres therapy as a treatment for ADHD.

Common Side Effects

The common side effects from Catapres include drowsiness (which may be helpful to counter the insomnia effects of stimulants when Catapres is given at bedtime), dry mouth, constipation, sedation, and dizziness. Less frequently, patients may report headaches, nausea and vomiting, weakness, nervousness, restlessness, agitation, and vivid dreams or nightmares. Side effects generally occur soon after the medication is started or when the dose is increased and then diminish with continued therapy.

Adverse Reactions and Precautions

Patients should not abruptly discontinue Catapres without consulting their physician. Catapres requires gradual dosage reduction over 2–4 days before stopping in order to avoid unpleasant symptoms. Sudden cessation may result in headaches, nervousness, agitation, tremor, and elevated blood pressure.

Catapres may induce **orthostatic hypotension,** which is associated with the medication's effect on blood pressure with postural changes. Catapres can block vasoconstriction that compensates for postural change, resulting in a momentary drop in blood pressure that can cause dizziness and fainting (orthostatic hypotension). Patients should be cautious when rising suddenly; from a lying position, the patient should first rise gradually to a sitting position before standing. If feeling lightheaded or dizzy, the individual should sit and wait for about 60 seconds before standing up, to allow the blood pressure to adjust.

Catapres may affect heart rate in some patients, resulting in strong and rapid beats (**palpitations**) for some patients and a relatively slow heart rate (**bradycardia**) for others. If these symptoms do not subside after onset, consult your physician.

In rare cases, there have been reports of sudden deaths and heart problems in children who received the combination of methylphenidate and clonidine. In review of these cases for the cause of death, no direct association with the drug combination was found. The combination of clonidine and methylphenidate is generally very safe. However, the reported fatalities prompted the recommendation of cardiac monitoring with ECG for children taking clonidine.

Use in Pregnancy and Breastfeeding: Pregnancy Category C

No well-controlled studies have been conducted in pregnant women to determine the safety of Catapres in pregnancy, and its effects on the developing fetus are unknown. Catapres should be used during pregnancy only if clearly indicated and when the physician and patient decide that the benefits outweigh the risks.

Catapres is excreted in human breast milk, and it is not recommended for nursing mothers.

Possible Drug Interactions

The significant medication interactions that have been reported with combinations of Catapres and some medications are summarized in the table below.

Beta-blockers (e.g., Inderal)	The combination of Catapres and a beta-blocker, such as Inderal, may decrease the antihypertensive effect of the beta-blocker. Closely monitor blood pressure after starting or discontinuing Catapres or a beta-blocker.
Tricyclic antidepressants (e.g., Elavil)	Tricyclic antidepressants, such as Elavil, may block the antihypertensive effects of Catapres. It is not known if the tricyclic antidepressant will oppose the action of Catapres when used for ADHD or Tourette's syndrome.
Verapamil (e.g., Calan, Isoptin)	The combination of Catapres and verapamil may have additive effects and cause toxicity, such as heart block (atrioventricular block) and severe hypotension.
Clozaril (clozapine), Geodon (ziprasidone), and Seroquel (quetiapine)	The combination of these second-generation antipsychotics and antihypertensive medications, such as Catapres (clonidine) and Inderal (propranolol), may increase the risk for orthostatic hypotension and exaggerate its effects.

Catapres may increase the central nervous system depressive effects of other sedative drugs, including alcohol, barbiturates, antihistamines, and other centrally acting medications. Combining Catapres with alcohol, for example, can increase drowsiness and sedation. Patients should exercise caution when driving or engaging in hazardous activities, such as operating machinery.

Catapres and some cardiovascular medications, such as digoxin, calcium channel blockers (e.g., Calan), and beta-blockers (e.g., Inderal), may potentially have the added effect of slowing heart rate. Patients should tell their physician about all of the medications they are taking.

Overdose

Clonidine overdose can be fatal, especially in young children. With an acute overdose, elevated blood pressure usually develops, followed by low blood pressure, slow heart rate, respiratory depression, weak vital signs, coma, and seizures. A suspected overdose requires immediate medical attention, and the person should be brought to the emergency room for evaluation and treatment. Bring the suspected bottles of medications to the emergency room with the patient, because the number of pills consumed can be estimated from the date when the medication was prescribed and the remaining number of pills in the bottle.

Special Considerations

- If you miss a dose, take it as soon as possible, within 2–3 hours of the scheduled dosing. If it is close to the next scheduled dose, skip the missed dose and continue on your regular dosing schedule. Do not take double doses.
- Catapres may be taken with or without food.
- Do not discontinue Catapres without consulting your physician. Catapres should be decreased gradually before stopping.
- The Catapres skin patch should be applied once a week. The patch is waterproof; bathing, showering, and swimming should not affect the patch. If the patch comes loose, apply an adhesive overlay, which comes with Catapres-TSS, over the patch to ensure that the patch stays on for a full 7 days. If you develop redness, itchiness, or rash, consult your physician.
- Store the medication in its originally labeled, light-resistant container, away from heat and moisture. Heat and moisture may precipitate breakdown of your medication, and the medication may lose its therapeutic effects.
- Keep your medication out of reach of children.

If you have any questions about your medication, consult your physician or pharmacist.

Notes

_____

_____

_____

_____

_____

_____

From Chew RH, Hales RE, Yudofsky SC: *What Your Patients Need to Know About Psychiatric Medications*, Second Edition. Washington, DC, American Psychiatric Publishing, 2009

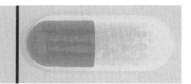

Strattera (atomoxetine)

Generic name: Atomoxetine
Available strengths: 10 mg, 18 mg, 25 mg, 40 mg, 60 mg,
    80 mg, 100 mg capsules
Available in generic: No
Drug class: Selective norepinephrine reuptake inhibitor

General Information

Strattera (atomoxetine) is the first in a new class of nonstimulant medications to be approved for the treatment of attention-deficit/hyperactivity disorder (ADHD). Its mode of action is unlike that of the stimulants, methylphenidate and amphetamines. Strattera therefore appears to have little or no abuse potential. Strattera's mechanism of action is to inhibit the reuptake of the neurotransmitter **norepinephrine.** Consequently, it is called a **selective norepinephrine reuptake inhibitor.**

An explanation of the process of **neurotransmission** may provide some understanding of how Strattera works. During neurotransmission, neurotransmitters are released by one neuron into the space between that neuron and the next neuron. The neurotransmitters come into contact with specific sites on the surface membrane of neurons called *receptors.* From there, the chemical signal is transformed into an electrical impulse that travels down the neuron, causing further release of neurotransmitters. This process of neurotransmission is repeated along a chain of neurons. During neurotransmission, after neurotransmitters are released and the chemical signal is transferred to neurons, the neurotransmitters are recaptured back into brain cells by a process known as *reuptake.* By blocking the neurotransmitters from going back into the neurons from where they were released, the antidepressant can amplify the effects of the neurotransmitter.

Through reuptake inhibition, Strattera boosts norepinephrine neurotransmission. Studies of patients with ADHD suggest that abnormal function of the norepinephrine and dopamine (another type of neurotransmitter) systems may in part be responsible for the inattention and hyperactivity problems seen with the disorder. ADHD and other mental disorders such as depression may be the result of abnormally low levels (or the abnormal neurotransmission) of neurotransmitters. The altered levels of the neurotransmitter may then cause changes in certain areas of the brain, which may produce the clinical signs and symptoms of a mental disorder such as ADHD, depression, or generalized anxiety disorder. When neurotransmission is improved by the medication, the affected areas of the brain are restored to normal functioning, reducing the symptoms of the illness.

Dosing Information

The starting dosage of Strattera for adults is 40 mg taken as a single dose in the morning. After a minimum interval of 3 days, the dosage may be doubled to 80 mg/day, administered as a single morning dose or in evenly divided doses in the morning and afternoon or early evening. The patient should be given a trial of 2–4 weeks at that dosage before any further increase. If the response is not adequate, the dosage may be increased to a maximum of 100 mg/day administered in morning and afternoon doses.

Common Side Effects

The common side effects from Strattera include jitteriness, nausea, sleepiness, nervousness, dizziness, headaches, decreased appetite, and insomnia. Side effects generally occur shortly after starting the medication or when increasing the dosage. If side effects become intolerable, the physician may decrease the dosage to allow the individual to adjust to the medication before increasing it again slowly. Strattera may cause urinary retention in some individuals.

Adverse Reactions and Precautions

Some patients taking normal dosages of Strattera may develop mild elevation of blood pressure (hypertension). At higher dosages, the incidence of Strattera-induced hypertension may be greater. The increase in blood pressure is usually modest, and very few patients have to discontinue Strattera because of hypertension. Generally, lowering the dosage will normalize blood pressure. For this reason, the patient's blood pressure should be checked before starting Strattera and routinely during therapy, especially for individuals with preexisting hypertension or those with a history of heart disease.

Strattera may cause drowsiness and sedation and impair physical coordination and mental alertness. Patients should avoid potentially dangerous activities, such as driving a car or operating machinery, until they are sure that these side effects will not affect their ability to perform these tasks.

Strattera may hinder the growth and weight of children. Some children taking Strattera may lag behind in weight and height for the first 9–12 months of treatment. The data from a group of treated children show that the lag in weight and height is generally minimal, and these children usually catch up to other children after about 12 months. Growth should be monitored while the child is taking Strattera, and therapy may need to be interrupted if he or she is not growing or gaining weight normally.

In rare cases, Strattera can cause liver injury. This finding came to light when two cases—out of the millions of patients who had taken Strattera—of liver injury were reported. Although liver injury caused by Strattera is very rare, patients should be alerted to the signs and symptoms of a liver problem. Patients should contact their physicians immediately when they develop any of the following: yellowing of the skin or whites of the eyes (jaundice), itchy skin (pruritus), dark urine, upper right-sided abdominal tenderness, and unexplained, prolonged flulike symptoms.

Strattera works in similar ways as antidepressants, even though it is used in the treatment of ADHD. There are concerns that antidepressants as a group may be associated with increased risk of suicidal thinking (ideation) in children and adolescents. In short-term studies, antidepressants were found to increase the risk of suicidal thinking and behavior in children and adolescents with major depression and other psychiatric disorders. On the basis of these findings, the U.S. Food and Drug Administration requires a warning in the package insert that prescribers must be aware of the suicide risks in their patients who are starting antidepressant therapy, especially in the pediatric population. Therefore, individuals, especially children and adolescents, should be closely observed for worsening signs of depression after antidepressant therapy is being started or changed.

Pregnancy and Breastfeeding: Pregnancy Category C

Strattera has not been tested in women to determine its safety in pregnancy. The effects of the medication on the developing fetus in pregnant women are unknown. Women who are pregnant or may become pregnant should discuss this with their physician.

Nursing mothers should not take Strattera, because small amounts will pass into breast milk and be ingested by the baby. If stopping Strattera is not an alternative, breastfeeding should not be started or should be discontinued.

Possible Drug Interactions

Strattera, like many other medications, is metabolized in the liver. The combined use of Strattera with certain other medications may result in adverse interactions because one medication may alter the blood levels of the other. Strattera should not be taken with antidepressants known as **monoamine oxidase inhibitors** (MAOIs), because the combination may trigger dangerously elevated blood pressure. This and other significant drug interactions reported with Strattera are summarized in the table below.

Ventolin (albuterol)	Strattera may increase the cardiovascular effects of Ventolin inhalers and inhalant solutions, including palpitations, rapid heart rate, and increased blood pressure.
Prozac (fluoxetine), Paxil (paroxetine), Tagamet (cimetidine), Wellbutrin (bupropion), Norvir (ritonavir)	These medications when combined with Strattera may inhibit its metabolism and increase the blood levels of Strattera, potentially increasing adverse side effects. Use of any of these medications may require lower dosages of Strattera.
Monoamine oxidase inhibitors (MAOIs) Nardil (phenelzine), Marplan (isocarboxazid), and Parnate (phenelzine)	Monoamine oxidase inhibitors should not be combined with Strattera. The combination may dangerously increase blood pressure.

Patients taking Strattera should avoid alcohol or consume it only in moderation.

Overdose

The effects of Strattera overdose are not fully known, because this medication was only recently introduced and clinical experience is limited. It is probably less dangerous in overdose than tricyclic antidepressants and MAOIs.

Any suspected overdose should be treated as an emergency. The person should be taken to the emergency room for observation and treatment. The prescription bottle of medication (and any other medication suspected in the overdose) should be brought as well, because the information on the prescription label can be helpful to the treating physician in determining the number of pills ingested.

Special Considerations

- **Warning:** Always let your physician or a family member know if you have suicidal thoughts. Notify your psychiatrist or family physician if you experience depressive symptoms while taking Strattera or whenever you feel unable to control suicidal urges and thoughts.
- If you miss a dose, take it as soon as possible, within 2–3 hours of the scheduled dose. If it is close to the next scheduled dose, skip the missed dose and continue on your regular dosing schedule. Do not take double doses.
- Strattera may cause dizziness, as well as drowsiness and sedation. Until you are certain that the medication does not affect your coordination, it is best to avoid driving and operating machinery.
- Do not take Strattera if you have a known allergy to it, or if you experienced a severe reaction after taking it.
- Strattera may be taken with food to decrease any gastrointestinal side effects.
- If Strattera is taken in divided doses, take the medication early in the morning and afternoon or early evening. Do not take the medication close to bedtime because it can interfere with sleep.
- Store the medication in its originally labeled, light-resistant container, away from heat and moisture. Heat and moisture may precipitate breakdown of your medication, and the medication may lose its therapeutic effects.
- Keep your medication out of reach of children.

If you have any questions about your medication, consult your physician or pharmacist.

Notes

_____

_____

_____

_____

_____

_____

_____

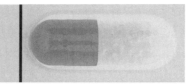

Tenex (guanfacine)

Generic name: Guanfacine
Available strengths: 1 mg, 2 mg tablets
Available in generic: Yes
Drug class: Adrenergic agonist

General Information

Tenex (guanfacine) was originally developed for the treatment of high blood pressure **(antihypertensive)**, but because of its unique action, it is effective in treating other conditions as well. The U.S. Food and Drug Administration, however, approved Tenex only for use as an antihypertensive. The use of a medication for its approved indications is called its *labeled use*. In clinical pratice, however, physicians often prescribe medications for *unlabeled* ("off-label") uses when published clinical studies, case reports, or their own clinical experiences support the efficacy and safety of those treatments. Tenex has also been found to be effective in the treatment of attention-deficit/hyperactivity disorder (ADHD), tic disorders, Tourette's syndrome, and other disorders.

How exactly Tenex works in ADHD is unknown. In the areas of the brain that regulate attention, **neurotransmitters** such as **norepinephrine** (nerve cells that utilize norepinephrine are called **adrenergic neurons**) and **dopamine** play a crucial role in maintaining attention and focus. Neurotransmitters are the chemicals in the brain that facilitate **neurotransmission**, the propagation of a signal to different neurons. ADHD may be due to the abnormal regulation of neurotransmission in the area of the brain that regulates attention and focus, and ADHD-associated impairments may be related to diminished levels of dopamine and norepinephrine. Medications that enhance levels of norepinephrine and dopamine, such as amphetamines and methylphenidate (stimulants), are effective in diminishing symptoms of ADHD. Tenex acts on the **receptors** (sites on the surface of nerve cells where neurotransmitters bind) of adrenergic neurons. Tenex is an **adrenergic agonist** because of its action on norepinephrine neurotransmission, which may explain its role in the treatment of ADHD.

Dosing Information

In the treatment of ADHD, Tenex is usually used in combination with a stimulant, such as Ritalin, but it may also be prescribed alone. The usual starting dosage is 0.5 mg/day, with the dosage increased by 0.5 mg every 3 days until an optimal clinical response or the maximum recommended dosage of 4 mg/day is reached.

Common Side Effects

Common side effects reported with Tenex include tiredness, sluggishness, headache, dizziness, drowsiness, dry mouth, constipation, sedation, and dizziness. These side effects are generally mild and become less bothersome after about a week. Side effects usually occur when the medication is being started or during dose increases and generally diminish with continued therapy.

Adverse Reactions and Precautions

Patients should not abruptly discontinue Tenex without consulting their physician. Tenex should be gradually reduced over 2–4 days before stopping in order to avoid unpleasant symptoms associated with abrupt withdrawal. Sudden cessation may result in headaches, nervousness, agitation, tremor, and elevated blood pressure.

Use in Pregnancy and Breastfeeding: Pregnancy Category B

No well-controlled studies have been conducted in pregnant women to determine the safety of Tenex in pregnancy. In animal studies, guanfacine did not produce any evidence of harm to the fetus. However, animal studies are not always predictive of human response, and the effects of Tenex on a human fetus are unknown. Tenex should be used during pregnancy only if the physician and patient both decide it is clearly indicated.

Tenex is not known to be excreted in human breast milk. However, it is not recommended that nursing mothers take Tenex.

Possible Drug Interactions

The drug interactions that have been reported with combinations of Tenex and some medications are summarized in the table below.

Dilantin	Dilantin (phenytoin) can lower the blood levels of Tenex and decrease its effectiveness.
Phenobarbital	Phenobarbital and other barbiturates can lower the blood levels of Tenex and decrease its effectiveness.
Tricyclic antidepressants (e.g., Elavil)	Tricyclic antidepressants, such as Elavil, may interfere with the action of Tenex and decrease its effectiveness.

Tenex may increase the central nervous system depressive effects of other sedative drugs, including alcohol, barbiturates, antihistamines, and centrally acting pain medications. Combining Tenex with alcohol, for example, can increase drowsiness and sedation. Patients should exercise caution when driving or engaging in potentially hazardous activities, such as operating machinery.

Overdose

An overdose of guanfacine can be potentially fatal, especially in younger children. With acute overdose, reported symptoms include sluggishness (**lethargy**), low blood pressure (**hypotension**), slow heart rate (**bradycardia**), and sedation.

Any suspected overdose should be treated as an emergency. The person should be taken to the emergency room for observation and treatment. The prescription bottle of medication (and any other medication suspected in the overdose) should be brought as well, because the information on the prescription label can be helpful to the treating physician in determining the number of pills ingested.

Special Considerations

- If you miss a dose, take it as soon as possible, within 2–3 hours of the scheduled dose. If it is close to the next scheduled dose, skip the missed dose and continue on your regular dosing schedule. Do not take double doses.
- Tenex may be taken with or without food.
- Do not discontinue Tenex without consulting your physician. Tenex should be decreased gradually before stopping.
- Exercise caution when driving or engaging in potentially hazardous activities, such as operating machinery, because Tenex may increase the central nervous system depressive effects of other sedative drugs, including alcohol, barbiturates, antihistamines, and centrally acting pain medications, and can increase drowsiness and sedation.
- Store the medication in its originally labeled, light-resistant container, away from heat and moisture. Heat and moisture may precipitate breakdown of your medication, and the medication may lose its therapeutic effects.
- Keep your medication out of the reach of children.

If you have any questions about your medication, consult your physician or pharmacist.

Notes

_____

_____

_____

From Chew RH, Hales RE, Yudofsky SC: *What Your Patients Need to Know About Psychiatric Medications*, Second Edition. Washington, DC, American Psychiatric Publishing, 2009

Cognitive Enhancers for Treatment of Alzheimer's Disease and Other Forms of Dementia

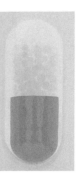

Aricept (donepezil)
Cognex (tacrine)
Exelon (rivastigmine)
Namenda (memantine)
Razadyne (galantamine)

Overview

Alzheimer's disease is the most common and well-known form of degenerative **dementia.** More than 50% of people who develop dementia have Alzheimer's disease, and it affects 2.4–4.5 million Americans. By definition, dementia is a syndrome—a cluster of symptoms—of impaired **cognition** affecting the individual's intellectual abilities, particularly memory, problem solving, judgment, awareness, and behavior. Alzheimer's disease is a progressive, irreversible brain disease involving a deterioration of brain cells that results in loss of intellectual functioning.

The cause of Alzheimer's disease is unknown, but symptoms of the disease may be associated with the selective loss of brain cells known as **cholinergic neurons** in affected areas of the brain. There are certain pathological hallmarks of Alzheimer's disease that are found at autopsy, including **senile plaques** (degenerating neurons twisted around a waxy protein-polysaccharide substance known as **amyloid**) and **neurofibrillary tangles** (helical threadlike tangles within neurons).

Cognitive enhancers are medications used for treating dementia. Commonly, they are used to treat mild-to-moderate dementia of Alzheimer's disease, with the exception of Namenda (memantine), which has an indication for treatment of moderate-to-severe Alzheimer's disease. Deterioration of cognition and memory in Alzheimer's disease, and perhaps in other forms of dementia, may be due to degeneration of cholinergic neurons. Cognitive enhancers improve function by inhibiting the breakdown of the neurotransmitter **acetylcholine,** thereby increasing brain acetylcholine levels and optimizing the function of intact cholinergic neurons. By blocking the **cholinesterase enzyme** that breaks down acetylcholine and thus inhibiting its destruction, these agents (except for Namenda), known as **cholinesterase inhibitors,** can improve memory and overall function.

Namenda (memantine) is distinct from the other cognitive enhancers. It represents a new class of medication with a mechanism of action that is quite different from the other cognitive agents for the treatment of Alzheimer's disease. Namenda works by blocking the receptors for the neurotransmitter **glutamate.** It is believed that glutamate plays an important role in the neural pathways associated with learning and memory. In brain disorders such as Alzheimer's disease, overexcitation of neurons produced by abnormal levels of glutamate may be associated with neuronal cell dysfunction (resulting in cognitive and memory deficits) and eventual cell death (leading to deterioration and collapse of intellectual functioning). By selectively blocking a type of glutamate receptor (the **NMDA receptor**) while allowing for normal neurotransmission, Namenda may help reduce the destructive, excitotoxic effects associated with abnormal transmission of glutamate. In addition, because Namenda works differently from other cognitive enhancers, it may be combined with other agents such as Aricept.

As research into new treatments for Alzheimer's disease continues, it is expected that new medications similar to Namenda may be introduced. Both Namenda and the cholinesterase inhibitors (Aricept, Cognex, Exelon, Razadyne [formerly Reminyl]) may improve the patient's overall function and delay worsening of symptoms, but neither class of medications can prevent the underlying progression of Alzheimer's disease. Research into the cause of Alzheimer's disease is as important as looking for new treatments. If the cause of the disease may be understood, then new measures to prevent it may also be discovered.

See also individual handouts for these medications. If you have any questions about your medication, consult your physician or pharmacist.

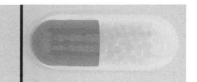

Aricept (donepezil)

Generic name: Donepezil
Available strengths: 5 mg, 10 mg tablets;
   5 mg, 10 mg orally disintegrating tablets;
   1 mg/mL oral solution
Available in generic: No
Drug class: Cognitive enhancer/cholinesterase inhibitor

General Information

Aricept (donepezil) is a cognitive-enhancing medication for treating mild-to-moderate dementia of Alzheimer's disease. Deterioration of cognition and memory in Alzheimer's disease, and in other forms of dementia, may be associated with degeneration of **cholinergic neurons.** Aricept inhibits the **cholinesterase enzyme** that breaks down **acetylcholine,** a neurotransmitter. This increases brain acetylcholine levels, optimizing the function of intact cholinergic neurons and improving memory and overall cognitive functioning.

Dosing Information

The starting dosage of Aricept is 5 mg once a day. The patient should receive 5 mg/day for 4–6 weeks before the dosage is increased to 10 mg/day. A trial period of 4–6 weeks allows the patient time to adjust to the medication and prevents the many frequent side effects associated with the higher dosage. Aricept should be taken shortly before retiring at nighttime. The dosage should not exceed 10 mg/day. Aricept orally disintegrating tablets or solution can be substituted for the tablets without a change in the dosage.

Common Side Effects

The most common side effects associated with Aricept are nausea, diarrhea, vomiting, insomnia, fatigue, muscle cramps, loss of appetite, and weight loss. These effects are more frequent at the 10 mg dosage, but in most cases the side effects are generally mild and transient and resolve after 1–3 weeks with continued therapy. Aricept may cause dizziness and drowsiness, especially during initiation of therapy.

Adverse Reactions and Precautions

Patients who are undergoing surgery should let their physician know that they are taking Aricept, because it can interact with any muscle-relaxing type of anesthesia that they may receive.

Aricept may have a slowing effect on heart rate. Patients who have a history of slow heart rate (bradycardia), who are taking medications for cardiac conduction problems, or who have a history of dizziness related to cardiac problems must be monitored closely while taking Aricept.

Aricept may cause seizures in susceptible individuals, although this adverse reaction is very rare. However, seizure activity may also be a manifestation of Alzheimer's disease.

Patients with a history of asthma or chronic obstructive pulmonary disease should be monitored closely while taking Aricept. Aricept may worsen these pulmonary diseases.

Aricept may increase gastric acid secretions. Patients who have a history of ulcers or who are taking nonsteroidal anti-inflammatory drugs (NSAIDs), such as ibuprofen or naproxen, should be monitored closely for signs of gastrointestinal bleeding.

Possible Drug Interactions

Few significant drug interactions are associated with Aricept. The clinically significant drug interactions reported with Aricept are summarized in the table below.

Anticholinergic agents (e.g., Cogentin)	Anticholinergic agents and Aricept, when used in combination, may oppose each other's action, reducing their effectiveness.
Nonsteroidal anti-inflammatory drugs (NSAIDs) (e.g., aspirin, ibuprofen, naproxen)	Because NSAIDs are associated with an increased risk of gastrointestinal ulcers and Aricept may increase gastric acid secretions, this combination may increase the risk of gastrointestinal bleeding.
Nizoral (ketoconazole) and Diflucan (fluconazole)	These antifungal agents may inhibit Aricept's metabolism and increase its blood levels and pharmacological actions, potentially producing adverse effects.

Patients taking Aricept should not consume alcohol because the combination may increase sedation and drowsiness. Moreover, the sedative effects of alcohol may act as a depressant, obscuring the therapeutic effects of Aricept and complicating treatment.

Overdose

Overdose with Aricept may result in a **cholinergic crisis** resulting from high levels of acetylcholine. The symptoms of a cholinergic crisis include severe nausea, vomiting, salivation, slow heart rate, sweating, low blood pressure, muscle weakness, respiratory depression, and convulsions. Overdose with Aricept can be life threatening.

Any suspected overdose should be treated as an emergency. The person should be taken to the emergency room for observation and treatment. The prescription bottle of medication (and any other medication suspected in the overdose) should be brought as well, because the information on the prescription label can be helpful to the treating physician in determining the number of pills ingested.

Special Considerations

- If you miss a dose, take it as soon as possible. If it is close to the next scheduled dose, skip the missed dose and continue on your regular dosing schedule. Do not take double doses.
- Aricept may be taken with or without food.
- It is best to take the medication at bedtime, shortly before retiring.
- Prolonged vomiting and diarrhea may result in dehydration and loss of electrolytes, and this can be dangerous, especially for seniors. Inform your physician when prolonged vomiting or diarrhea occurs for more than 1 day.
- Aricept may cause dizziness and drowsiness, especially during initiation of therapy, and may impair your alertness. Use caution when driving or performing tasks that require alertness.
- Store the medication in its originally labeled, light-resistant container, away from heat and moisture. Heat and moisture may precipitate breakdown of your medication, and the medication may lose its therapeutic effects.
- Keep your medication out of reach of children.

If you have any questions about your medication, consult your physician or pharmacist.

Notes

_____

_____

_____

_____

_____

From Chew RH, Hales RE, Yudofsky SC: *What Your Patients Need to Know About Psychiatric Medications*, Second Edition. Washington, DC, American Psychiatric Publishing, 2009

Cognex (tacrine)

Generic name: Tacrine
Available strengths: 10 mg, 20 mg, 30 mg, 40 mg capsules
Available in generic: No
Drug class: Cognitive enhancer/cholinesterase inhibitor

General Information

Cognex (tacrine) is a cognitive-enhancing medication for treating mild-to-moderate dementia of Alzheimer's disease. Deterioration of cognition and memory in Alzheimer's disease, and in other forms of dementia, may be associated with degeneration of **cholinergic neurons.** Cognex inhibits the **cholinesterase enzyme** that breaks down **acetylcholine,** a neurotransmitter. This increases brain acetylcholine levels, optimizing the function of intact cholinergic neurons and improving memory and overall cognitive functioning.

Dosing Information

The usual starting dosage of Cognex is 10 mg four times a day (40 mg/day). The patient should receive this dosage for a minimum of 4 weeks before the dosage is increased. Laboratory tests should be obtained to monitor liver function in the fourth week after initiation of therapy and then every other week for the next 4 months. If the results of liver function tests are normal, the dosage may be increased to 20 mg four times a day (80 mg/day). In another 4–6 weeks, the dosage may be increased to 30 mg four times a day (120 mg/day) and again in 4–6 weeks, if tolerated, to 160 mg/day. The optimal target dosage is 120–160 mg/day, but the daily dosage should not exceed 160 mg/day.

Common Side Effects

The most common side effects associated with Cognex are nausea, vomiting, diarrhea, indigestion, insomnia, tremors, muscle cramps, loss of appetite, and weight loss. These effects are more frequent at the higher dosages, but in most cases the side effects are generally mild and transient and resolve after 1–3 weeks with continued therapy. Cognex may cause dizziness and drowsiness, especially during initiation of therapy,

Adverse Reactions and Precautions

Cognex is associated with liver toxicity. Individuals with a history of liver disease should not receive Cognex but may benefit from one of the other cognitive enhancers. Therapy with Cognex requires close monitoring of liver function. Blood tests to measure liver enzymes (called **transaminase** levels) are necessary for detecting early signs of liver toxicity. Elevation of liver transaminase enzymes provides an indication of liver injury. Blood tests are obtained to measure liver enzymes 4 weeks after initiation of Cognex, and the tests are repeated every other week for the next 4 months. Thereafter, transaminase levels are obtained every 3 months for as long as the patient continues to receive Cognex. Elevated liver enzymes or other abnormal liver function test results may require reduction of the daily dosage of Cognex or discontinuation of therapy.

Patients who are undergoing surgery should let their physician know that they are taking Cognex, because it can interact with any muscle-relaxing type of anesthesia that they may receive.

Cognex may have a slowing effect on heart rate. Patients who have a history of slow heart rate (bradycardia), who are taking medications for cardiac conduction problems, or who have a history of dizziness related to cardiac problems must be monitored closely while taking Cognex.

Cognex may cause seizures in susceptible individuals, although this adverse reaction is very rare. However, seizure activity may also be a manifestation of Alzheimer's disease.

Patients with a history of asthma or chronic obstructive pulmonary disease should be monitored closely while taking Cognex. Cognex may worsen pulmonary diseases.

Cognex may increase gastric acid secretions. Patients who have a history of ulcers or who are taking nonsteroidal anti-inflammatory drugs (NSAIDs), such as ibuprofen or naproxen, should be monitored closely for signs of gastrointestinal bleeding.

Possible Drug Interactions

Few significant drug interactions are associated with Cognex. The clinically significant drug interactions reported with Cognex are summarized in the table below.

Anticholinergic agents (e.g., Cogentin)	Anticholinergic agents and Cognex, when used in combination, may oppose each other's action, reducing their effectiveness.
Nonsteroidal anti-inflammatory drugs (NSAIDs) (e.g., aspirin, ibuprofen, naproxen)	Because NSAIDs are associated with an increased risk of gastrointestinal ulcers and Cognex may increase gastric acid secretions, this combination may increase the risk of gastrointestinal bleeding.
Tagamet (cimetidine)	Tagamet may inhibit the metabolism of Cognex and increase its blood levels and pharmacological actions, potentially producing adverse effects.

Patients taking Cognex should not consume alcohol because the combination may increase sedation and drowsiness. Moreover, the sedative effects of alcohol may act as a depressant, obscuring the therapeutic effects of Cognex and complicating treatment.

Overdose

Overdose with Cognex may result in a **cholinergic crisis** resulting from high levels of acetylcholine. The symptoms of a cholinergic crisis include severe nausea, vomiting, salivation, slow heart rate, sweating, low blood pressure, muscle weakness, respiratory depression, and convulsions. Overdose with Cognex can be life threatening.

Any suspected overdose should be treated as an emergency. The person should be taken to the emergency room for observation and treatment. The prescription bottle of medication (and any other medication suspected in the overdose) should be brought as well, because the information on the prescription label can be helpful to the treating physician in determining the number of pills ingested.

Special Considerations

- If you miss a dose, take it as soon as possible. If it is close to the next scheduled dose, skip the missed dose and continue on your regular dosing schedule. Do not take double doses.
- To be effective, Cognex should be taken at regular intervals during waking hours, separated by 3–4 hours. For example, take the medication at mealtimes and bedtime.
- Take Cognex with food to avoid stomach upset.
- Prolonged vomiting and diarrhea may result in dehydration and loss of electrolytes, and this can be dangerous, especially for seniors. Inform your physician when prolonged vomiting or diarrhea occurs for more than 1 day.
- Cognex may cause dizziness and drowsiness, especially during initiation of therapy, and may impair your alertness. Use caution when driving or performing tasks that require alertness.
- Store the medication in its originally labeled, light-resistant container, away from heat and moisture. Heat and moisture may precipitate breakdown of your medication, and the medication may lose its therapeutic effects.
- Keep your medication out of reach of children.

If you have any questions about your medication, consult your physician or pharmacist.

Notes

_____

_____

_____

_____

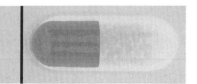

Exelon (rivastigmine)

Generic name: Rivastigmine

Available strengths: 1.5 mg, 3 mg, 4.5 mg, 6 mg capsules;
  2 mg/mL oral solution;
  4.6 mg/24 hr, 9.5 mg/24 hr topical patch

Available in generic: Yes, except the patch

Drug class: Cognitive enhancer/cholinesterase inhibitor

General Information

Exelon (rivastigmine) is a cognitive-enhancing medication for treating mild-to-moderate dementia of Alzheimer's disease and dementia of Parkinson's disease. Deterioration of cognition and memory in Alzheimer's disease and Parkinson's disease, and in other forms of dementia, may be associated with degeneration of **cholinergic neurons.** Exelon inhibits the **cholinesterase enzyme** that breaks down **acetylcholine,** a neurotransmitter. This increases brain acetylcholine levels, optimizing the function of intact cholinergic neurons and improving memory and overall cognitive functioning.

Dosing Information

The recommended starting dosage of Exelon is 1.5 mg twice a day (3 mg/day). The patient should receive this dosage for a minimum of 2 weeks. If it is tolerated, the dosage may be increased to 3 mg twice daily (6 mg/day). If needed, the subsequent higher dosages are 4.5 mg twice a day (9 mg/day) followed by 6 mg twice a day (12 mg/day). The dosage should be adjusted only after a minimum of 2 weeks at the lower dosage. The maximum dosage is 12 mg/day.

With the topical patch, the patient can be started with a 4.6 mg/24 hours patch. The patient should stay at this dosage for a recommended period of 4 weeks of treatment before increasing to the higher dosage of 9.5 mg/24 hours. If the physician is switching the patient from oral to topical dosing, the patient taking a total daily dose of less than 6 mg can be switched to the 4.6 mg/24 hours patch. The patient whose total daily dose is 6–12 mg can use the 9.5 mg/24 hours patch.

Common Side Effects

The most common side effects associated with Exelon are dizziness, nausea, vomiting, diarrhea, abdominal cramps, fatigue, loss of appetite, and weight loss. These effects are more frequent at the higher dosages, but in most cases the side effects are generally mild and transient and resolve after 1–3 weeks with continued therapy. Exelon may cause dizziness and drowsiness, especially during initiation of therapy

Adverse Reactions and Precautions

Patients who are undergoing surgery should let their physician know that they are taking Exelon, because it can interact with any muscle-relaxing type of anesthesia that they may receive.

Exelon may have a slowing effect on heart rate. Patients who have a history of slow heart rate (bradycardia), who are taking medications for cardiac conduction problems, or who have a history of dizziness related to cardiac problems should be monitored closely while taking Exelon.

Exelon may cause seizures in susceptible individuals, although this adverse reaction is very rare. However, seizure activity may also be a manifestation of Alzheimer's disease.

Patients with a history of asthma or chronic obstructive pulmonary disease should be monitored closely while taking Exelon. Exelon may worsen these pulmonary diseases.

Exelon may increase gastric acid secretions. Patients who have a history of ulcers or who are taking nonsteroidal anti-inflammatory drugs (NSAIDs), such as ibuprofen or naproxen, should be monitored closely for signs of gastrointestinal bleeding.

Possible Drug Interactions

Few significant drug interactions are associated with Exelon. The clinically significant drug interactions reported with Exelon are summarized in the table below.

Anticholinergic agents (e.g., Cogentin)	Anticholinergic agents and Exelon, when used in combination, may oppose each other's action, reducing their effectiveness.
Nonsteroidal anti-inflammatory drugs (NSAIDs) (e.g., aspirin, ibuprofen, naproxen)	Because NSAIDs are associated with an increased risk of gastrointestinal ulcers and Exelon may increase gastric acid secretions, the combination may increase the risk of gastrointestinal bleeding.

Patients taking Exelon should not consume alcohol because the combination may increase sedation and drowsiness. Moreover, the sedative effects of alcohol may act as a depressant, obscuring the therapeutic effects of Exelon and complicating treatment.

Overdose

Overdose with Exelon may result in a **cholinergic crisis** resulting from high levels of acetylcholine. The symptoms of a cholinergic crisis include severe nausea, vomiting, salivation, slow heart rate, sweating, low blood pressure, muscle weakness, respiratory depression, and convulsions. Overdose with Exelon can be life threatening.

Any suspected overdose should be treated as an emergency. The person should be taken to the emergency room for observation and treatment. The prescription bottle of medication (and any other medication suspected in the overdose) should be brought as well, because the information on the prescription label can be helpful to the treating physician in determining the number of pills ingested.

Special Considerations

- If you miss a dose, take it as soon as possible. If it is close to the next scheduled dose, skip the missed dose and continue on your regular dosing schedule. Do not take double doses.
- Exelon may be taken with or without food.
- It is best to take Exelon in the morning and at bedtime, shortly before retiring.
- Prolonged vomiting and diarrhea may result in dehydration and loss of electrolytes, and this can be dangerous, especially for seniors. Inform your physician when prolonged vomiting or diarrhea occurs for more than 1 day.
- Exelon may cause dizziness and drowsiness, especially during initiation of therapy, and may impair your alertness. Use caution when driving or performing tasks that require alertness.
- When applying Exelon topical patches, you should rotate the application site daily to minimize skin irritation. Remember to change the patch after 24 hours. If you or the caretaker forgets to apply a new patch at the usual time, change the patch immediately and apply the next patch at the usual time. The skin patch can be applied to the upper arm or chest, to an area of the skin that is dry, clean, hairless, and not red or inflamed. Do not apply over areas of the skin after applying lotions or creams. When properly applied, the patch stays intact even with bathing or sweating.
- If more than several days have elapsed between treatments, consult your physician. Sometimes the patient may need to restart the medication at a lower dose.
- Store the medication in its originally labeled, light-resistant container, away from heat and moisture. Heat and moisture may precipitate breakdown of your medication, and the medication may lose its therapeutic effects.
- Keep your medication out of reach of children.

If you have any questions about your medication, consult your physician or pharmacist.

Notes

From Chew RH, Hales RE, Yudofsky SC: *What Your Patients Need to Know About Psychiatric Medications*, Second Edition. Washington, DC, American Psychiatric Publishing, 2009

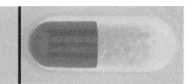

Namenda (memantine)

Generic name: Memantine
Available strengths: 5 mg, 10 mg tablets; 2 mg/mL oral solution
Available in generic: No
Drug class: Cognitive enhancer/NMDA receptor antagonist

General Information

Namenda (memantine) is a cognitive-enhancing medication for treating moderate-to-severe dementia of Alzheimer's disease. Namenda is distinct from the other cognitive enhancers because it represents a new class of medications with a mechanism of action that is very different from that of other cognitive-enhancing agents. Namenda works by blocking the receptors for the neurotransmitter **glutamate.** It is believed that glutamate plays an important role in the neural pathways associated with learning and memory. In brain disorders such as Alzheimer's disease, overexcitation of neurons produced by abnormal levels of glutamate may be associated with neuronal cell dysfunction (resulting in cognitive and memory deficits) and eventual cell death (leading to deterioration and collapse of intellectual functioning). By selectively blocking a type of glutamate receptor (the **NMDA receptor**) while allowing for normal neurotransmission, Namenda may help reduce the destructive, excitotoxic effects associated with abnormal transmission of glutamate. In addition, because Namenda works differently from other cognitive enhancers, it may be combined with other cognitive-enhancing agents such as Aricept. In one short-term (24 weeks) clinical study, patients who took a combination of Namenda and Aricept scored better on measures of cognition, daily activities, and overall functioning than individuals who took Aricept alone, but the study did not provide data on the long-term benefits of the combination.

Dosing Information

The starting dosage of Namenda is 5 mg once a day. The dosage is increased in increments of 5 mg/day, separated by a minimum interval of 1 week. After 1 week, for example, the dosage is increased to 5 mg twice a day (10 mg/day). Dosage adjustments are based on the patient's response and tolerance to the medication. The recommended target dosage is 10 mg twice a day (20 mg/day). Patients with impairment of kidney (renal) function may need lower dosages because renal excretion of Namenda is diminished.

Common Side Effects

Namenda is generally well tolerated. The most frequent side effects reported with Namenda include dizziness, headache, confusion, constipation, sleepiness, fatigue, and general body ache and pain. These adverse effects were more frequent at the 20 mg/day dosage, but in most cases side effects are mild and transient and resolve after 1–3 weeks with continued therapy. Namenda may cause dizziness and drowsiness, especially during initiation of therapy

Adverse Reactions and Precautions

In clinical trials, patients receiving Namenda had a higher incidence (4%) of high blood pressure than did patients who received placebo (2%). It is not clear whether Namenda is associated with a risk of inducing high blood pressure. Patients should routinely check their blood pressure while taking Namenda.

Namenda is primarily excreted from the body by the kidneys. The excretion of Namenda from the kidneys may be significantly reduced when the urine is alkaline (basic), which may reduce Namenda clearance by about 80%. Medical conditions (e.g., urinary tract infections), medications (e.g., Diamox [acetazolamide], sodium bicarbonate), or diets that alkalinize urine would be expected to reduce excretion of Namenda from the body, which may lead to accumulation of the medication and may potentially increase adverse effects.

Namenda is associated with causing dizziness. This is particularly worrisome in seniors who may be susceptible to falling. At the initiation of therapy and at higher dosages, patients and caregivers should be aware of this potential adverse effect and the risk of falling.

Agitation and aggression were observed with Namenda during clinical trials. Caregivers of patients with Alzheimer's disease should keep in mind that aggressive behavior or agitation may not necessarily be symptoms of dementia but may be the result of an adverse effect of the medication. Family members should report any significant change in the patient's behavior to his or her physician.

Possible Drug Interactions

Few significant drug interactions are associated with Namenda. Because it is not metabolized extensively by the liver but excreted primarily by the kidneys unchanged, other medications do not play a significant role in the metabolism of Namenda. However, medical conditions, medications, or diets that influence the condition of urine, making it more alkaline, may affect the excretion of Namenda. Medications known as carbonic anhydrase inhibitors, including Diamox and Neptazane (methazolamide), prescribed as diuretics and for treatment of glaucoma, may alkalinize urine and decrease the excretion of Namenda. Sodium bicarbonate, found in baking soda and Alka-Seltzer, is also an alkalinizing agent.

Patients taking Namenda should not consume alcohol because the combination may increase sedation and drowsiness. Moreover, the sedative effects of alcohol may act as a depressant, obscuring the therapeutic effects of Namenda and complicating treatment.

Overdose

There are few documented cases of overdose with Namenda, and the information for management of overdose is continually evolving. In a reported case of overdose with 400 mg (forty 10-mg tablets) of Namenda, the patient experienced restlessness, agitation, psychosis, visual hallucinations, somnolence, stupor, and loss of consciousness. The patient recovered from the overdose.

Any suspected overdose should be treated as an emergency. The person should be taken to the emergency room for observation and treatment. The prescription bottle of medication (and any other medication suspected in the overdose) should be brought as well, because the information on the prescription label can be helpful to the treating physician in determining the number of pills ingested.

Special Considerations

- If you miss a dose, take it as soon as possible. If it is close to the next scheduled dose, skip the missed dose and continue on your regular dosing schedule. Do not take double doses.
- Namenda may be taken with or without food.
- It is best to take the medication in the morning and at bedtime, shortly before retiring.
- Prolonged vomiting and diarrhea may result in dehydration and loss of electrolytes, and this can be dangerous, especially for seniors. Inform your physician when prolonged vomiting or diarrhea occurs for more than 1 day.
- Namenda may cause dizziness and drowsiness, especially during initiation of therapy, and may impair your alertness. Use caution when driving or performing tasks that require alertness.
- Store the medication in its originally labeled, light-resistant container, away from heat and moisture. Heat and moisture may precipitate breakdown of your medication, and the medication may lose its therapeutic effects.
- Keep your medication out of reach of children.

If you have any questions about your medication, consult your physician or pharmacist.

Notes

_____

_____

_____

_____

_____

_____

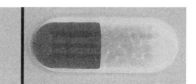

Razadyne (galantamine)

Generic name: Galantamine
Available strengths: 4 mg, 8 mg, 12 mg tablets;
    8 mg, 12 mg, 16 mg extended-release capsules (Razadyne ER);
    4 mg/mL oral solution
Available in generic: Yes, except Razadyne ER
Drug class: Cognitive enhancer/cholinesterase inhibitor

General Information

Razadyne (galantamine) is a cognitive-enhancing medication for treating mild-to-moderate dementia of Alzheimer's disease. Deterioration of cognition and memory in Alzheimer's disease, and in other forms of dementia, may be associated with degeneration of **cholinergic neurons.** Razadyne inhibits the **cholinesterase enzyme** that breaks down **acetylcholine,** a neurotransmitter. This increases brain acetylcholine levels, optimizing the function of intact cholinergic neurons and improving memory and overall cognitive functioning.

Dosing Information

The starting dosage of Razadyne is 4 mg twice a day (8 mg/day). The patient should receive this dosage for a minimum of 4 weeks before any dosage adjustment. If tolerated, the dosage may be increased to 8 mg twice daily (16 mg/day). If needed, the dosage may be increased after 4 weeks to 12 mg twice a day (24 mg/day). Dosages higher than 24 mg/day are not recommended. If Razadyne is stopped and therapy interrupted for several days or longer, the patient should start treatment again at the lowest dosage, and the dosage should be increased slowly to the original dosage.

    The recommended starting dosage of Razadyne ER is 8 mg once a day. To allow time to evaluate response and tolerability, the physician should not increase the dosage to the next higher dosage of 16 mg/day without a minimum trial of 4 weeks. It is not recommended that the dosage exceed a maximum of 24 mg/day. Razadyne ER should be taken in the morning, preferably with food.

Common Side Effects

The most common side effects associated with Razadyne are dizziness, nausea, diarrhea, vomiting, fatigue, loss of appetite, and weight loss. These effects are more frequent at the higher dosages, but in most cases the side effects are generally mild and transient and resolve after 1–3 weeks with continued therapy. Razadyne may cause dizziness and drowsiness, especially during initiation of therapy.

Adverse Reactions and Precautions

Patients who are undergoing surgery should let their physician know that they are taking Razadyne, because it can interact with any muscle-relaxing type of anesthesia that they may receive.

Razadyne may have a slowing effect on heart rate. Patients who have a history of slow heart rate (bradycardia), who are taking medications for cardiac conduction problems, or who have a history of dizziness related to cardiac problems must be monitored closely while taking Razadyne.

Razadyne may cause seizures in susceptible individuals, although this adverse reaction is very rare. However, seizure activity may also be a manifestation of Alzheimer's disease.

Patients with a history of asthma or chronic obstructive pulmonary disease should be monitored closely while taking Razadyne. Razadyne may worsen these pulmonary diseases.

Razadyne may increase gastric acid secretions. Patients who have a history of ulcers or who are taking nonsteroidal anti-inflammatory drugs (NSAIDs), such as ibuprofen or naproxen, should be monitored closely for signs of gastrointestinal bleeding.

Possible Drug Interactions

Few significant drug interactions are associated with Razadyne. The clinically significant drug interactions reported with Razadyne are summarized in the table below.

Anticholinergic agents (e.g., Cogentin)	Anticholinergic agents and Razadyne, when used in combination, may oppose each other's action, reducing their effectiveness.
Nonsteroidal anti-inflammatory drugs (NSAIDs) (e.g., aspirin, ibuprofen, naproxen)	Because NSAIDs are associated with an increased risk of gastrointestinal ulcers and Razadyne may increase gastric acid secretions, the combination may enhance the risk of gastrointestinal bleeding.
Nizoral (ketoconazole) and Diflucan (fluconazole)	These antifungal agents may inhibit Razadyne's metabolism and increase its blood levels and pharmacological actions, potentially producing adverse effects.
Tagamet (cimetidine)	Tagamet may inhibit the metabolism of Razadyne and increase its blood levels and pharmacological actions, potentially producing adverse effects.

(continued)

Erythromycin	Erythromycin may inhibit the metabolism of Razadyne and increase its blood levels and pharmacological actions, potentially producing adverse effects.
Paxil (paroxetine)	Paxil may inhibit the metabolism of Razadyne and increase its blood levels and pharmacological actions, potentially producing adverse effects.

Patients taking Razadyne should not consume alcohol because the combination may increase sedation and drowsiness. Moreover, the sedative effects of alcohol may act as a depressant, obscuring the therapeutic effects of Razadyne and complicating treatment.

Overdose

Overdose with Razadyne may result in a **cholinergic crisis** resulting from high levels of acetylcholine. The symptoms of a cholinergic crisis include severe nausea, vomiting, salivation, slow heart rate, sweating, low blood pressure, muscle weakness, respiratory depression, and convulsions. Overdose with Razadyne can be life threatening.

Any suspected overdose should be treated as an emergency. The person should be taken to the emergency room for observation and treatment. The prescription bottle of medication (and any other medication suspected in the overdose) should be brought as well, because the information on the prescription label can be helpful to the treating physician in determining the number of pills ingested.

Special Considerations

- If you miss a dose, take it as soon as possible. If it is close to the next scheduled dose, skip the missed dose and continue on your regular dosing schedule. Do not take double doses.
- Razadyne may be taken with or without food. Razadyne ER should be taken preferably with food.
- It is best to take Razadyne in the morning and at bedtime, shortly before retiring. Razadyne ER should be taken in the morning (preferably with food).
- Prolonged vomiting and diarrhea may result in dehydration and loss of electrolytes, and this can be dangerous, especially for seniors. Inform your physician when prolonged vomiting or diarrhea occurs for more than 1 day.
- Razadyne may cause dizziness and drowsiness, especially during initiation of therapy, and may impair your alertness. Use caution when driving or performing tasks that require alertness.
- Store the medication in its originally labeled, light-resistant container, away from heat and moisture. Heat and moisture may precipitate breakdown of your medication, and the medication may lose its therapeutic effects.
- Keep your medication out of reach of children.

If you have any questions about your medication, consult your physician or pharmacist.

Notes

_____

_____

_____

_____

_____

_____

_____

_____

_____

_____

_____

_____

Medications for Treatment of Alcohol Dependence

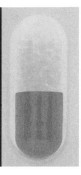

Antabuse (disulfiram)
Campral (acamprosate)
ReVia (naltrexone) and
Vivitrol (naltrexone injection)

General Information

Alcohol dependence, or alcoholism, is one of the most serious health care issues in the United States today. In 2006, the Centers for Disease Control and Prevention ranked alcohol third among the leading preventable causes of death in this country. In the United States, the estimated annual cost of alcohol-related problems, including the loss of productivity, is $185 billion. The destructive toll of alcoholism is widespread—alcoholism affects not only the afflicted individual but families and society as well.

Alcohol dependence is characterized by the following criteria: **craving**—a persistent, strong urge to drink; **tolerance**—the need to drink more alcohol to get high or intoxicated; **loss of control**—inability to stop drinking once started; **significant impairment in the person's life**—neglect of occupational, social, and family activities due to alcohol use; and **physical dependence**—marked by withdrawal symptoms such as nausea, sweating, nervousness, and shakiness. The severity of impairment, of course, varies with the degree of alcohol abuse.

Treatment of alcohol dependence incorporates support groups, psychotherapy, and medications to achieve sobriety. Support groups such as Alcoholics Anonymous (AA) have helped countless alcohol-dependent individuals. It has been shown that the combination of medication with psychosocial support results in higher rates and longer periods of alcohol abstinence.

There are four medication options to treat alcohol dependence: Antabuse (disulfiram), Campral (acamprosate), ReVia (naltrexone), and Vivitrol (naltrexone injection). All four medications are approved by the U.S. Food and Drug Administration (FDA) for the treatment of alcohol dependence. ReVia and Vivitrol are the same drug, naltrexone: ReVia is in tablet form, and Vivitrol is in a long-acting, injectable form.

Antabuse (disulfiram) was the first medication approved by the FDA to treat alcohol dependence. Antabuse blocks an enzyme in the liver that breaks down alcohol (ethanol), causing the metabolite **acetaldehyde** to accumulate. Acetaldehyde accumulation produces symptoms such as flushing, nausea, vomiting, headache, and rapid heartbeat. When a person takes Antabuse daily, consumption of any alcohol, intentionally or unintentionally, can trigger these symptoms, also known as a **disulfiram reaction.** The potential of this adverse reaction discourages the person from drinking and reinforces abstinence.

Naltrexone, in ReVia and Vivitrol, acts in the central nervous system to block **opiate (narcotic) receptors** in order to decrease the craving for alcohol. Receptors are sites on nerve cells (**neurons**) that interact with **neurotransmitters** (the chemicals of the nervous system that are responsible for propagating the signal to other neurons) to produce a specific change in the nerve cell. Naltrexone is an opiate receptor antagonist in the brain, but how it works in treating alcohol dependence is not completely understood. One possible explanation is that opiate receptors interact with **dopamine neurons** and enhance dopamine neurotransmission, especially in the area of the brain called the **nucleus accumbens.** Dopamine neurotransmission has been linked to reinforceable behaviors, such as pleasure-seeking behaviors. By blocking the opiate receptors and reducing dopamine neurotransmission, naltrexone blunts the reward system and the pleasure that occurs with drinking. Reducing the pleasure that occurs with drinking diminishes the cravings.

Campral (acamprosate) was approved in 2004 by the FDA for maintenance treatment of alcohol dependence. Campral works differently from naltrexone and affects different neural systems. How Campral works in maintaining alcohol abstinence is not completely understood. One possible explanation is that the balance between the inhibitory and excitatory neural systems in the brain is affected by chronic alcohol abuse. **Gamma-aminobutyric acid (GABA)** is the **inhibitory neurotransmitter** contained in those neurons that inhibit, or slow, the brain, and **glutamate** is the **excitatory neurotransmitter** in those neurons that excite, or activate, the brain. Campral is structurally similar to GABA, and it potentiates the action of GABA but antagonizes the action of glutamate. It is possible that through this action, Campral restores the GABA–glutamate balance and thus reduces cravings and the need for drinking.

Medications alone to treat alcohol dependence have limited success in achieving long-term abstinence. Research has shown that individuals who receive a combination of psychosocial support and medication therapy show higher rates and longer periods of abstinence than do individuals who receive monotherapy.

See also individual handouts for these medications. If you have any questions about your medication, consult your physician or pharmacist.

From Chew RH, Hales RE, Yudofsky SC: *What Your Patients Need to Know About Psychiatric Medications*, Second Edition. Washington, DC, American Psychiatric Publishing, 2009

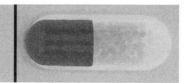

Antabuse (disulfiram)

Generic name: Disulfiram
Available strength: 250 mg
Available in generic: No
Drug class: Agent for treatment of alcohol dependence

General Information

Antabuse (disulfiram) was the first medication approved by the U.S. Food and Drug Administration for treatment of alcohol dependence. Currently, there are three other medications approved in the United States for alcohol dependence. Antabuse should be used only for select individuals who clearly understand that it induces an enforced state of sobriety and for those who are highly motivated to stay abstinent. By no means does Antabuse provide a cure for alcoholism. It must be used in conjunction with a program that includes group support therapy and counseling in order to have any impact on the drinking pattern of the chronically alcoholic individual.

Antabuse blocks an enzyme in the liver that breaks down alcohol (ethanol), causing the metabolite **acetaldehyde** to accumulate. Acetaldehyde accumulation produces symptoms such as flushing, nausea, vomiting, headache, and rapid heartbeat. When a person takes Antabuse daily, consumption of any alcohol, intentionally or unintentionally, can trigger these symptoms, also known as a **disulfiram reaction.** The potential of this adverse reaction discourages the person from drinking and reinforces abstinence.

Before prescribing Antabuse, the physician should obtain a complete medical history from the patient. If the patient has any history of liver disease, cardiovascular disease, stroke, diabetes mellitus, or seizures, the patient should not receive Antabuse. The physician must provide the patient with a clear understanding of a disulfiram reaction; family members or caretakers should receive this information as well. It is highly recommended that the patient sign an informed consent form, documenting that he or she understands the consequences of ingesting alcohol and assumes the responsibility of avoiding all alcohol intake.

Dosing Information

Antabuse should not be started or taken until the patient has abstained from alcohol for at least 12 hours. The usual dosage is 250 mg once a day, in the morning. The patient may take the dose at bedtime if daytime sedation is a problem. Some physicians may initiate Antabuse at 500 mg/day for 1–2 weeks and then decrease the dosage. The maintenance dosage can range from 125 mg/day to 500 mg/day and should not exceed 500 mg/day.

Common Side Effects

In the absence of alcohol, Antabuse produces few side effects. Infrequently, patients have complained of mild drowsiness, sedation, tiredness, headache, nausea, metallic aftertaste, or acne. Usually, these side effects are mild and subside with continued therapy or dosage reduction.

Adverse Reactions and Precautions

The ingestion of alcohol, even in small amounts, in the presence of Antabuse can trigger a reaction not unlike a very bad hangover. Symptoms include nausea, intense vomiting, palpitations, throbbing headache, flushing, sweating, dizziness, shortness of breath, and low blood pressure (**hypotension**). The intensity and duration of the reaction depend on the amounts of Antabuse in the system and of alcohol ingested. The reaction can last 30–60 minutes or for several hours in more severe reactions. In rare and very severe reactions, Antabuse can induce heart attacks, arrhythmias, convulsions, and death.

Patients must also be aware that foods and medications may contain alcohol, though it may not always be obvious. Always read the label before consuming any products that may contain alcohol. For example, many liquid cold and cough preparations contain an alcohol base, and in the usual dose it is enough to trigger a disulfiram reaction.

There have been reported cases of liver toxicity associated with taking Antabuse. In some cases, the liver failures were fatal. While the patient is taking Antabuse, the physician will monitor the patient's liver function through laboratory tests and stop the medication if there is any indication that Antabuse is affecting the liver. The patient should report any signs or symptoms of a liver problem to the physician, including fatigue, nausea, vomiting, yellowing of the eyes or skin (jaundice), or dark urine. These may be indicative of a liver problem.

Use in Pregnancy and Breastfeeding: Pregnancy Category C

Studies have not been conducted in pregnant women to determine the safety of Antabuse in pregnancy. Antabuse should not be given to women who are pregnant or who plan to become pregnant. A disulfiram reaction may endanger the lives of the fetus and mother.

It is not known if Antabuse is excreted in breast milk. Nursing mothers should not take Antabuse.

Possible Drug Interactions

Antabuse may interfere with the metabolism of some medications. When taken in combination, Antabuse may elevate the plasma levels of the affected drugs and possibly cause toxicity. The table on the next page provides information on medications that may interact with Antabuse.

Patients should consult their physician or pharmacist before taking any over-the-counter medications or herbal supplements.

Patients should inform their physician when they relapse and resume drinking, but they should not stop taking Antabuse without consulting their physician.

Coumadin (warfarin)	The anticoagulant effect of Coumadin may be increased by Antabuse. Closely monitor anticoagulation, and adjust Coumadin if needed. Watch for signs of bleeding or bruising.
Benzodiazepines	With some benzodiazepines (e.g., Valium, Librium, Xanax), Antabuse may inhibit their metabolism and increase the sedative effect. Coadministration may require a lower dose of the benzodiazepine.
Dilantin (phenytoin)	Antabuse can interfere with the metabolism of Dilantin, resulting in elevated levels of plasma phenytoin and possible Dilantin toxicity.
Flagyl (metronidazole)	Coadministration of Antabuse and Flagyl has been reported to cause confusion and acute psychosis. These two medications should not be taken together.
Theophylline (e.g., Theo-Dur)	Antabuse may interfere with the metabolism of theophylline and potentially increase its toxic effects. Monitor theophylline closely, and adjust the dosage if necessary.
Tricyclic antidepressants (e.g., Elavil)	Coadministration of Antabuse and tricyclic antidepressants has been reported to cause impaired mental function, with disorientation, confusion, and psychosis. The elderly may be particularly susceptible to this reaction when taking a tricyclic antidepressant and Antabuse.

Overdose

An Antabuse overdose can be potentially dangerous. The severity of toxicity depends on the amount ingested, the age and weight of the person, and if the person also ingested other medications. The safety of Antabuse overdose in children is unknown.

Any suspected overdose should be treated as an emergency. The person should be taken to the emergency room for observation and treatment. The prescription bottle of medication (and any other medication suspected in the overdose) should be brought as well, because the information on the prescription label can be helpful to the treating physician in determining the number of pills ingested.

Special Considerations

- Antabuse is usually taken once a day or as directed by a physician. If you miss a dose, take it as soon as possible. If it is close to the next scheduled dose, skip the missed dose and continue on your regular dosing schedule. Do not take double doses.
- Always check for alcohol content in foods and medications. Even alcohol in topical products (e.g., aftershave lotion) sometimes can be absorbed through the skin and induce a disulfiram reaction.
- Antabuse has been shown to lead to maintenance of abstinence only when total treatment includes group support therapy and counseling.
- If relapse occurs, do not get discouraged; discuss your drinking with your physician, counselor, or therapist. Continue taking Antabuse as directed, and consult your physician as soon as possible.
- If you experience any symptoms of depression, particularly with suicidal thoughts, contact your physician, counselor, or therapist immediately.
- Store the medication in its originally labeled, light-resistant container, away from heat and moisture. Heat and moisture may precipitate breakdown of your medication, and the medication may lose its therapeutic effects.
- Keep your medication out of reach of children.

- The following Web sites can provide you and your family members with additional information:
  - Alcoholics Anonymous: www.alcoholics-anonymous.org
  - National Institute on Alcohol Abuse and Alcoholism: www.niaaa.nih.gov
  - National Clearinghouse for Alcohol and Drug Information: www.ncadi.samhsa.gov
  - National Organization on Fetal Alcohol Syndrome: www.nofas.org
  - American Council on Alcoholism (locate treatment program and support groups in your area): www.aca-usa.org

If you have any questions about your medication, consult your physician or pharmacist.

Notes

From Chew RH, Hales RE, Yudofsky SC: *What Your Patients Need to Know About Psychiatric Medications*, Second Edition. Washington, DC, American Psychiatric Publishing, 2009

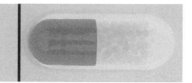

Campral (acamprosate)

Generic name: Acamprosate
Available strength: 333 mg
Available in generic: No
Drug class: Agent for treatment of alcohol dependence

General Information

Campral (acamprosate) was approved in 2004 by the U.S. Food and Drug Administration for the treatment of alcohol dependence. It is indicated for the maintenance of alcohol abstinence and not for treatment of alcohol withdrawal. Campral should be used in conjunction with a program that includes group support therapy and counseling in order to have any substantive effect on the drinking pattern of the chronically alcoholic individual.

Dosing Information

Treatment with Campral should begin shortly after alcohol detoxification when the individual achieves abstinence. The recommended starting dosage of Campral is two 333 mg tablets, or 666 mg, taken three times a day. Campral may be taken without regard to meals, but taking it with food may reduce the side effects of nausea and gastrointestinal irritation, and the mealtime schedule can be a helpful reminder to take the medication. There is generally no need to increase the dose beyond the starting dose. A lower dosage, a 333 mg tablet three times a day, may be effective for some individuals. Patients with moderate kidney impairment should *not* take more than 333 mg three times daily, and those with severe kidney impairment should not take Campral.

Common Side Effects

Diarrhea is the most frequent side effect associated with Campral. Other, less frequent side effects reported with Campral include nausea, constipation, gas, abdominal pain, dizziness, insomnia, nervousness, and depression. These side effects generally subside as patients develop tolerance to the medication. It is unlikely that any of these side effects are related to alcohol withdrawal symptoms. Campral taken at the recommended dosages has not been shown to produce any evidence of withdrawal symptoms.

Adverse Reactions and Precautions

Like other centrally acting medications, Campral may impair thinking and coordination, especially early in the course of therapy. The effects of Campral may become more pronounced if Campral is taken with other centrally acting medications. Patients are cautioned about the hazards of driving and operating machinery when taking Campral.

Patients should inform their physician when they relapse and resume drinking. Patients should not stop taking Campral without consulting their physician. Campral does not produce an adverse reaction with alcohol as Antabuse does.

In clinical trials, Campral-treated patients had statistically higher rates of suicidal thinking and suicide attempts than did the individuals in the placebo group (who received sugar pills). Many of these cases were related to alcohol relapse. Depression is frequently associated with alcohol dependence, and suicidality is higher in individuals with untreated depression. During the early phase of therapy, patients should be monitored closely for clinical signs of depression, especially for suicidal thinking and behavior.

Use in Pregnancy and Breastfeeding: Pregnancy Category C

Studies have not been conducted in pregnant women to determine Campral's safety in pregnancy. In animal studies, Campral was found to cause malformations in the fetuses. The effects of Campral on the developing human fetus are unknown. Campral should not be used during pregnancy unless the physician and patient decide the benefits of treatment outweigh the risks.

It is not known if Campral is excreted in human breast milk. Because many drugs are excreted in breast milk, nursing mothers should not take Campral. Women taking Campral should always inform their physician if they plan to nurse.

Possible Drug Interactions

There are no significant drug interactions known with Campral. Campral is excreted primarily by the kidneys and does not undergo metabolism in the liver. Intake of alcohol with Campral does not alter the levels or excretion of either substance. Campral is not an opiate (narcotic) antagonist and will not produce opioid withdrawal symptoms as naltrexone will. Campral does not interact with antianxiety medications (e.g., benzodiazepines such as Valium) or any sleep medications.

Overdose

In the few reported cases of acute overdose with Campral, diarrhea was the only associated symptom. However, it should not be assumed that a Campral overdose is always benign. The severity of toxicity depends on the amount ingested, the age and weight of the person, and whether the person also ingested other medications. The safety of a Campral overdose in children is unknown.

Any suspected overdose should be treated as an emergency. The person should be taken to the emergency room for observation and treatment. The prescription bottle of medication (and any other medication suspected in the overdose) should be brought as well, because the information on the prescription label can be helpful to the treating physician in determining the number of pills ingested.

Special Considerations

- Campral is usually taken three times a day, or as directed by your physician. If you miss a dose, take it as soon as possible. If it is close to the next scheduled dose, skip the missed dose and continue on your regular dosing schedule. Do not take double doses.
- Campral has been shown to lead to maintenance of abstinence only when total treatment includes group support therapy and counseling.
- If relapse occurs, do not get discouraged; discuss your drinking with your physician, counselor, or therapist. Continue taking Campral as directed, and consult your physician as soon as possible.
- If you experience any symptoms of depression, particularly with suicidal thoughts, contact your physician, counselor, or therapist immediately.
- Campral may impair thinking and coordination, especially early in the course of therapy. The effects of Campral may become more pronounced if Campral is taken with other centrally acting medications, such as alcohol. Use caution when driving or performing tasks that require alertness, and be aware of the hazards of driving and operating machinery.
- Store the medication in its originally labeled, light-resistant container, away from heat and moisture. Heat and moisture may precipitate breakdown of your medication, and the medication may lose its therapeutic effects.
- Keep your medication out of reach of children.
- The following Web sites can provide you and your family members with additional information:
  - Alcoholics Anonymous: www.alcoholics-anonymous.org
  - National Institute on Alcohol Abuse and Alcoholism: www.niaaa.nih.gov
  - National Clearinghouse for Alcohol and Drug Information: www.ncadi.samhsa.gov
  - National Organization on Fetal Alcohol Syndrome: www.nofas.org
  - American Council on Alcoholism (locate treatment program and support groups in your area): www.aca-usa.org

If you have any questions about your medication, consult your physician or pharmacist.

Notes

_____

_____

_____

_____

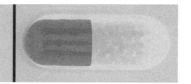

ReVia (naltrexone) and Vivitrol (naltrexone injection)

Generic name: Naltrexone
Available strengths: 50 mg tablets (ReVia); 380 mg/vial,
    long-acting injection (Vivitrol)
Available in generic: Yes, but only ReVia
Drug class: Agents for treatment of alcohol dependence

General Information

ReVia (naltrexone) is approved by the U.S. Food and Drug Administration (FDA) for treatment of alcohol dependence and narcotic addiction; **Vivitrol (naltrexone)** long-acting injection is approved only for treatment of alcohol dependence. Both forms of naltrexone are indicated for the maintenance of alcohol abstinence. ReVia and Vivitrol should be used in conjunction with a program that includes group support therapy and counseling in order to have any substantive effect on the drinking pattern of the chronically alcoholic individual.

Dosing Information

The patient should not start ReVia until after alcohol detoxification and after the individual has achieved abstinence. In addition, the patient should not have taken any narcotic (opioid) medications for the past 7–10 days. The recommended dose for ReVia is a 50 mg tablet taken once a day in the morning, which is an effective dose in treating most patients for alcohol dependence. Patients with acute hepatitis or active liver disease should not take naltrexone.

Naltrexone can also be given in an injectable form. The patient should be given a trial of oral naltrexone before being switched to Vivitrol, a long-acting injection of naltrexone. However, pretreatment with oral naltrexone is not an absolute requirement before using Vivitrol. Vivitrol should be administered by a health care provider. A single vial containing 380 mg is reconstituted and administered intramuscularly every 4 weeks.

Common Side Effects

Frequent side effects of ReVia and Vivitrol at the recommended doses are headache, nausea, abdominal pain, and dizziness. With Vivitrol, pain and tenderness at injection sites are also frequently reported. These side effects generally subside with continued therapy. It is unlikely that any of these side effects are related to alcohol withdrawal symptoms.

Adverse Reactions and Precautions

Naltrexone has not been shown to produce alcohol withdrawal symptoms. However, in opioid-dependent individuals, ReVia and Vivitrol can precipitate opioid withdrawal symptoms because of naltrexone's blocking action. To prevent acute withdrawal symptoms, patients must be opioid-free for a minimum of 7–10 days.

In clinical studies, naltrexone was found to cause elevation of liver enzymes at higher doses, suggesting that it can cause liver injury when given in excessive doses, although no cases of liver failure or fatality have been reported. At the recommended dosage (50 mg/day), naltrexone did not appear to cause an elevation of liver enzymes. In light of this finding, the FDA imposed a labeling requirement to warn that naltrexone should not be used in patients with acute hepatitis or liver failure, and its use in patients with active liver disease (e.g., cirrhosis) must be carefully weighed against the risk of potential hepatotoxicity.

Patients must be aware that ReVia and Vivitrol are potent opioid (narcotic) antagonists. Naltrexone has been shown to negate the euphoric effects of opioid drugs and so may pose a risk to individuals who self-administer larger amounts of a narcotic to attain the desired effects; doing so may lead to a fatal overdose. Naltrexone should not be combined with narcotic medications, unless it is prescribed under the close supervision of a physician.

Depression is frequently associated with alcohol dependence and substance abuse, and suicidality is higher in individuals with untreated depression. During the early phase of therapy, patients should be monitored closely for clinical signs of depression, especially for suicidal thinking and behavior.

Use in Pregnancy and Breastfeeding: Pregnancy Category C

Studies have not been conducted in pregnant women to determine the safety of naltrexone in pregnancy. The effects of naltrexone on the developing human fetus are unknown. Naltrexone should not be used during pregnancy unless clearly indicated.

It is not known if naltrexone is excreted in human breast milk. Because many drugs are excreted in breast milk, nursing mothers should not take ReVia or receive Vivitrol injections.

Possible Drug Interactions

There are no significant drug interactions known with naltrexone. Naltrexone is excreted primarily by the kidneys and does not undergo metabolism in the liver. ReVia and Vivitrol do not interact with antianxiety medications (e.g., benzodiazepines such as Valium) or any sleep medications. Naltrexone, however, can oppose the action and benefits of narcotic medications, such as cough preparations containing codeine, antidiarrheal preparations, and opioid analgesics.

Overdose

The clinical experience with naltrexone overdose is limited. In one study, patients who received 800 mg/day for 1 week showed no signs of toxicity. However, it should not be assumed that an overdose of naltrexone is always benign. High doses of naltrexone may cause liver injury. The severity of toxicity depends on the amount ingested, the age and weight of the person, and whether the person also ingested other medications. The safety of naltrexone in overdose in children is unknown.

Any suspected overdose should be treated as an emergency. The person should be taken to the emergency room for observation and treatment. The prescription bottle of medication (and any other medication suspected in the overdose) should be brought as well, because the information on the prescription label can be helpful to the treating physician in determining the number of pills ingested.

Special Considerations

- ReVia is usually taken once a day or as directed by your physician. If you miss a dose, take it as soon as possible. If it is close to the next scheduled dose, skip the missed dose and continue on your regular dosing schedule. Do not take double doses. Vivitrol is administered intramuscularly every 4 weeks by your health care provider.
- ReVia and Vivitrol have been shown to lead to maintenance of abstinence only when total treatment includes group support therapy and counseling.
- If relapse occurs, do not get discouraged; discuss your drinking with your physician, counselor, or therapist. Continue taking ReVia or receiving Vivitrol injections as directed, and consult your physician as soon as possible.
- If you experience any symptoms of depression, particularly with suicidal thoughts, contact your physician, counselor, or therapist immediately.
- Store ReVia in its originally labeled, light-resistant container, away from heat and moisture. Heat and moisture may precipitate breakdown of your medication, and the medication may lose its therapeutic effects.
- Keep your medication out of reach of children.
- The following Web sites can provide you and your family with additional information:
  - Alcoholics Anonymous: www.alcoholics-anonymous.org
  - National Institute on Alcohol Abuse and Alcoholism: www.niaaa.nih.gov
  - National Clearinghouse for Alcohol and Drug Information: www.ncadi.samhsa.gov
  - National Organization on Fetal Alcohol Syndrome: www.nofas.org
  - American Council on Alcoholism (locate treatment program and support groups in your area): www.aca-usa.org

If you have any questions about your medication, consult your physician or pharmacist.

Notes

From Chew RH, Hales RE, Yudofsky SC: *What Your Patients Need to Know About Psychiatric Medications*, Second Edition. Washington, DC, American Psychiatric Publishing, 2009

Index

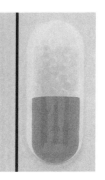

Page numbers printed in **boldface** type refer to tables or figures.